D1524327

21ST CENTURY GLOBAL HEALTH DIPLOMACY

Global Health Diplomacy

ISSN: 2010-0493

Series Editors: Thomas E. Novotny *(San Diego State University, USA)*
Ilona Kickbusch *(Graduate Institute of International and Development Studies, Switzerland)*

Published:

Vol. 1: Innovative Health Partnerwships: The Diplomacy of Diversity
edited by Daniel Low-Beer

Vol. 2: Negotiating and Navigating Global Health: Case Studies in Global Health Diplomacy
edited by Ellen Rosskam and Ilona Kickbusch

Vol. 3: 21st Century Global Health Diplomacy
edited by Thomas E. Novotony, Ilona Kickbusch and Michaela Todd

GLOBAL HEALTH DIPLOMACY – Vol. 3

21ST CENTURY GLOBAL HEALTH DIPLOMACY

Editors

Thomas E. Novotny
San Diego State University, USA

Ilona Kickbusch
Graduate Institute of International and Development Studies, Switzerland

Michaela Told
Graduate Institute of International and Development Studies, Switzerland

World Scientific

NEW JERSEY • LONDON • SINGAPORE • BEIJING • SHANGHAI • HONG KONG • TAIPEI • CHENNAI

Published by

World Scientific Publishing Co. Pte. Ltd.

5 Toh Tuck Link, Singapore 596224

USA office: 27 Warren Street, Suite 401-402, Hackensack, NJ 07601

UK office: 57 Shelton Street, Covent Garden, London WC2H 9HE

Library of Congress Cataloging-in-Publication Data
21st century global health diplomacy / [edited by] Thomas E. Novotny, Ilona Kickbusch, Michaela Told.
    p. ; cm. -- (Global health diplomacy vol. 3)
    Twenty-first century global health diplomacy
    Includes bibliographical references and index.
    ISBN 978-9814355155 (hardcover : alk. paper)
    I. Novotny, Thomas E. II. Kickbusch, Ilona, 1950– III. Told, Michaela. IV. Title: Twenty-first century global health diplomacy. V. Series: Global health diplomacy vol. 3.
    [DNLM: 1. World Health. 2. International Cooperation. WA 530.1]
    RA418
    362.1--dc23

                                  2013011741

British Library Cataloguing-in-Publication Data
A catalogue record for this book is available from the British Library.

Typeset by Stallion Press
Email: enquiries@stallionpress.com

Printed by FuIsland Offset Printing (S) Pte Ltd Singapore

Foreword

Twenty-First Century Health Diplomacy

Sir George Alleyne, MD, FRCP, FACP (Hons), DSc (Hons)*

From time immemorial, as long as there were groups of human beings separated spatially — or, rather, territorially — the demands of commerce and communication between them necessitated the use of emissaries for negotiation about sensitive issues. Negotiations of important issues could not take place through group interaction. Even today, in certain cultures, the ultimate sensitive issue — that of arranging a marriage — is initially addressed through emissaries. This process must be the origin of the class of persons who were trained and trusted to negotiate and to arrive at an agreement that was acceptable to the involved parties. The development of other, more sophisticated forms of social organization led to better categorization of the skills and practices of those emissaries. The open diplomacy of classical Greece, with its many diplomatic missions, public elaboration of policy, and strict orders to emissaries, is well described as an example of the better organization of the diplomatic culture. Later European history, especially that of Italy, is replete with examples of the development of the functions of diplomats with their large retinues and their precise order of precedence, with pride

---

*Chancellor, University of the West Indies, Director Emeritus, Pan American Health Organization.

of place going to the diplomats from the Vatican. After the 1648 Peace of Westphalia, which is credited as the origin of direct international relations between sovereign nation-states, a better definition of territoriality and forms of domestic government arose, and that development concretized some of the fundamental canons of the practice of diplomacy as integral to the practice of foreign policy, which is one of the central themes of this book.

Tom Novotny and Ilona Kickbusch have parlayed their impeccable credentials as pioneers in the codification of heath diplomacy as a discipline into assembling a remarkable group of authors to explore further the relevance of diplomacy to health concerns of the 21st century. This book is a fascinating study of much of the background to health diplomacy; right from the beginning, the authors emphasize that the basic purpose of foreign policy and the diplomacy that served it was the protection of the territory of the nation-state from external threats, of which military aggression is the greatest concern. Health — if it was considered at all — figured rather poorly in diplomatic considerations. This omission is being corrected, and a recent significant advance has been the attention paid by the United Nations in a series of resolutions that recognize the close relationship — even interdependence — between foreign policy and global health.

The chapters of this book analyze the various aspects of global health that are of critical importance to foreign policy and explore the nature of the interactions between nations that are fundamental to achieving health nationally and globally. Diplomacy is treated as a craft practiced within the ambit of a country's foreign policy, and some of the instruments that will be critical for practice of this craft are detailed. For example, an elegant taxonomy of health diplomacy instruments is described, with many of those institutions having peculiar relevance to the functions and operation of the World Health Organization.

It is not being trite to point out that the main tool is really information, or what might be referred to in diplomatic parlance as "intelligence." Traffic in data and information remains a hallmark of the work of diplomats in service to their country, as the recent WikiLeaks exposure showed so clearly. Access to information about the national and global state of health is critical for adequate representation and negotiation. As the book points out, however, access to and use of information are in themselves not enough, but adequate preparation for the studied practice of negotiation represents an important tool that the 21st century diplomat will use consistently. It was refreshing to see reference to that standard text, *Getting to Yes*, by Fisher, which presents one of the finest and simplest approaches to conducting principled negotiation.

For several reasons, including the increasing interconnectedness that is a feature of modern globalization, there has been a shift of understanding about human security from a focus on preservation of territorial integrity and the sufficiency of the personal environment to concern for human well-being. In addition, there is general acceptance of the view that health is essential to the capacity of the individual to so expand choice as to achieve that well-being. It is good to point out, however, that the nature of health threats to human security is changing. Whereas the threat of communicable diseases and the fear of contagion previously were sufficient to create public apprehension and subsequent response to the health threat, the situation has changed. Chronic noncommunicable diseases, such as hypertension, diabetes, heart disease, cancer, and chronic respiratory disease, are now the major cause of death worldwide; even in developing countries, they represent a significant challenge for the poor, and the difference between the rich and the poor in their capacity to cope is an egregious manifestation of inequity.

But health is only one of the capacities needed for well-being. There can be no hubristic proposal for the preeminence or dominance of the health capability, and the health diplomat has to be aware of the actions of other sectors in providing human security. In this context, intersectoral collaboration will be critical, and the primacy of health in achieving human security within a foreign policy paradigm must include the health diplomat's awareness of the need to pay attention to those other capacities and the roles they may play. Thus, a description of interdepartmental, interministerial collaboration is a welcome addition to the discussion on health diplomacy. Health diplomacy within foreign policy has to be an aspect of what has been described as "international health statecraft."

A more critical issue addressed in various parts of the book is the relationship between national and global health. Global health is the health of the world's people irrespective of where they live, and the critical issue of today is the health inequity that condemns so many to ill health. Inequity does not respect national borders. The reduction of inequity is traditionally seen as the province of the state, and the mechanisms by which national action can reduce the inequity among nations or within foreign nations are among the more vexing questions in public health. To date, the only mechanism available for addressing this conundrum is that of the international health organizations, but some neofunctionalists have taken the position that such organizations have not fully used the normative instruments at their disposal to reduce the global inequity. Diplomats with a national allegiance in spite of having a remit in health have not in general been able to cut this knot. It is still not clear how health diplomacy will address the national inequity that has to be considered if the objective of global health is the health of all people. As Kickbusch points out, "[F]oreign policy needs to be driven by the new mindset, which accepts a double responsibility, for one's own country and for the global community. This is the challenge for health diplomacy at the beginning of the 21st century." Meeting this challenge may very well entail consideration of the kind of interventionist foreign policy that hitherto has been reserved for threats to security other than health.

If one accepts responsibility for one's own country as well as for other countries with respect to addressing global health, then one has to accept the responsibility for reducing inequity globally as well as nationally. As mentioned repeatedly in this volume, national action in health is normally within the responsibility of the state. Therefore, it would seem that health diplomacy has to have a national expression as well. The means of negotiation at the national level to reduce inequities in health are clear, and they have been seen as the domain of internal politics, not as a concern of foreign policy, and, ergo, not as a concern of diplomats. But there may indeed be situations in which the health of other countries and the inequities in those countries can profoundly affect the health of one's own country. In that sense, foreign policy that has an impact on external factors affecting the security of one's own country can properly involve health diplomacy. Such a situation is seen acutely in matters related to trade and agricultural policy, wherein the actions of other countries have an impact on domestic health. This concept of global responsibility, touching on global citizenship, has been a frequent theme in Kickbusch's work.

The problem of domestic state action brings to the fore an issue that is highlighted throughout this volume. The question is: Can the old forms of international health governance accommodate the new roles of health diplomacy and address the new health challenges? In the era immediately following the Treaty of Westphalia, the state and the government were for all purposes coterminous. But the recent steady growth of political pluralism has been such that there are now several powerful nongovernmental actors in many nations, such as civil society and the private sector, that claim legitimacy in negotiations that were formerly the exclusive province of governments. The ability of these nongovernmental actors to influence the health policy that has been taken to be an aspect of foreign policy is growing apace, and any construct that has states as the critical actors in international politics must consider that the modern state is no longer a unipolar structure. The question is: How will the practice of health diplomacy evolve as a part of foreign policy, and be able to affect the decisions that are taken in organizations whose governance reflects the growing political pluralism? The day will come when the current organizations — which are really intergovernmental and not truly international — have to recognize officially, rather than in the current, unofficial manner, the need for these other, nongovernmental actors to be part of the formal decision-making process in global health. The political home of health diplomacy at that stage and the nature of the international statecraft that shapes foreign policy will be of considerable interest.

This book is not a compendium of platitudes about the magnitude of health and suffering and the need for the world as a whole to be concerned. The well-argued discussions presented here not only propose possible solutions but implicitly or explicitly pose some questions that will be central to diplomatic practice in health in the 21st century. This volume is a welcome addition to the discourse and debate on the nature and practice of health diplomacy. Its contents can be seen as a partial response to the most recent UN resolution on global health and foreign policy, which "[e]ncourages member states, the UN system, academic institutions, and networks to further increase their capacity for the training of diplomats and health officials, in particular those from developing countries, on global health and foreign policy, by developing best practices and guidelines for training and open source information and education and training resources for this purpose." All who have a stake in the health of the people of the world and who view that health as one of our few nonrenewable resources should read this book.

Contents

List of Contributors

(in alphabetical order, including editorial team)

Vincanne Adams
University of California, San Francisco
Anthropology, History & Social Medicine
3333 California Street, suite 485
PO Box 0850
San Francisco, CA 94143 – 0850
USA
adamsv@dahesm.ucsf.edu

Santiago Alcázar
SQN 206 Bloco D
Apt 103 Asa Norte
Brasilia, DF 70844-040
Brazil
alcazar3@hotmail.com

Sir George A.O. Alleyne
Pan-American Health Organization
525 23rd St., NW
Washington, DC 20037
alleyned@paho.org

Kristofer Bergh
Stockholm International Peace Research Institute
Signalistgatan 9
SE-169 70 Solna
Sweden
bergh@sipri.org

Ebony Rose Bertorelli
McGill University | Université McGill
McGill World Platform For Health and Economic Convergence
845, Sherbrooke Street West
Montreal, Quebec
Canada H3A 0G4
ebony.bertorelli@gmail.com

Eugene V. Bonventre
2109 12th Pl NW
Washington, DC 20009
bonventre@yahoo.com

Paulo Marchiori Buss
FioCruz–Fondação Oswaldo Cruz
Center of Global Health
Av. Brazil, 4365
Manguinhos
Rio de Janeiro
Brazil
buss@fiocruz.br

Col Valérie Denux
57, rue de Clichy
75009 Paris
France
valeriedenux@aol.com

Nick Drager
Global Health Programme
Graduate Institute of International and Development Studies
PO Box 136
1211 Geneva 21
Switzerland
dragern@gmail.com

Harley Feldbaum
Director for Global Health, International Economics
National Security Council
The White House
1600 Pennsylvania Avenue NW
Washington, DC 20500
harley.feldbaum@gmail.com

Bates Gill
Stockholm International Peace Research Institute
Signalistgatan 9
SE-169 70 Solna
Sweden
gill@sipri.org

Wolfgang Hein
GIGA Institut für Lateinamerika-Studien
Neuer Jungfernstieg 21
20354 Hamburg
Germany
hein@giga-hamburg.de

Sebastian Kevany
Aghern Military Road
Killiney, Co
Dublin
Ireland
Sebastian.Kevany@ucsf.edu

Ilona Kickbusch
Global Health Programme
Graduate Institute of International and Development Studies
PO Box 136
1211 Geneva 21
kickbusch@bluewin.ch

Kelley Lee
Simon Fraser University
Faculty of Health Sciences (FHS)
Blusson Hall, Room 11300
8888 University Drive
Burnaby, B.C.
Canada V5A 1S6
kelley_lee@sfu.ca
Kelley.Lee@lshtm.ac.uk

Thomas E. Novotny
Graduate School of Public Health
San Diego State University
5500 Campanile Drive, Hardy Tower
119 San Diego
California, 92182
USA
tnovotny@mail.sdsu.edu

Valerie Percival
Carleton University
1125 Colonel By Drive
Ottawa, Ontario
K1S 5B6 Canada
valerie_percival@carleton.ca

Gaudenz Silberschmidt
Ch. des Pétoleyres 22
1110 Morges
Switzerland
gaudenz@silberschmidt.ch

Steven A. Solomon
World Health Organization
Avenue Appia 20
1211 Geneva 27
Switzerland
solomons@who.int
stevensolomon@yahoo.com

Michaela Told
Global Health Programme
Graduate Institute of International and Development Studies
PO Box 136
1211 Geneva 21
michaela.told@graduateinstitute.ch

Thomas Zeltner
Gerechtigkeitsgasse 31
CH 3011 Bern
Switzerland
t.zelt@bluewin.ch

1

21st Century Health Diplomacy: A New Relationship Between Foreign Policy and Health

*Ilona Kickbusch, PhD**

Introduction

In 2009, a new concept of global health diplomacy (GHD) was adopted by United Nations General Assembly (UNGA) Resolution 63/33[1] and reaffirmed by UNGA Resolutions 64/108,[2] 65/95,[3] and 66/115.[4] All of these resolutions recognize the strong interface between foreign policy and global health. According to the Secretary-General's Note, "Global health interacts with the core functions of foreign policy: achieving security, creating economic wealth, supporting development in low-income countries, and protecting human dignity" (Ref. 5, para. 5). This statement draws attention to "making the relationship between global health and foreign policy an increasingly important issue for the United Nations, the World Health Organization, many intergovernmental organizations and processes, and national governments" (Ref. 5, para. 58).

However, although these proclamations hark back to the origins of health diplomacy over the past 160 years, it is only in the past decade that the technical areas of global health have been explicitly linked to

*Adjunct Professor, Graduate Institute of International and Development Studies, Geneva, Switzerland; Director, Global Health Programme, Graduate Institute, Geneva, Switzerland.
E-mail: kickbusch@bluewin.ch

the sphere of diplomacy. This linkage primarily results from shifts in the global political environment, the emergence of new epidemics, and the greater need for international cooperation in health. In today's globalized world, nations need, now more than ever, to cooperatively address mutual threats. As former UN Director-General Kofi Annan stated in 2004, "No state, no matter how powerful, can by its own efforts alone make itself invulnerable to today's threats."[6] In 2011, UN Secretary-General Ban Ki-moon highlighted in his remarks to the General Assembly after being appointed for a second term that "[W]e live in an era of integration and interconnection, a new era [in which] no country can solve all challenges on its own."[7]

The Origins of Health Diplomacy

The Multilateral Health Conference

Transboundary challenges in the 19th century put to use the diplomatic tool known as the "multilateral conference." Its construct was both simple and revolutionary: a group of countries would meet *ad hoc* to reach agreements "on a common policy with regard to a common problem," and then would later meet again to see whether these policies had been implemented and to determine whether adjustments to the agreements were needed. These meetings developed into a cycle of international conferences, the first of which was established in 1815 as the Central Commission for the Navigation of the Rhine. The objective of this commission was to bind states to a common purpose — in this case, to adopt rules on how to navigate the river Rhine in order to promote economic development and free trade.[8]

  With similar aspirations, the first meeting of the International Sanitary Conference (ISC) in 1851 brought 12 states together to "render important services to trade and shipping."[9] Today, the ISC's successor organization is the World Health Organization (WHO), which brings together 193 countries to debate and formulate policies and agreements on common health threats, including those of a transboundary nature. These include diverse issues such as addressing health workforce migration, intellectual property and health, tobacco control, virus-sharing in response to infectious disease epidemics, and destruction of the smallpox virus. Increasingly, each of these issues involves critical political and economic dimensions related to national security interests, geopolitical power shifts, and international trade. For example, the latest version of the International Health Regulations (IHR), adopted in 2005, states in Article 2 that the purpose and scope of the IHR are "to prevent, protect against, control, and provide a public health response to the international spread of disease in ways that are commensurate with and restricted to public health risks and [that] avoid unnecessary interference with international traffic and trade" (Ref. 10, Article 2). These links have put health back on the foreign policy agenda.

None of this would surprise an observer from the mid-19th century. As the French Foreign Minister stated during the opening ceremony of the first ISC in 1858,[9] that period in history was "so fruitful of new and great things." It enabled modern international commerce, but it also witnessed the rapid spread of infectious diseases. The beginning of the ISC, then, was a "cosmopolitan moment," which called for international cooperative action to address infectious diseases while preserving trade.[11] The term *cosmopolitan moment* implies the recognition that it requires joint political action by sovereign states to avert a global risk: it becomes "an unprecedented resource for consensus and legitimation, nationally and internationally."[12] Cosmopolitan moments create new political spaces and enable or oblige new actors to join in global diplomatic instruments such as the IHR.[13]

Increased movement of goods and people led to new types of organizations and agreements. Already in 1843 the Egyptian Quarantine Board was established in Alexandria, based on the Conseil Supérieure de Santé de Constantinople, which had been created in 1839 to regulate the sanitary control of foreign shipping in Ottoman ports. It was composed of the Ottoman health council and delegates of the maritime powers. In 1851, an unprecedented six million visitors attended the First Great International Exhibition, in London. It presented to the world a new age of optimism supported by great trust in science and technology: infectious diseases, and the poverty and destitution caused by them, were to be things of the past. However, the national policies and instruments available to control the spread of infectious diseases (such as quarantine) had failed to contain several epidemics. For example, cholera pandemics struck Europe in 1821 and 1851; they led to significant loss of life, in particular among the poorest communities in London, Paris, and St. Petersburg.[9] Merchants also suffered great financial burdens and bore the brunt of quarantine measures imposed without compensation for loss of trade revenue. In the face of tough global competition among states, there was political concern that quarantine measures were, in fact, applied by some in order to achieve unfair trade advantage. It was after the second pandemic, in 1851, then, that the new organization, the ISC, helped level the playing field for trade amid the very real health concerns at that time.

One hundred and fifty years later, in 2003, a cosmopolitan moment was again provoked by the epidemic of severe acute respiratory syndrome (SARS) and its global economic impact. This event convinced nations to act so that economies could be protected from the effects of disease spread in the 21st century's borderless world.[14–18] Because of "the growth in international travel and trade, and the emergence or re-emergence of international disease threats and other public health risks, the 48th WHA [World Health Assembly] called for a substantial revision of the Regulations adopted in 1969."[10] History had repeated itself.

Although the history of international health agreements includes some negotiations that were concluded in record time, many other such negotiations dragged on for long periods, because of the lack of political will or of easy consensus on multinational actions. Much has been written about the delayed outcomes of the ISCs.[9,14,17,18] Achieving consensus proved difficult in these meetings because of major disagreements on the causes and modes of cholera transmission and subsequently on the measures that were needed to contain the epidemics. Ten conferences took place over about 50 years, and they often were marked by heated debates among different scientific schools of thought on the causation of cholera. In fact, because of the vicious nature of these controversies, diplomats in charge of negotiations at one point excluded scientists from some of the deliberations. The first convention document was signed in 1892, after 41 years of debate. This delay is remarkable, given that Filippo Pacini (in 1854) and Robert Koch (in 1883) had discovered *Vibrio cholera*, the causative agent of cholera. With these discoveries, the medical establishment finally accepted the fact that micro-organisms — and not simply filth — had caused the illness. Science-based cholera control efforts were undertaken during the building of the Suez Canal (1892) and later supported by sanitary conventions during the Haj pilgrimage to Mecca (1894) and in the international response to plague (1897).[18]

Learning by Doing

Such negotiations at the interface of diplomacy and science had not previously been conducted. Political leaders, diplomats, and scientific experts had to familiarize themselves with new demands for health diplomacy and negotiations at the multilateral rather than at the bilateral level, where most diplomacy had been conducted until then. Initially, countries joining the ISC put concerns for trade at the center of their discussions, and thus these conferences focused on possible treaties to protect trade in the face of health threats. Over time, the meetings also became an international forum at which to present advances in science and to discuss a wide range of public health and medical issues. This process ultimately led countries to recognize the need for structured international health cooperation and laid the groundwork for the subsequent institutionalization of such cooperation. These processes also shifted some responsibility away from diplomats and onto health experts, because the focus of negotiations moved from political agreements and treaties to more technical issues based on the rapidly expanding medical and public health knowledge. Many health and political leaders felt that effective outcomes could only be ensured through a more stable governance mechanism, and thus the idea of a permanent international health agency was raised at the 1874 ISC in Vienna. However, it took another 30 years to establish the first such international agency (in 1907), as the Office International d'Hygiène Publique (OIHP). In the Americas, the Pan American Sanitary Bureau had been established in 1902 as the first regional international health structure.

One might contrast this slow, multinational bureaucratic process with the creation, also in the mid-19th century, of the International Committee of the Red Cross (ICRC; a voluntary organization) in just five years. This rapid startup was facilitated by Henry Dunant, a charismatic individual who witnessed the death and abandonment of more than 40,000 wounded soldiers following the 1859 Battle of Solferino in the Austro-Sardinian War. The international response he was able to mobilize — a shocked general public pushed states into voluntary humanitarian cooperation[19] — is not dissimilar to the global response to the HIV/AIDS epidemic at the end of the 20th century.

Diplomatic Revolutions

Diplomacy is the art and practice of negotiation and relationship building within different contexts and on many different subjects. States assert foreign policy priorities through diplomacy, and thus diplomacy is essentially a political activity.[20] When we refer to diplomacy, we mean both specific methods for reaching compromise or consensus and a system of organization for representation, communication, and the negotiating process. Former US Secretary of State Henry Kissinger described this interface as "the adjustment of differences through negotiation... in a legitimate international order."[21] Diplomacy as a method has been practiced between states for centuries through the assignment of envoys and the establishment of resident missions. Over time, as the environment within which diplomacy functions has changed, both the methods and the system of diplomacy had to adapt to a new international order of nations, to changing international governance structures, and to a wide range of new organizational roles in foreign policy.

The Modern System of Diplomacy

The modern system of diplomacy emerged in 15th century Europe within the Italian city-states and was further developed through the establishment of national foreign ministries and the function of the resident ambassador. "By the early 18th century, most of the machinery of modern diplomacy was in place."[22] It is intricately linked to the emergence of the sovereign nation-state. The treaty called the Peace of Westphalia in 1648 introduced a new political order in central Europe, based upon the concept of state sovereignty over lands, people, and agents abroad. This proved to be the basis of all later diplomatic efforts — the legitimate order that Kissinger refers to — and gave impetus to the pursuit of national interests within a basically bilateral system of representation and negotiation. The first foreign ministry was created in France in 1626 by Cardinal Richelieu. The priority given to diplomacy in France was only achieved by most other countries in the course of the 19th century.

The 19th century then saw the emergence of multilateral diplomacy. After the Napoleonic Wars the diplomatic innovation of the peacetime conference was turned into a "cabinet of the great powers" or, as it was sometimes called, the "concert of Europe." These meetings not only allowed simultaneous negotiations among states, a necessary approach to areas of common concern in the age of colonial expansion and rapid economic growth, it also led to a sharing of international authority and provided the mechanism for continuous management of the problems at hand. What followed was an "explosion in multilateral diplomacy" which was characterized by the creation of regular committees and conferences and by an increase in the number of intergovernmental organizations with their own secretariats.[20,23]

After the First World War, with the establishment of the League of Nations (the League) in the early 20th century, yet another completely novel form was added to the diplomatic system: the universal membership organization, open to all states and committed to "open diplomacy." This "new diplomacy" brought with it that negotiations were conducted not only simultaneously but in international assemblies modeled on a parliamentary process. This structure both allowed the participation of smaller countries and was designed to reach political solutions with transparency and accountability — the ideal was a universal association of nations. These organizations were run by a secretariat, i.e. a new corps of international civil servants who were, in principle, beholden to the international organization and not to their nation of origin. Very few countries had resident missions to interact with these organizations, and governments would send high-level representatives to attend the assemblies. The old-type conference diplomacy continued in parallel. After World War II these international structures were further elaborated through the establishment of the United Nations System,[23] with the aim of providing it (through the Security Council) with more power.

Increasingly, they required a country's presence (a permanent delega-tion) at the seat of the organization and new forms of representation and accreditation. Countries established high-level diplomatic positions such as Ambassador to the United Nations or Representative to the World Trade Organization. The delegations to multilateral organizations might further involve not only diplomats but also specific issue experts from ministries of health, environment, labor, or defense — raising the issue of the relationship between generalist and specialist diplomats. In view of the many dimensions of diplomacy, the Vienna Convention on Diplomatic Law was agreed in 1961 to guide countries and provide rules to be adhered to.

21st Century Diplomacy

Twenty-first century diplomacy is adapting to a globalized world com-munity. Global challenges such as the environment and health and the growing awareness of global interdependence have transformed the very essence of diplomacy. At present, describing foreign policy as "the strat-egy or approach chosen by the national government to achieve its goals in relation with external entities"[24] seems insufficient. A career UK diplomat, Robert Cooper, stated that the goal of foreign policy is increasingly "taken to be peace and prosperity rather than power and prestige."[25] Similarly, the UN Secretary-General defined the core functions of foreign policy as "achieving security, creating economic wealth, supporting development in low income countries, and protecting human dignity."[4] Others maintain that the role of the diplomat now includes a double responsibility: to represent both the interests of his or her country and the interests of the global community.[26] This new role requires that global public goods for health be ensured and that trade and economic development regimes need to be complemented by binding agreements that ensure health and envi-ronmental safety.[27,28]

Some analysts assert that the "management of the global system on a continuous basis" is increasingly the task of the modern diplomat.[29,30] The day-to-day work of representatives to international organizations seems to underscore this assertion; specifically, technical experts (e.g. experts on the environment or health) are now routinely included in negotiating teams and, increasingly, there are technically qualified diplomats working alongside foreign policy generalists. Member state support for international organizations is often dependent on how well these organizations manage the complexity of negotiating global health, trade, agricultural, or intellectual property regimes.

The 21st Century System and Method of Diplomacy

In the 21st century, the system of diplomacy makes use of bilateral and multilateral diplomatic processes that have been developed over the past two centuries. The unstructured pluralism reflected in this system has two dimensions: on the one hand, it offer the flexibility necessary for conducting complex negotiations on complex subjects, including testing the reception of negotiating positions in different fora; on the other hand, it allows an "*à la carte*" multilateralism, in which new forms of dialogue and "coalitions of the willing" are created to avoid obligations based on agreements reached in international organizations. The great power conferences have been reborn as the Group of Seven, Group of Eight, and Group of Twenty (G-7, G-8, and G-20).[31] Summit meetings, which first became popular in the post-WWII period, have increased in number rapidly at regional and global levels and as regional rather than global negotiations.[20] In fact, multilateral, *ad hoc* conferences have become the primary mechanism by which environmental and climate change agendas are advanced,[32] while the development of health treaties has been repositioned under the WHO.[33]

Membership in some international membership organizations may be conditional. For example, gaining membership to the World Trade Organization (WTO) is in itself a process of negotiation; any state or customs territory having full autonomy in trade policies may join ("accede to") the WTO, but WTO members must agree on the terms of accession.

Other new fora are now part of the diffusion of the diplomatic system; for example, regular high-level gatherings such as the World Economic Forum in Davos, Switzerland; board meetings of public–private partnerships (such as the Global Fund for AIDS, Tuberculosis, and Malaria and the GAVI Alliance); and an increasing number of regional groups have become critical parts of the response to global health challenges. Finally, as will be argued below, health diplomacy has itself become an accepted form of diplomacy, a form that is integral to the practice of foreign policy; it is now part of the diplomatic arsenal of countries as diverse as the United States, China, Norway, and Brazil. In fact, health was described as a "pillar of foreign policy" by the US Institute of Medicine in 2008.[34]

The method of diplomacy — the practice of the art — is also changing. Sucharipa[35] has outlined an entirely new set of skills for the 21st century diplomat. He stated that the diplomat will need, first and foremost, to be an expert who works with a new diplomatic mind frame. This perspective embraces openness instead of secrecy, defines diplomacy as a "service industry," redefines professional roles as network-based rather than hierarchical and, in the information age, requires well-developed analytical skills. The practice of diplomacy has also changed through the ease of travel and the introduction of new technologies, such as electronic communication and new forms of knowledge management. Geoffrey Wiseman,[36] in his study "Polylateralism and New Modes of Global Dialogue," proposed that "traditional state-centered bilateral and multilateral diplomatic concepts and practices need to be complemented with explicit awareness of a further layer of diplomatic interaction and relationships. Accordingly, the diplomat of the future will need to operate at the bilateral level, the multilateral level, and, increasingly, the polylateral level (relations between states and other entities)." In addition, the health diplomat in the 21st century will increasingly be female.[35]

In summary, some of the defining features of the new 21st century diplomacy in a globalized world are that it:

• Needs to function within a multipolar world and within a multi-level and multi-dimensional global governance structure, which increasingly includes a regional level.
• Is no longer conducted only by traditional, professional diplomats.
• Is challenged to manage not only the relations between states (bilateral and multilateral) but also the relations between states and other actors (polylateral); it manages these relationships at various diplomatic venues and by using a wide range of instruments.
• Is increasingly engaged in public diplomacy *vis-à-vis* an informed public and many new actors at home and abroad.

- Is involved in and contributes to a host of international issues which require global coordination under conditions of interdependence, such as security, health, the environment, global finance, and climate change.
- Needs to consider a much closer interface between domestic and international policies and cooperation with national ministries.[33–41]

These factors constitute the backdrop to global health diplomacy (GHD), as will be discussed below.

Health Diplomacy: Broadening the Scope of Foreign Policy and Diplomacy

When we speak of GHD, we aim to capture particularly those multilevel and multi-actor negotiation processes that shape and manage the global policy environment for health in health and non-health fora. Ideally, GHD is conducted in the spirit of a common endeavor to ensure health as a human right and a global public good, and it is based on the double responsibility of the diplomat to serve both national and global interests. It brings together a range of disciplines, including public health, international affairs, management, development, law, and economics. Its broadest focus is on health issues and health determinants that cross national boundaries, that are global in nature, and that require global agreements to address them.[54]

If well-conducted, GHD results in: (1) better health security and population health outcomes for each (and all) of the countries involved and an improved global health situation; (2) improved relations between states and a commitment of a wide range of actors to work together to improve health; and (3) outcomes that are deemed fair and that support the goals of reducing poverty and increasing equity.

As described above, health diplomacy can look back on a history of nearly 160 years. It is notable that international health negotiations have had an institutionalized mechanism for more than 100 years. Using the definitions of diplomacy introduced earlier, health diplomacy at the multilateral level can be considered as a method for reaching compromise and consensus in matters pertaining to health, usually in the face of other interests related to international politics, economic interests, and ethical values. Health diplomacy is — like all other forms of diplomacy — essentially a political process (see the chapter by Feldbaum in this volume); it involves negotiation but also much relationship building and is part of the management of global affairs. As health becomes more politically relevant in domestic and foreign policy, health diplomacy plays an increasingly important global role. This change clearly is an expression of changes in the dynamic relationship between the health and diplomacy fields. Alcazar maintains that a "Copernican shift" in global health is underway. He says: "Globalization takes the issue of health from the relative obscurity in which it found itself, especially in developing countries, and brings it to the front page where it is featured not as health as we know it, but as global health in combination with foreign policy, which we are still struggling to define."[41]

The multilevel nature of health diplomacy is well illustrated in a presentation to an international audience by the Chinese Minister of Health, Professor Zhu Chen, who in 2009 introduced the following list of health diplomacy activities and relationships in which China engages:

- Multilateral: the WHO; the World Bank; the Association of Southeast Asian Nations; the Shanghai Cooperation Organization; the Global Fund for AIDS [acquired immune deficiency syndrome], Tuberculosis, and Malaria; and the UN Programme on HIV [human immunodeficiency virus]/AIDS (UNAIDS).
- Bilateral: 300 cooperation agreements with 89 countries.
- South–South: China–Africa Cooperation (Chinese medical teams).
- South–North: 11 regular ministerial dialogues with the United States, France, and other countries.
- Public–Private: the Clinton Foundation, the Bill and Melinda Gates Foundation, the China Medical Board, and Project Hope.

The Dynamics of Health and Foreign Policy

The changing dynamics between health and foreign policy can be illustrated if we assume a continuum with two endpoints — one (A) in which foreign policy neglects or even hinders health and another (D) in which foreign policy serves health (as represented in the Oslo Declaration on global health[40]). Along the continuum, we can observe several different

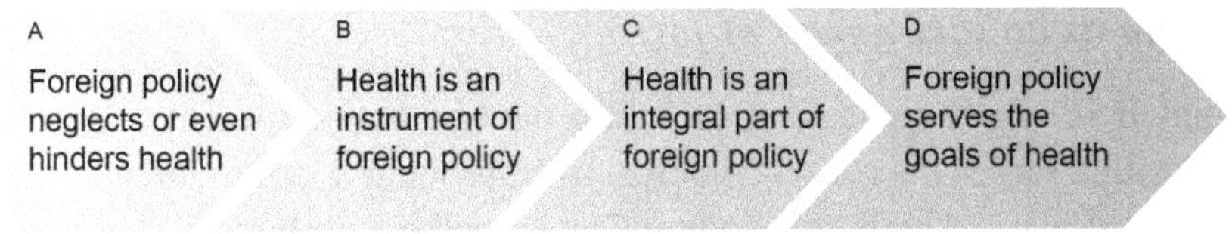

A	B	C	D
Foreign policy neglects or even hinders health	Health is an instrument of foreign policy	Health is an integral part of foreign policy	Foreign policy serves the goals of health

Fig. 1. The continuum of the relationship between health and foreign policy. Adapted with permission from Kickbusch.[44]

interactions between health and foreign policy, two of which are of particular importance: (B) health as an instrument of foreign policy and (C) health as an integral part of foreign policy (Fig. 1).

All four points along the continuum in Fig. 1 serve foreign policy goals that are not necessarily distinct; they all serve the national interest, but they do so to various degrees. As one approaches point D, the dual responsibility — serving national interests as well as the global community — is particularly evident as a political commitment to health objectives. Indeed, the Oslo Declaration speaks of health objectives "as a point of departure" for foreign policy. A short review of the four types of interactions between health and foreign policy may help illustrate this perspective.

Foreign policy neglects or even hinders health outcomes

At point A in Fig. 1, public health may be severely endangered when diplomacy fails, and hard-power interventions might ensue. These interventions could include military actions and increasingly economic actions — for example, economic sanctions or agreements on trade or intellectual property that neglect the effect of the agreements on public health. They also could include a lack of agreement in such areas as climate change, as evidenced at the 2009 UN Climate Change Conference in Copenhagen.[45] Currently, policies and agreements that are negotiated internationally or that are part of regional and bilateral agreements are seldom reviewed for their public health impact. Indeed, powerful countries often seek bilateral agreements specifically to avoid or circumvent multinational agreements that might constrain their actions in trade, economic development, and security matters.

Health as an instrument of foreign policy

Point B in Fig. 1 indicates that health may be an instrument of foreign policy that serves the national interest by improving relations among states in several ways. The long-standing Cuban medical diplomacy program is a typical example,[46] as are the many health projects that form part of the agreements between China and African states.[47] In 2003, at the height of the Iraq war, the US president launched the President's Emergency Plan for AIDS Relief (PEPFAR), the largest international health initiative in history for a single disease (initially US$15 billion for 5 years, now US$51 billion for 6 years). The signals that these foreign policy initiatives send are intended not only for recipient countries but also for the global community overall; they are part of public diplomacy. In many cases, national governments support global health initiatives to improve their image at home and abroad; in particular, many of the smaller European nation-states (such as those of Scandinavia) use the health arena to demonstrate their commitment to the multilateral systems that provide them with a voice and allow them a leading role on the global stage.

In the Western countries, this use of health within foreign policy goals is often looked at critically by development agencies, public health organizations, and health activists, who argue that programs should be established "for health's sake" — not for other motives — and that they should be based on criteria of need and equity, not political expedience. As a consequence, international development agencies — or, as is sometimes the case, ministries of development — are often at odds with ministries of foreign affairs over priorities and approaches, because the agencies do not want to be instrumentalized for goals other than health development. Many of the newly founded South–South initiatives in health, in contrast, support the new geopolitical positioning of the emerging economies toward Africa, which has been called "the continent of the future," and countries such as China are considering the establishment of a development agency to structure and strengthen their level of influence in Africa. This approach has been termed "soft power," which aims to bind developing countries to centers of power in a multipolar environment through means other than coercion.[48] Lee *et al.* recently illustrated the use of this approach in the case of Brazil and the Framework Convention on Tobacco Control (FCTC).[49]

Finally, in the Iraq and Afghanistan wars, health assistance has been used in parallel with military intervention in an effort to "win the hearts and minds" of the people in those countries.[50] In part, this approach builds on the experiences gained by the Pan American Health Organization in Central America in the 1980s, when temporary cease-fires were negotiated to allow for vaccination programs. This type of initiatives came to be termed "Health as a Bridge for Peace" or described as "vaccine diplomacy," and they also were used in the aftermath of the Balkan conflicts.[51] The term "humanitarian diplomacy" is also gaining ground — and health is an important dimension of this approach.

Health as an integral part of foreign policy

An important part of the shift in the relationship between health and foreign policy indicates that some dimensions of health have now become an integral part of foreign policy (point C in Fig. 1) in many countries. There is of course a fluid line from using health as an instrument of foreign policy to integrating it into foreign policy strategies — this is sometimes termed "smart power." Health as a part of 21st century foreign policy is reflected in approaches to "heath security," which is similar to the involvement of foreign ministries in environmental diplomacy. Cooper[25] underlined this by pointing out: "In the past, it was enough for a nation to look after itself — today, that is no longer sufficient." The realizations that disease knows no borders and that pandemics and bioterrorist attacks can endanger national security have become a concern of foreign policy and security specialists, and have pulled health experts into these realms. In the United States in the 1990s, health issues, particularly human immunodeficiency virus (HIV) and acquired immune deficiency syndrome (AIDS), were of concern to the National Security Council and were a regular feature of national intelligence reports.[49] Many other countries, as well as the European Union (EU), consider health issues to be part of their national security strategies. It was such a perspective that led to the rapid agreement by numerous countries on the revision of the IHR, despite the fact that the IHR transcends individual national sovereignty in some of its provisions.

Foreign policy serves the goals of health

Finally, we may see the increasing trend of foreign policy serving the goals of health (point D in Fig. 1). GHD and civil society advocacy have been extraordinarily successful in inserting health into the many negotiations underway in the general foreign policy environment. Health has become integral to the meetings of the G-7, G-8, G-20, and Group of 77; it is the subject of regular summit meetings as well as a myriad of multilateral *ad hoc* conferences; new UN-based health organizations have been created; new organizational forms, such as global funds, alliances, and initiatives, are being established; and regional bodies and fora deliberate on health matters. Two major health negotiations were conducted within the WHO, and within a very short time two major international agreements were approved: the FCTC (2003)[53] and the revised IHR (2005).[10] These negotiations were chaired and headed by senior diplomats (such as the IHR revision[54]). Health is squarely on the UN agenda, for example as a central component of the Millennium Development Goals (MDGs) and most recently the high-level UN meeting on noncommunicable disease prevention and control. Particularly in the UN context, most negotiations of relevance to health are conducted by diplomats.

A group of seven ministers of foreign affairs have expressed this development in the Oslo Declaration, as follows: "In today's era of globalization and interdependence, there is an urgent need to broaden the scope of foreign policy.... We believe that health is one of the most important, yet still broadly neglected, long-term foreign policy issues of our time.... We believe that health as a foreign policy issue needs a stronger strategic focus on the international agenda. We have therefore agreed to make [the] impact on health a point of departure and a defining lens that each of our countries will use to examine key elements of foreign policy and development strategies, and to engage in a dialogue on how to deal with policy options from this perspective."[43]

The Changing System of Health Diplomacy

Health diplomacy has its own *system of organization* (i.e., a range of dedicated health agencies) ... first and foremost, the WHO and the approaches and mechanisms of representation and negotiation that have emerged as health has become a more important dimension of diplomacy. The role of health as both an instrument and an integral part of foreign policy and the challenge of the "double responsibility" of the modern diplomat have led to the need for adjustment in both the system of diplomacy, which now includes health issues and health experts in new ways, and the health arena, which now needs to accommodate and make use of diplomatic expertise in new ways.

These adjustments are reflected in new types of relationships between ministries of health and ministries of foreign affairs at the national level, which sometimes take the form of official policy documents, as in Switzerland and the United Kingdom.[56] They are also mirrored in the composition of many diplomatic representations in which an increasing number of health attachés and health experts serve and in the inclusion of health in the training of diplomats. The departments of international and global health in the ministries of health are growing in importance (but not necessarily in resources) and, in some cases, ministries of foreign affairs have also established units on global health that interact with or supersede the technical ministries. Regional bodies are moving in the same direction and, in May 2010, the Foreign Affairs Council of the EU adopted Council Conclusions on the Union's role in global health.[57] Special ambassadors have been appointed by countries or by the UN Secretary-General to negotiate on specific disease challenges. US Ambassador to the UN Eric Goosby serves as the United States Global AIDS Coordinator, leading all US government international HIV/AIDS efforts,[60] and the UN Secretary-General has appointed a UN System Influenza Coordinator.[5]

In the first years of this new century, as the number of health actors has greatly expanded, this system of "health negotiation in a legitimate international order" is being politically challenged with regard to representation, recognition, legitimacy, and transparency. As in other periods of historical change, health diplomacy must be shaped to fit the new environment. We have indicated above how the International Sanitary Conferences moved from a political process of health negotiations to an increasingly technical undertaking; to some extent the diplomacy system has come full circle — back to an increased interface of health and politics. The following rough outline of the phases of institutionalization of health diplomacy focuses on the move toward a universal health organization. However, we must not forget that, even in the early stages of health diplomacy, the field of health diplomacy included many actors, not just states. Two of these actors deserve special mention: the ICRC (founded in 1863), which pioneered a new ethics of impartiality and neutrality in relation to health in humanitarian settings, and the Rockefeller Foundation (founded in 1913), which has been in the vanguard of foundation activity for health beyond borders. From its beginnings the foundation was so active throughout the world and in working with the health office of the League of Nations that, in 1928, it created its own international health division at its headquarters in New York.[9,59] Its financial investments at the time compare with those of the Bill and Melinda Gates Foundation today.

Phases of Institutionalization of Health Diplomacy

The first phase of institutionalization of health diplomacy (1907–1919) led to the establishment of the Office International d'Hygiène Publique OIHP in Paris in 1907, by an agreement signed by 12 states (Belgium, Brazil, Egypt, France, Italy, the Netherlands, Portugal, Russia, Spain, Switzerland, the United Kingdom, and the United States). The regional Pan American Sanitary Bureau, which is often described as the first international health organization, had already been working since 1902, and a number of other international/regional health organizations were already in existence or were beginning to be established at that time. By 1914, the OIHP had grown to include nearly 60 countries and colonies, and its main concern — following the International Sanitary Convention — continued to be international quarantine; in one of its most important early acts, it prepared the ISC in 1926, which added smallpox and typhus to cholera, plague, and yellow fever. It also adopted measures of notification, requiring governments to inform the OIHP immediately of any outbreak of plague, cholera, or yellow fever or of the appearance of smallpox or typhus in epidemic form. Disease surveillance has remained a key issue of health security and is a key component of the revised IHR 2005.

In the second phase of institutionalization of health diplomacy (1919–1948), health became part of the remit of the first multilateral and multipurpose organization. The League of Nations was created in 1919 by

44 states; its establishment marked the beginning of a new phase of diplomacy for settling international disputes, ensuring peace, and solving problems common to all by taking an "institutionalized" approach to international affairs.[60] As one of the problems common to all, health was included in the Covenant of the League; Article XXIII(f) provides that members would "endeavor to take steps in matters of international concern for the prevention and control of diseases." This provision led to the creation of a health office within the League of Nations. For health, the hope was that the broad multilateral platform of the League would provide the means for dealing with the scale and urgency of health problems after WWI. For example, the great influenza pandemic of 1918–1919 was estimated to have killed 15–20 million people and, in 1919, almost 1.6 million people died in the former Russian Empire as a result of a typhus epidemic. Death and disease in the colonies were not yet a priority of the Member States of the League, even though the first institutes of tropical medicine had been established to conduct research, develop therapeutics, and preserve the economic viability of colonial enterprises through health interventions.[61]

Action was hampered from the start by the fact that the United States did not join the League of Nations but continued to work through the OIHP on quarantine issues. The League developed a permanent epidemiology office to collect and disseminate data on the status of international epidemics (through the *Weekly Epidemiological Record*) and created technical commissions on malaria, cancer, typhus, leprosy, and biological standardization. Between the two world wars, the world had two international health offices — both of them weak and not well-resourced and, for political reasons, not well-coordinated — as well as some important regional bodies such as the Pan American Sanitary Bureau. During WWII, the work of the two health organizations was rendered impossible. The devastation during and the health challenges following WWII led the UN Economic and Social Council, at its first meeting in 1946, to call an international conference to consider the establishment of a single health organization under the UN. The intention was that such an organization would prove to be more effective if it was not subsumed under the political UN as an office, but if instead it worked as an independent, specialized technical agency with its own governing body, the World Health Assembly (WHA).

The third phase of institutionalization of health diplomacy (1948–1996) was decisive in its evolution. The International Health Conference convened under the auspices of the UN in New York on June 19, 1946.[9] It adopted a most forward-looking constitution for the WHO, which would carry on the functions previously performed by the League and the OIHP. The WHO constitution would balance technical expertise and political decision-making by differentiating the functions assigned to the WHO's Executive Board (a meeting of experts) and its Assembly (a meeting of states). A cosmopolitan moment, i.e. a major disease outbreak — a cholera epidemic in Egypt — again helped push the agenda forward, and the number of countries ratifying the WHO's constitution grew quickly. The first WHO assembly convened in Geneva in June 1948; for the first time in history, there was a single international organization with the broad mandate to "act as the directing and coordinating authority on international health work." A new, permanent venue for health diplomacy had been established in Geneva, bringing together all nation-states as members with equal representation (one country, one vote), which gave the organization a high level of legitimacy. The range of countries and their equal representation, as well as its broad mandate, differentiated the WHO from all other previous health organizations and underlies its convening power. For nearly 50 years, it remained at the center of all international health work.

The representation of countries in this new body gradually moved from diplomats to representatives from ministries of social affairs and then to ministries of health, which were increasingly important within the governments of Member States. The trans-boundary vision that had driven the International Health Conferences emerged in the successful drive to eradicate smallpox by 1976, but it became increasingly difficult to overcome national interests to reach other joint global goals. WHO Member States instituted important political commitments, such as the Health For All Strategy, adopted in 1977, but health remained very much a purely national rather than global concern, as health systems were established, colonies won their independence, and the industrialized countries celebrated the "victory" over infectious diseases. Many debates were hampered by the ideological positions of the two blocs of Cold War adversaries, which juxtaposed socialized medicine with the system of private health care. Furthermore, the opportunity provided in the WHO constitution to develop health treaties was not utilized; the organization came close only when, as a remarkable exception, the WHA adopted, in 1981, The International Code of Marketing of Breast-Milk Substitutes.[62] The International Sanitary Regulations (inherited from the OIHP) remained the sole binding instrument for international health agreements. They were adopted, revised, consolidated, and renamed The International Health Regulations in 1969. Further amendments followed in 1973. In 1995, the WHO and its Member States agreed on the need to revise the IHR because of their inherent limitations, but no agreement could be reached to move forward until the 2003 SARS epidemic, as described above.

Whereas the ISCs had been created because of a heightened awareness of the pressures of globalization in the 19th century and the recognition of interdependence, 100 years later it seemed to many that the existing organization, the WHO, could no longer meet the political and technical challenges of a new era.[63] The diplomatic community was focused on the new global challenge of the environment, with major negotiations being conducted within the 1997 Kyoto Protocol. In the period of transition from international to global health,[64] health came into focus at other venues, such as the World Trade Organization and the World Bank. A quantum leap made health move up the ladder to become a prime concern of social justice and international development — the cosmopolitan moment drove the emergence of the global movement to fight a new and deadly disease, HIV/AIDS.

The period of the diversification of health diplomacy began. The new health diplomats were the AIDS activists and the representatives of the development agencies. For them, the institutionalized forum of the WHO did not deliver what was necessary — neither the capacity to implement programs nor the political clout to effect changes in attitudes or in funding. At this point, the 20th century system of health diplomacy was in crisis, and the technical and the political world of health were out of touch with each other. Major powers were no longer committed to universal membership organizations or to multilateralism, and the world's expert body for health, the WHO, had not been able to respond adequately to the AIDS crisis. It was deeply symbolic of this crisis that the WHO's program on HIV/AIDS was shut down, and a new agency, UNAIDS, was established in 1996.

What has followed is the fourth phase of institutionalization (1996 to the present), which can be described as the establishment of an "unstructured pluralism" of agencies and actors in what had become a global health arena. This phase could also be considered one of transition, within which GHD has not yet found a functional architecture. Thus, an institutional form needs to be identified for the polylateral health diplomacy of the 21st century.[65] In the late 1980s and the 1990s, there was a move away from the state-centric approach of the international organizations to mechanisms that could act more rapidly, could generate more resources, were more accountable, and allowed the inclusion of other actors. The private sector was promoted as being more effective and efficient in action, and this led to the creation of new types of organizations and mechanisms, such as public–private partnerships, involving large philanthropic organizations. The ability to achieve results — to "deliver" and to provide "more health per dollar spent" — became a key concept. As Bull and McNeill wrote, "Market multilateralism brought the norms of multilateralism and the interest of market actors together."[66] Such approaches were new for the health sector, but had been practiced conceptually in the field of environmental diplomacy from the very beginning of global negotiations on these issues.

At the same time, civil society and the social justice agenda became central in the global health arena. For a short period, analysts saw the system of diplomacy changing drastically toward a "post-Westphalia" world, in which states were increasingly losing power and multilateral organizations that had been built on state sovereignty were outdated. New organizations were created to take their place or to take on governance functions required in the new environment. In this phase, reference would frequently be made to the global environmental issue, which had made it to the top of the international agenda and was taken very seriously by heads of state. The global environmental agenda involved a host of international agreements, treaties, protocols, and advocates, and it had significant economic implications for trade, development, and long-term human security. Yet it did not have an intergovernmental organization such as the WHO to act as an organ of policy-making and debate. Questions were raised as to whether the institutional form of the state-based, universal, multilateral health organization was still workable, and an extensive debate on global health governance was conducted in order to search for alternatives in the global health architecture.[39,40,67,68]

Major Factors in Environmental Diplomacy

The environment is often referred to as an exercise in global governance, having emerged in the latter part of the 20th century. It moved ahead, while GHD seemed to stagnate. Young[33] emphasized that the challenges at hand were addressed with innovative approaches to regime formation; these approaches did not require the establishment of new centralized, international, state-based organizations. Instead, mechanisms were developed that included both civil society and the private sector in agenda-setting, negotiation, and operationalization of policies. This development meant that the environmental agenda was not hampered by state-centric rules. The 1992 Earth Summit and the 1997 Kyoto Protocol became symbols for the new global practice of diplomacy and indicators of what it can achieve.

A description of the rationale for environmental diplomacy from 1998 captures the essence of this new field of diplomatic activity: "Environmental policy has become one of the pillars of international cooperation in the post-Cold War era. Environmental regimes are intertwined with other areas of cooperation such as the international trade system and global financial institutions. The relationship between international environmental regimes and other multilateral treaties and institutions is characterized by conflict as well as by cooperation. In the past, economic interests have often prevailed over environmental considerations."[69] Environmental diplomacy set out to change the economic perspectives in favor of the environment and, for the health sector, this change was also necessary.

US Ambassador Richard Benedick, in his classic analysis of environmental diplomacy,[70] described the multilateral negotiations that addressed global environmental issues. These negotiations began with the 1985 Vienna Convention on Protecting the Ozone Layer and reached their pinnacle at the 1992 UN Conference on Environment and Development (UNCED) in Rio de Janeiro, also known as the "Earth Summit." UNCED was the largest gathering of heads of state ever held; nearly 180 nations participated, including 118 at head-of-state level. In addition, there were dozens of UN organizations and other intergovernmental organizations, plus thousands of observers who represented hundreds of nongovernmental organizations (NGOs), as well as extensive media representation.

The Kyoto Protocol, an international agreement linked to the UN Framework Convention on Climate Change, was adopted in on December 11, 1997, and it entered into force on February 16, 2005. It is generally seen as an important first step toward a truly global environmental regime, and it provides the essential architecture for any future international agreement on climate change. Its major feature is that it sets binding targets for 37 industrialized countries and the European community for reducing greenhouse gas emissions; whereas the Convention encouraged industrialized countries to stabilize these emissions, the Protocol commits them to do so. The Kyoto Protocol places a heavier burden on developed nations under the principle of "common but differentiated responsibilities."

UNCED 1992 was a watershed: not only did it set the precedent for other global conferences and negotiations that were to follow, but it also shifted the responsibility for negotiations on environmental issues to the ministries of foreign affairs. Furthermore, it began to engage many other sectors of government, notably finance, economics, science, energy, agriculture, and development. This pattern was to repeat itself as global health gained in political importance. It became clear that these increasingly complicated negotiations required not only expertise in complex subject matters but also insights into the impact of health on the economy, agriculture, and human security. This complexity requires knowledge of international law and its instruments, an understanding of global power dynamics, and a well-honed set of negotiation skills. Benedick highlighted the five major factors that distinguish the new environmental diplomacy: (1) the nature of the subject matter; (2) the role of science and scientists; (3) the complexity of the negotiations; (4) the unique equity issues involved; and (5) the innovative features and approaches.[70] These factors can clearly be applied to GHD.

Factors that Characterize Global Health Diplomacy

Five factors characterize GHD and are of a very similar nature to those described for environmental diplomacy:

(1) *The nature of the subject matter.* That is to say, health is a transboundary concern for all nations, and it requires joint action.

(2) *The role of science and scientists.* That is to say, the response to the spread of disease is heavily dependent on an understanding of the causes of the disease, and the productive interface between diplomats and health experts is critical to successful health negotiations.

(3) *The complexity of the negotiations.* That is to say, the interface between diplomacy and science, the multilevel, multifactor, and multi-actor negotiations and the repercussions for trade and commerce, power relations, and values all make for complicated negotiations.

(4) *The unique equity issues involved.* That is to say, equity has been a driving force of the global health agenda since its inception, but it has gained force with the adoption of the MDGs, and a range of global health strategies deal with equity issues in specific ways, such as differential pricing.

(5) *The innovative features and approaches which characterize global health.* That is to say, throughout its history, in each institutional phase, health diplomacy has been highly innovative in developing methods, instruments, and organizational forms.

Many of the experiences gained in the field of environmental diplomacy have informed and inspired approaches to global health in its fourth institutional phase: involvement of the private sector, regime building through framework conventions, differentiated responsibilities, and strong involvement of civil society. The greatest difference between environment and global health negotiations lies in the difference in institutionalization and in the extent of the involvement of the private sector. The Kyoto Protocol, for example, allows for market-based mechanisms, such as emissions trading, and encourages the stimulation of green investment. With respect to global health, there has been a more critical approach to the private sector, and only recently have market-based approaches to global health investments gained broader acceptance. These include private–public partnerships, economic incentives for essential medicines, and negotiated agreements on drug pricing and technology transfer.

The Copenhagen Climate Summit in 2009, which served as a followup to Kyoto, raised questions about the kind of multilateral negotiation system that can bring results.[71] Copenhagen clearly was a diplomatic failure; it could be argued that an experienced secretariat and an accepted set of rules of procedure might have provided a better framework than the *ad hoc* multilateral conference approach that was taken. Surely, the summit would not have authorized a separate "Big Power conference" within the 170-member assembly; this exclusivity was a slap in the face of the "open diplomacy" on which the creators of the multilateral system in 1919 had pinned their hopes. It ignored the power shifts in global health and environmental leadership that have become so important to 21st century diplomacy.

Defining Features of 21st Century Health Diplomacy

As outlined above, the beginning of the 21st century has seen great changes in diplomacy, and global health is one of the areas in which this transition is most visible. The rules, norms, and expectations of the global health system are in a period of rapid transition.[39,40] They can best be summarized as three parallel power shifts.

Three Parallel Power Shifts

The first of these power shifts is that between nations. It marks the transition to a multipolar world, in which an increasing number of power centers exist. There is an ever-growing presence in the global health policy arena of low- and middle-income countries, such as Kenya, Mexico, Brazil, China, India, Thailand, and South Africa.[72] The second power shift marks a transition beyond nations. Although states remain strong and important players, various non-state actors from the private sector and civil society have entered the global health field and have radically changed the global architecture. The third of the power shifts takes place within nations, and it has to do with the continua between domestic and foreign policies and between hard- and soft-power issues. Health is now part of economic and foreign policies, and foreign policy agreements on health can have a significant impact on national health systems.[13] These power shifts correspond directly to the three defining features of 21st century diplomacy.

The power shift between nations

Health diplomacy functions within a multipolar world and within a multi-level and multidimensional global governance structure, which increasingly includes the regional level. The more power centers there are, the more important the consultation, negotiation, and coalition-building become. As more and more countries learn to take advantage of the decision-making and political power of international platforms, multilateral organizations acquire new strength. Together with the emergence of new economic powers, bridge-building roles become increasingly important at multilateral venues. The new multilateralism promises success to those who are most able to show commitment, gather broader support, and form coalitions. In this context, health can be viewed as an instrument for deepening the relationships between different nations and as a stable basis for building alliances.

This multipolar world order influences the dynamics of health diplomacy. In an interconnected world, in which diseases can spread faster than ever before but also in which a growing understanding of the responsibilities of a global community exists, countries become increasingly aware of the need to cooperate on global health. They do so, however, in changing constellations within which they aim to find their place and their spheres of influence in what is often referred to as a "geopolitical marketplace."[73] A new geography of power emerges, and common challenges can develop new groupings of nation-states or divide earlier groupings.

The new global health arena is marked by the growing influence of emerging economies such as Brazil, Russia, India, China, and South Africa (known as "the BRICS"); they have reached a tipping point of power in relation to global agendas.[74] With growing discursive and resource-based power, they use their diplomatic influence to include health in their strategic arsenal. China, for example, has more than 300 bilateral cooperation agreements with more than 89 countries and has provided medical teams in Africa since the 1960s. Brazil is "successfully leveraging its model fight against HIV/AIDS into expanded South–South assistance and leadership," in service of its own foreign policy objectives for reform of the UN Security Council and a louder voice in the international monetary system.[74,75]

At the same time, low- and middle-income countries are increasingly discovering and using the opportunities provided by regional and broader international platforms. The thinking in terms of well-defined North–South divides is more frequently challenged, as discussed during the UN High-Level Conference on South–South Cooperation in Nairobi in December 2009. The 4th Summit of the India–Brazil–South Africa (IBSA) Dialogue Forum in April 2010 illustrated the enhanced role of developing countries and the increasing dialogue among them. The IBSA facility fund, with US$3 million targeted annually for South–South development, is exemplary for leading the changing roles in South–South cooperation. The Africa–South America (created in 2006) and Africa–India (from 2008) summits also are illustrative of this development. Since 2011 the BRICS countries have also organized their own health summits.

The past two decades have also seen an increasing role for regionalism. Regional actors such as the EU, the African Union, the Common Market of the Southern Cone, the Shanghai Cooperation Organization, the Association of Southeast Asian Nations, the Asia–Pacific Economic Cooperation program, the Asia–Africa Summit/Focus on China–Africa Cooperation, the Union of the South American Nations, and the Central Asia Regional Economic Cooperation program are all expanding their program of work and at the same time putting health issues on their agendas.[3] Cooperative activities include intergovernmental meetings and common declarations and strategies on health; the goals of the activities include addressing the social determinants of health, supporting access to medicines, enhancing human resources for health, and creating new surveillance, response, and pharmaceutical capabilities. The EU Member States have, for example, created the European Centre for Disease Prevention and Control. The African Union scaled up its activities on health issues, as reflected in the annual reports on the MDGs, the development of human resources for health, and the Global Health Workforce Alliance. The Asia–Pacific Economic Cooperation program established a Health Task Force in 2003, which became a Health Working Group in 2007, with the mandate to implement health-related activities agreed upon by the organization. However, the consequences of this expanded dialogue and increased cooperation go much further than health. They create habits of communication and, where possible, cooperation among countries, and thus they provide a basis for improved relationships overall.

The power shift beyond nations

Health diplomacy is no longer conducted only by professional diplomats; and it is challenged to manage not only the relations between states but also the relations between states and other actors. It is unique, in that it has a universal, multilateral organization with treaty-making power at its disposal.

In the rapidly changing international context of the 21st century, diplomacy engages a very large number of players. In the words of Haas,[76] "a world dominated by dozens of actors, processing and exercising various kinds of power" has begun to take shape. Today, the practice of diplomacy no longer resides solely with traditional diplomats but also involves a wide range of other actors.[33] A growing and increasingly diverse group beyond the nation-states has emerged and profoundly changed the global health landscape. On the global health stage, an ever-greater variety of civil society and NGOs, private firms, and private philanthropists work along with (and sometimes challenge) traditional actors such as national ministries and the WHO.[72] The increased importance of global health has captured a growing interest among philanthropic foundations, advocacy networks, think thanks, and academic institutions. The new public–private partnerships, donors, funding organizations, and other actors have all contributed to the diversification of global health activities. For example, more than 200 public–private partnerships now work on global health issues.[77] In less than a decade, 60,000 NGOs have focused their work only on HIV/AIDS.[78] In 2010, there were 185 accredited NGOs in official relationships with the WHO.[79,a]

Besides the fact that there has been a marked increase in the number of non-state actors that are prominent in the area of global health, the role of these actors has grown and can be linked to all stages of the policy process. They have won a firm place in providing high-quality expertise, conducting research, providing policy analysis, and engaging

---

[a] According to the WHO document entitled "Principles Governing Relations with Nongovernmental Organizations," NGOs in official relationships with the WHO "shall be in conformity with the spirit, purposes, and principles of the Constitution of WHO, shall center on development work in health or health-related fields, and shall be free from concerns which are primarily of a commercial or profit-making nature." For more information, see http://www.who.int/civilsociety/relations/principles/en/index.html.

in advocacy. They have been instrumental in providing educational opportunities and designing training programs, and they are particularly useful for efforts to bridge the capacity gap in low- and middle-income countries. Mobilizing resources and establishing field capacity has proven to be among their strengths in the fight against HIV/AIDS, malaria, polio, and many other global health challenges. NGOs also have provided expertise in program monitoring and evaluation, activities that increasingly are required in the era of private–public partnerships and new business-like models for health investment. Such capacities may influence different stages of the global decision-making process. The negotiations for the WHO Global Code of Practice on the International Recruitment of Health Personnel and the FCTC provide a clear example of the increasingly important role of NGOs in 21st century health diplomacy. From "outsiders," NGOs are turning into "insiders," which have strong influence on the traditional state-centric multinational organizations and even on national governments. The outcomes of this development have not yet been sufficiently analyzed.

The diversification of players on the global level is accompanied by changing relationships among them. Innovative forms of governance are emerging to accommodate the increasingly complex interplay among the public sphere, the private sphere, and civil society. As Held *et al.* wrote, "Nation-states have become enmeshed in and functionally part of a larger pattern of global transformations and global flows."[80] Much has been written on the hybrids of global entities and financing mechanisms that have emerged in the past decade. The key characteristic of these hybrids is probably that of the "interface,"[81] which refers to the recurrent interaction and influence through discursive, organizational, legal, and resource transfers that take place in many transnational fora. Attracting resources and public attention, non-state actors have brought huge commitments to global health in terms of money, human resources, and expertise beyond what was expected a few decades ago. The global health enterprise has provided opportunities for innovation, creativity, entrepreneurship, rapid action, flexible alliances, and new types of partnerships.[13] The challenges now are to address the structural implications of the (over)crowded field of global health and to ensure coherence in policy, actions, and financial sustainability.

With the evolution of the new context for GHD and the exponential increase in global health actors, the role of the WHO has often been challenged. In spite of the huge financial power that single non-state actors such as the Bill and Melinda Gates Foundation may bring, however, the WHO still provides the legitimacy for global collective action. It has universal membership that is open to all nation-states; its annual assembly is an unparalleled forum for discussion among the 193 Member States; and that forum provides a venue at which large and small countries can debate on an equal basis. The wide range of governance instruments at its disposal, including its treaty-making power, reinforces the leadership role that the WHO must play in global health. It is the agency tasked with ensuring global health stewardship, country support, and global health governance, albeit at the cost of a high degree of bureaucratization and politicization.[39] Yet, the WHO needs to seriously consider how to better engage non-state players in a more transparent and rules-based approach to the negotiations that are conducted at the WHO.

The power shift within nations

For GHD, the intersection between the national and global levels becomes increasingly important. It encompasses a much closer interface between domestic and foreign policy and demands cooperation among a wide range of national sectoral ministries.

As Slaughter wrote, "Understanding 'domestic' issues in a regional or global context must become part of doing a good job. Increasingly, the optimal solution to these issues will depend on what is happening abroad, and the solutions to foreign issues, in a corresponding measure, [will depend on] what is happening at home."[82] National systems are core components of the global system.[40,56] This shift also applies to health: global health begins and ends "at home."[57]

In response to the need to address the interface between national and global health issues, countries are exploring new mechanisms for policy coherence. Consistency is sought in two directions: first, across government sectors and the work of different ministries and, second, between national interests and global responsibilities. Switzerland[83] and the United Kingdom[84] provide clear examples of such approaches. Other countries are preparing similar strategies and exploring other mechanisms to build the basis for coherence in the national approaches to global health. A more consistent approach to health policy on the national level and the improved coordination among the ministries are key to addressing global health challenges. Such an approach guarantees that national interests and international responsibility are balanced. It also helps ensure that any agreements reached on the international level will have the required political support within the country, so that they may be successfully implemented.

Conclusion

As stated at the beginning of this chapter, the UNGA Resolutions on Global Health and Foreign Policy[1-4] have ushered in a new phase of Global Health Diplomacy. Ministers of foreign affairs have affirmed the political realm of global health and, in the process, reinforced the significance of multilateral organizations as a platform for negotiations on global health. Of most interest is the question of how to balance the health agenda between the UNGA as the global political body and the WHO as the global technical organization. Politics and technical capacity have come together under the rubric of GHD as never before.

To some extent, however, health diplomacy has come full circle. In 160 years, it has moved from a political arena to a technical agenda and then back to a political arena of negotiation; it has also returned to the UN and to "open diplomacy," not as an operational institution, but as a political priority at the highest level of the UN. The UN Security Council and the UNGA deliberate on health, as illustrated by UNGA Resolutions 63/33,[1] 64/108,[2] 65/95,[3] and 66/115,[4] of 2008, 2009, 2010, and 2011. As a result, the UN Secretary-General appointed a UN System Influenza Coordinator, and the UNGA devoted special sessions to HIV/AIDs and, in 2011, conducted a special session on noncommunicable diseases. Health is also at the heart of the MDGs, the leading framework for UN efforts to advance human development. Health is the specific subject of three of these goals and forms "a critical precondition for progress on most of them."[85]

In addition, the UN Secretary-General has identified the challenge of making people's lives healthier to be a touchstone for the effectiveness of UN reforms (Ref. 5, para. 49). Health has also become a major issue for many other multinational bodies, such as the World Bank Group, the WTO, the World Intellectual Property Organization, the UN Children's Fund (UNICEF), the UN Environment Programme, and the UN Commission on Human Rights.

The deeper relevance of the UN Resolutions on Global Health and Foreign Policy is that they emphasize both the core relationship between health and foreign policy in the 21st century and the dynamic role of diplomacy in supporting health. This perspective suggests the direction that the new phase of institutionalization of global health must take: health must become an integral part of foreign policy. In addition, foreign policy needs to be driven by the new mindset that accepts the diplomatic corps' double responsibility: that for one's own country and that for the global community. These responsibilities are the challenge for health diplomacy at the beginning of the 21st century.

References

1. United Nations. (2008) Resolution A/Res/63/33. Global Health and Foreign Policy. Available at www.who.int/trade/events/UNGA_RESOLUTION_ GHFP_63_33.pdf (accessed November 30, 2011).
2. United Nations. (2009) Resolution A/Res/64/108. Global Health and Foreign Policy. Available at daccess-dds-ny.un.org/doc/UNDOC/GEN/N09/468/31/ PDF/N0946831.pdf?OpenElement (accessed November 30, 2011).
3. United Nations. (2010) Resolution A/Res/65/95. Global Health and Foreign Policy. Available at daccess-dds-ny.un.org/doc/UNDOC/GEN/N10/518/24/ PDF/N1051824.pdf?OpenElement (accessed November 30, 2011).
4. United Nations. (2011) Resolution A/66/115. Global Health and Foreign Policy. Available at http://daccess-ods.un.org/TMP/7261011.60049438.html (accessed February 26, 2012).
5. United Nations. (2010) Global health and foreign policy: Strategic opportunities and challenges. Note by the Secretary-General A/64/365. Available at daccess-dds-ny.un.org/doc/UNDOC/GEN/N09/522/15/PDF/N0952215. pdf?OpenElement (accessed November 30, 2011).

6. United Nations. (2004) A more secure world: Our shared responsibility. Report of the Secretary-General's High-level Panel on Threats, Challenges and Change. UN Doc A/59/565. Available at http://www.un.org/secureworld/report.pdf

7. UN Secretary-General. (2011) Remarks to the General Assembly after being appointed for a second term, New York, June 21, 2011. Available at http://www.un.org/apps/sg/sgstats.asp?nid=5365 (accessed November 30, 2011).

8. Reinalda B. (2008) The performance of international organizations and questions for organization theory. Prepared for the International Studies Association Annual Convention (San Francisco, CA; March 26–29, 2008).

9. World Health Organization. (1958) The first 10 years of the World Health Organization. World Health Organization.

10. World Health Organization. (2005) International Health Regulations (2005). World Health Organization. Available at http://whqlibdoc.who.int/publications/2008/9789241580410_eng.pdf

11. Beck U. (2007) *Weltrisikogesellschaft. Auf der Suche nach der verlorenen Sicherheit* ("World at Risk: the Search for Lost Security"). Suhrkamp, Frankfurt a.M., Germany.

12. Beck U. (2008) Risk Society's "Cosmopolitan Moment." Presentation held on November 12, 2008, at Harvard University.

13. Kickbusch I. (2009) Moving global health governance forward. In: Buse K, Hein W, Drager N (eds.), *Making Sense of Global Health Governance — A Policy Perspective*. Palgrave Macmillan, Basingstoke, UK, pp. 320–339.

14. Fidler D. (2005) From International Sanitary Conventions to global health security: The new International Health Regulations. *Chin J Int Law* **4:** 325–392.

15. Goddard NL, Delpech VC, Watson JM, *et al.* (2006) Lessons learned from SARS: The experience of the Health Protection Agency, England. *Public Health* **120(1):** 27–32.

16. World Health Assembly. (2003) Resolution 56.29. Severe acute respiratory syndrome (SARS). Available at www.who.int/csr/sars/en/ea56r29.pdf (accessed November 30, 2011).

17. Birn AE. (2009) The stages of international (global) health: Histories of success or successes of history? *Global Public Health* **4(1):** 50–68.

18. Howard-Jones N. (1975) The scientific background of the International Sanitary Conferences 1851–1938. World Health Organization.
19. International Committee of the Red Cross. (2004) From the battle of Solferino to the eve of the First World War. Available at www.icrc.org/eng/resources/documents/misc/57jnvp.htm (accessed November 30, 2011).
20. Berridge GR. (2005) *Diplomacy: Theory and Practice*, 3rd edn. Palgrave Macmillan, Basingstoke, UK.
21. Kissinger H. (1994) *Diplomacy*. Simon and Schuster, New York, pp. 17–28.
22. Hamilton K, Langhorne R. (1995) *The Practice of Diplomacy: Its Evolution, Theory and Administration*. Routledge, New York.
23. Kennedy P. (2006) *The Parliament of Man: The Past, Present, and Future of the United Nations*. Vintage Books (Random House), New York.
24. Hudson VM. (2008) The history and evolution of foreign policy analysis. In: Smith S, Hadfield A, Dunne T (eds.), *Foreign Policy: Theories, Actors, Cases*. Oxford University Press, New York, pp. 11–30.
25. Cooper R. (2004) *The Breaking of Nations: Order and Chaos in the 21st Century*, revised and updated edition. Atlantic Books, London.
26. Muldoon J Jr, Sullivan E, Aviel JF, Reitano R. (2005) *Multilateral Diplomacy and the United Nations Today*, 2nd edn. Westview Press, Boulder, CO.
27. Kaul I, Le Goulven K. (2003) Financing global public goods: A new frontier of public finance. In: Kaul I, Conceicao P, Goulven K, Mendoza R (eds.), *Providing Global Public Goods: Managing Globalization*, Oxford University Press, New York, pp. 329–370.
28. Kaul I, Grunberg I, Stern MA (eds.). (1999) *Global Public Goods: International Cooperation in the 21st Century*. Oxford University Press, New York.
29. Kurbalija J (ed.). (2002) Knowledge and diplomacy. UN Development Programme. 1999 Conference on Knowledge and Diplomacy (University of Malta). Available at http://www.diplomacy.edu/resources/books/knowledge-and-diplomacy
30. Kurbalija J, Katrandjiev V (eds.). (2006). Multistakeholder diplomacy. Challenges and opportunities. DiploFoundation, Mdiga, Malta. Available at http://textus.diplomacy.edu/textusbin/env/scripts/Pool/GetBin.asp?IDPool=956
31. Støre JG. (2010) Time for G-20 to address its legitimacy. *The Straits Times* (Manila, the Philippines), April 6, 2010. Available at www.regjeringen.no/en/

dep/ud/whats-new/Speeches-and-articles/speeches-foreign.html?id=450637 (accessed November 30, 2011).

32. Young OR (ed.). (1997) *Global Governance: Drawing Insights from the Environmental Experience.* MIT Press, Cambridge, MA.

33. Kickbusch I. (2010) *Globale Gesundheitspolitik* ("Global health politics"). *Internationale Politik* **4**: 46–52.

34. Committee on the US Commitment to Global Health (Board on Global Health and the Institute of Medicine). 2009. The US commitment to global health: Recommendations for the new administration. The National Academies Press, Washington, DC.

35. Sucharipa E. (2000) 21st century diplomacy. Available at campus.diplomacy. edu//lms/pool/BD materials/Sucharipa.htm (accessed November 30, 2011).

36. Wiseman G. (2004) "Polylateralism" and new modes of global dialogue. In: Jönsson C, Langhorne R (eds.), *Diplomacy,* Vol. III. Sage, London, pp. 36–57.

37. Barston RP. (2006) *Modern Diplomacy*, 3rd edn. Longman (Pearson Education), Harlow, UK.

38. Heine J. (2006) On the manner of practising the new eiplomacy. Centre for International Governance Innovation (CIGI) Working Paper #11. Available at www.cigionline.org/publications/2006/10/manner-practising-new-diplomacy (accessed November 30, 2011).

39. Moon S, Szlezák NA, Michaud CM, *et al.* (2010) The global health system: Lessons for a stronger institutional framework. *PLoS Med* **7(1)**: e1000193. doi: 10.1371/journal.pmed.1000193.

40. Frenk J. (2010) The global health system: Strengthening national health systems as the next step for global progress. *PLoS Med* **7(1)**: e1000089. doi: 10.1371/journal.pmed.1000089.

41. Alcazar S. (2008) The Copernican shift in global health. Working Paper No. 3. Global Health Program Graduate Institute, Geneva. Available at graduateinstitute.ch/webdav/site/globalhealth/shared/1894/GHD/Working Papers–003-WEB new version 15062009.pdf (accessed November 30, 2011).

42. Feldman H. (2012) Health diplomacy in the 21st century. In: Novotny TE, Kickbusch I, Told M (eds.), *21st Century Global Health Diplomacy*, World Scientific, Singapore.

43. Ministers of foreign affairs of Brazil, France, Indonesia, Norway, Senegal, South Africa, and Thailand. (2007) Oslo Ministerial Declaration — Global health: A pressing foreign policy issue of our time. *Lancet* **369**: 1373–1378.

44. Kickbusch I. (2011) Global health diplomacy: How foreign policy can influence health. *BMJ* **342:** d3154.
45. Fidler DP. (2010) The Challenges of Global Health Governance. Working Paper. Council on Foreign Relations. International Institutions and Global Governance Program. Council on Foreign Relations, New York.
46. Spiegel J M. (2006) Commentary: Daring to learn from a good example and break the "Cuba taboo." *Int J Epidemiol* **35:** 825–826.
47. Ministry of foreign affairs of the People's Republic of China. (2006) China's Africa policy, Part IV. Enhancing all-round cooperation between China and Africa. Available at www.china.org.cn/english/features/focac/183721.htm (accessed November 30, 2011).
48. Nye JS Jr. (2004) *Soft Power: The Means to Success in World Politics*. Public Affairs (Perseus Books Group), New York.
49. Lee K, Chagas LC, Novotny T. (2010) Brazil and the Framework Convention on Tobacco Control: Global health diplomacy as soft power. *PLoS Med* **7(4):** e1000232. doi:10.1371/journal.pmed.1000232.
50. Vanderwagen W. (2006) Health diplomacy: Winning hearts and minds through the use of health interventions. *Mil Med* **171(10 Suppl):** 3–4.
51. McInnes C, Lee K. (2006) Health, security, and foreign policy. *Rev Int Stud* **32:** 5–23.
52. Garrett L. (2005) HIV and national security: Where are the links? A Council on Foreign Relations Report. Available at www.cfr.org/national-security-and-defense/hiv-national-security-links/p8256 (accessed November 30, 2011).
53. World Health Organization. (2003) Framework Convention on Tobacco Control. World Health Organization.
54. Whelan M. (2008) Negotiating the International Health Regulations. Working Paper No. 1. Global Health Programme Graduate Institute, Geneva. http://graduateinstitute.ch/webdav/site/globalhealth/shared/1894/Working%20Papers_001_WEB%20new%20version%2024112009.pdf
55. Novotny T, Kickbusch I, Leslie H, Adams V. (2008) Global health diplomacy — A bridge to innovative collaborative action. *Global Forum Update on Research for Health* **5:** 41–45. Available at graduateinstitute.ch/webdav/site/globalhealth/shared/1894/GHD-a bridge to innovative collaborative action.pdf (accessed November 30, 2011).
56. Silberschmidt G, Zeltner T. (2012) Global health begins at home: Policy conference. In: Novotny TE, Kickbusch I, Told M (eds.), *21st Century Global Health Diplomacy*. World Scientific, Singapore.

57. Council of the European Union. (2010) EU Council Conclusions on the EU role in global health. No. prev. 9505/10. Available at www.europa-eu-un.org/articles/en/article_9727_en.htm (accessed November 30, 2011).
58. The United States President's Emergency Plan for AIDS Relief. (2009) Ambassador Eric Goosby, US Global AIDS Coordinator. Available at http://www.pepfar.gov/press/125262.htm (accessed November 30, 2011).
59. Farley J. (2004) To cast out disease: A history of the International Health Division of the Rockefeller Foundation, 1913–1951. Oxford University Press, New York.
60. Kennedy D. (1987) The move to institutions. *Cardozo Law Rev* **8(5):** 841–988.
61. Adams V. (2012) A history of international health encounters: Diplomacy in transition. In: Novotny TE, Kickbusch I, Told M (eds.), *21st Century Global Health Diplomacy*, World Scientific, Singapore.
62. WHO. (1981) International Code of Marketing of Breast-Milk Substitutes. World Health Organization. http://www.who.int/nutrition/publications/code_english.pdf
63. Godlee F. (1994) WHO in crisis. *BMJ* **309:** 1424–1428.
64. Brown TM, Cueto M, Fee E. (2006) The World Health Organization and the transition from "international" to "global" public health. *Am J Public Health* **96:** 62–72.
65. Hein W, Kickbusch I. (2010) Global health, aid effectiveness and the changing role of the WHO. *GIGA Focus Int Ed* **2010(3):** 1–8.
66. Bull B, McNeill D. (2007) *Development Issues in Global Governance: Public–Private Partnerships and Market Multilateralism.* Routledge (Warwick Studies in Globalisation), Abingdon, UK.
67. Gostin LO, Mok EA. (2009) Grand challenges in global health governance. *Br Med Bull* **90:** 7–18.
68. Fidler D. (2002) Global health governance: Overview of the role of international law in protecting and promoting global public health. World Health Organization and London School of Hygiene and Tropical Medicine. Available at www.who.int/trade/GHG/en/index.html (accessed November 30, 2011).
69. Müller-Kraenner S (ed.). (1998) Environmental diplomacy. American Institute for Contemporary German Studies, The Johns Hopkins University, Washington, DC. Available at http://www.aicgs.org/documents/environmentaldiplomacy.pdf (accessed November 30, 2011).

70. Benedick R. (1998) Diplomacy for the environment. In: Müller-Kraenner S (ed.). (1998) *Environmental Diplomacy*. American Institute for Contemporary German Studies, The Johns Hopkins University, Washington, DC, pp. 3–12.

71. Hufbauer G, Kim J. (2010) Reaching a global agreement on climate change: What are the obstacles? *Asian Econ Policy Rev* **5:** 39–58.

72. Szlezák NA, Bloom BR, Jamison DT, *et al.* (2010) The global health system: Actors, norms, and expectations in transition. *PLoS Med* **7(1):** e1000183. doi: 10.1371/journal.pmed.1000183.

73. Khanna P. (2008) *The Second World: Empires and Influence in the New Global Order*. Random House, New York.

74. Gomez E. (2009) Brazil's blessing in disguise: How Lula turned an HIV crisis into a geopolitical opportunity. *Foreign Policy,* July 22. Available at www.foreignpolicy.com/articles/2009/07/22/brazils-blessing-in-disguise (accessed November 30, 2011).

75. Feldbaum H, Michaud J. (2010) Health diplomacy and the enduring relevance of foreign policy interests. *PLoS Med* **7(4):** e1000226. doi:10.1371/journal.pmed.1000226.

76. Haas RN. (2008) The age of non-polarity. What will follow US dominance? *Foreign Aff* **87(3):** 44–56.

77. Kickbusch I, Hein W, Silberschmidt G. Addressing global health governance challenges through a new mechanism: The proposal for a Committee C of the World Health Assembly. *J Law Med Ethics* **38(3):** 550–563.

78. Garrett L. (2007) The challenge of global health. *Foreign Aff* **86:** 14–38.

79. World Health Organization. (2010) English/French list of 185 NGOs in official relations with WHO reflecting decisions of EB 126 January 2010. Available at http://www.who.int/civilsociety/relations/ngolisteb120.pdf (accessed November 30, 2011).

80. Held D, McGrew A, Goldblatt D, Perraton J. (1999) *Global Transformations: Politics, Economics and Culture*. Polity, Cambridge, UK.

81. Bartsch S, Hein W, Kohlmorgen L. (2007) Interfaces: A concept for the analysis of global health governance. In: Hein W, Bartsch S, Kohlmorgen L (eds.), *Global Health Governance and the Fight Against HIV/AIDS*. Palgrave Macmillan, Basingstoke, UK, pp. 30–32.

82. Slaughter AM. (2004). *A New World Order*. Princeton University Press.

83. Swiss Federal Department of Home Affairs and Federal Department of Foreign Affairs. (2006) Swiss foreign health policy: Agreement on foreign health policy objectives. Swiss Government, Bern.

84. HM Government (UKHG Annex). (2008) Health is global: A UK government strategy 2008–2013. Annexes. HM Government, London. Available at http://www.dh.gov.uk/en/Publicationsandstatistics/Publications/Publications PolicyAndGuidance/DH_088702

85. Economic and Social Council of the United Nations. (2009) Theme of the annual ministerial review: Implementing the internationally agreed goals and commitments in regard to global public health. Report of the Secretary-General (E/2009/81). Available at daccess-dds-ny-un.org/doc/UNDOC/GEN/N09/343/76/PDF/N0934376.pdf?OpenElement (accessed November 30, 2011).

2

A History of International Health Encounters: Diplomacy in Transition

Vincanne Adams, PhD*

Introduction

The notion that health and politics are intertwined is certainly not new to the 21st century or to the advent of what we call in this volume "global health diplomacy." Health and politics have a long and deeply intertwined history. One could trace the rise and fall of ancient societies and civilizations to the consequences of political actions in relation to health, whether in terms of augmenting or preventing the spread of epidemics, mortality from tribal warfare, the building of aqueducts and sewage systems, pronatalism and infant survival, and even the social regulation of marital relations.[1-3] Empires have grown and societies have survived, in part because of the health afforded by politics, whether in tribes, chiefdoms, kingdoms, early or modern states. Political negotiations and governing infrastructures have enabled things like agricultural development, trade, traditional healing, and even the growth of modern medical science. In some instances, medical power is even constituted as political power, whether in the work of the shaman (in rural Nepal) or the Surgeon General (in the United States).

---

*University of California, San Francisco, Anthropology, History & Social Medicine, 3333 California St., Ste. 485, San Francisco, CA 94143-0850, USA. Tel.: (415) 502-6483. E-mail: adamsv@dahsm.ucsf.edu

For the purposes of this volume, I offer a cursory glimpse into some of the dynamics emergent in the relationships between health and politics that are visible in recent history or what Emmanuel Wallerstein[4] identified as the era of the World System — the economic and political exchanges that from at least the 17th century have connected most regions of the world into a global whole. Although instances of deliberate health politics are found long before the 17th century, history after the birth of the World System marks the advent of the distinctly modern effort to think about how to manage health in and through institutions of state-based and global governance. The material presented here is not an exhaustive but rather a thematic overview of tensions between health and politics that make "health diplomacy" a dynamic push and pull between two potentially competing agendas: the attempt to navigate health by way of politics and the attempt to navigate politics by way of health.

The first agenda, referred to as the *politics of health*, proposes that health needs to be addressed only to the extent that it will further or perhaps interfere with a political goal. Here, health serves the interests of politics. We see this today in the notions that national security may be achieved through health security; that health care will reduce the poverty burden and thus make a nation more politically stable; and that epidemic surveillance and even medical relief require strategic rather than humanitarian interventions for the purposes of advancing political goals.[5] Under this agenda, health diplomacy is organized around the idea that political outcomes are achieved by way of rhetorical and actual use of health goals — health is both a tool and bargaining chip in political battles. When politics needs health, it is a focus for political investment (for example, federal support for humanitarian relief post-disaster along partisan lines in an election year). When politics sees health as an obstacle to its own goals (for example, warfare), health is augmented (by increasing combat activities) or decreased (by ending combat) or vice-versa, on political rather than medical grounds, thus enabling politics to trump health.

The second agenda reverses this equation. *Health politics* focuses on the idea that politics can and should be used to further global health goals. Here, politics serves the interests of health as a global public good that surpasses political end points. International conventions on health, whether to reduce tobacco use, distribute medicines, or even to allow military forces to provide medical relief, are intended primarily to put health goals above those of politics, even when some sovereign interests must be overcome for such agreements to be enacted. In health politics, health diplomacy advances the possibility that politics can serve the goals of health and simultaneously work against the tendency for politics to get in the way of or impede health. Yet, diplomats in the world of health politics must for this very reason work within political arenas, calling for policies and practices that transcend conflicting political interests while also catering to these same specific interests to achieve positive health outcomes.

Looking historically at the intertwining of health and politics, one can see that sometimes these agendas have come together, whereas, in other instances, they have competed with one another. In almost all cases, they are intertwined. In what follows, I explore some of the dynamics of health and politics, from key 19th century social theorists and the work of missionary, colonial, and tropical medicine, all the way to contemporary theories of biopolitics, health, and therapeutic citizenship in an era of global health sciences. A survey over time may be instructive in delineating what has and what has not been accomplished in the delicate marriage of global health and politics as well as what health diplomacy might add to this relationship.

Nineteenth Century Health Politics

Philosophers and humanitarians of the European world early on identified the important role that politics could play in furthering health. In 1861, for example, the pathologist and anthropologist Rudolf Virchow, who eventually held office in the Prussian parliament, noted that political reform was necessary for improving the health of the public.[6] Likening the sociopolitical infrastructure of a nation to that of the physiognomy of the human body, he argued that health on a "cellular" level in the body was like the health of a nation — dependent upon the vital and healthy political functioning of all of its "molecular" or civil sectors. Offering some of the earliest insights into health politics, Virchow coined the now-famous aphorism "Politics is nothing but medicine on a grand scale." For him the analogy was metaphorical: bodies were like societies, and the health of the body was like the health of the state. But, in his conceptualization, the metaphor was also literal: political reforms were not only able to cure what crude treatments of the physicians of his day could not (by ending poverty and increasing the circulation of clean water, food and wealth) but were also the cure for corrupt and ineffective governance that made people suffer. It was the job of the politician to ensure the health of the public, not just the job of the physician. Virchow's insights created a political template for health activism that has persisted into the 21st century in the form of "social medicine."[7]

Karl Marx and Frederic Engels, near contemporaries of Virchow, one of whom was from Prussia as well, identified the health conditions of the working class as a problem that called for political solutions.[8] The notion that, without political reform, there could be no improvement in the basic conditions of the poorest sectors of modern industrial society has had a huge impact far beyond the European context in which the notion was developed. Marx's and Engels's particular insights into the links between health and politics — between psychological alienation, poor health, impoverished living conditions and entrenched social inequality brought about by specific political–economic infrastructures — were used as a platform in several revolutionary contexts, both large (the Soviet Union and China) and small (Cuba and Nepal).[9,10] In these contexts, calls for political reform in the name of health were articulated through entirely different political agendas, including communist, socialist, and demo-cratic. More recently, even Egypt's Arab Spring made use of medicine and health as platforms for revolutionary action with the aim of advancing democratic freedoms. In these contexts, we witness a blurring of *health politics* with a *politics of health*, as political efforts become articulated in and through mandates that place health at the center of reformist agendas and make health and politics simultaneous and mutually dependent goals. The radical theories of these 19th century social theorists continue to inform the leftist health politics of many industrialized nations today, particularly in those nations that have attempted to establish strong public health and socialized medicine programs,[11,12] despite the absence of a revolutionary ideology that was a hallmark of their predecessors.

It is interesting that, even while political reformers of the 19th and early 20th century took up political action as a means of improving health for the masses, larger forces that were aligned with a different sort of relationship between health and politics had long been at work in some nations. The early history of mercantilism and colonialism offers examples of how a *politics of health* was at work, making health a handmaiden to the political and economic success of mercantile and colonial regimes. Humanistic health reformers of the 19th century witnessed social inequalities in their home nations, but they were also exposed to more egregious forms of inequality in the form of late-stage extractive colonial capitalism.[13] The roots of tropical medicine are themselves complex, dating back to the time of missionary, mercantile, and colonial regimes, and thus they are worth exploring as a starting point for early relationships between global health and politics.

Politics of Health: Missionaries, Mercantilism, and the Colonial Health Imperative

The relationships between politics and health under early missionary, mercantile, and colonial eras are best characterized as a mixture of interests and infrastructures. Imperialism and mercantilism paved the way for some development of international medical care by the mid-17th century. Colonial doctors who worked for the British and Dutch East India companies, for example, set up clinical services in remote outposts and port cities of southern Africa and India.[14,15] From these posts, physicians primarily attended to the care of Europeans who ran these companies and served in colonial administrations, but they also treated natives and used those opportunities to observe and develop a rudimentary scientific inventory of the health conditions found in what would later become colonized regions.[13,16,17]

Missionary medical teams who worked alongside or in opposition to mercantile and colonial infrastructures offered opportunities for native populations to receive medical care, sometimes in exchange for conversion to Christianity.[16] Saving souls continued to be thought of as a means of saving lives among those missionaries and colonial humanitarians for whom social Darwinism explained social inequality — and (for some) it justified colonialism — up through the early 20th century. The varied perspectives of colonial medicine entailed different political investments.

Missionary medicine was driven by a humanitarian ethic, but it was usually accompanied by pressure for cultural (as well as religious) conversion, which, in turn, was often seen by natives as political since religious leadership usually challenged local tribal and chiefly infrastructures of governance. Missionary work was at times seen as oppositional to the work of mercantile and colonial interests, with missionary medicine addressing some of the spoils of economic pillage.[18] For some, missionary medicine was considered a means of atoning for the sins of colonialism (as was the case for Albert Schweitzer and many others). In other locales, missionary medicine served to assist colonial governance[19] and helped acquiescence to colonial regimes.[16] It also ensured the health of the native labor force working in the extractive industries under unhealthy conditions, including mining, textile production, and tea growing.[19] Whether one placed political or economic goals above those of health might be best seen as a conundrum for health professionals working in colonial settings, with a good deal of conflict resulting from both the humanitarian and economic mandates.

Nineteenth century international public health interventions focused largely on the control or prevention of infectious diseases — efforts that were as much about keeping colonials in place as about keeping natives healthy. Eliminating smallpox, syphilis, tuberculosis, malaria, yaws, yellow fever, cholera, and trachoma, for example, was important because it was not just native populations that they affected. Colonials were exposed and vulnerable to the same diseases as natives and, thus, to ensure the livelihoods, well-being, and productivity of the native labor force was to ensure the well-being of the colony as well. Still, colonial medicine indisputably supported colonial commerce and industry in ways that had impacts far beyond elite communities.[13] In the eyes of the colonizer, public health efforts and political rule were surely intertwined. Colonial medicine allowed more peaceful governance and successful businesses, in some instances a route to quelling discontent among the natives.[19,22]

For colonized populations, obtaining medical care was often fraught with the political contestations accompanying colonialism. Fanon[20,21] described the resistance among Algerians to receiving modern medical care arising not because natives could not understand or accept the effectiveness of modern medicine, but because this medicine represented the medicine of the colonizers. To accept this care signaled acquiescence to political oppression. Brown[22] identified similar problems with early efforts by the Rockefeller Foundation, in which public health campaigns were identified by local populations as being more about the population's productivity than about their actual health status.[23] In some critical analyses, these medical efforts were seen as an advance guard for American and European economic imperialism.[13,22]

By the time that colonial infrastructures were installed in Africa, the Americas, and India, efforts to build on existing medical resources had led to larger programs in public health and hygiene. In some regions, the involvement of colonial states in health affairs came after a century or more of health activities by missionaries.[16] Hospitals and clinics established by missionaries and humanitarian organizations became resources for public health campaigns launched by colonial governments in the early 20th century, both to care for colonialists and to improve the health of the native populations. As a result, a cadre of trained colonial physicians and health care workers emerged to help establish schools of tropical medicine and hygiene in Europe and Britain.[17,24]

Under colonial governance, motivations to promote health were formed under a larger rubric of colonial ideology, in which it was understood that what the colonial, or the missionary, could bring far surpassed what the natives already had or did in relation to health. Thus, even when not allied with the spoils of colonialism, such as in the work of missionary medical teams, medicine and public health efforts at this time indirectly worked to make colonialism possible. Under the infrastructures of colonialism, we see early examples of health diplomacy. Colonial administrations were not dealing with foreign governments as much as with internal colonial relations. Thus, the need for "diplomacy" in health had more to do with convincing the natives to "use" colonial health care resources than with negotiating between the colonial powers. Efforts to get natives to use medicines or health interventions correctly, or legislating that they do so, even when these efforts entailed a good deal of coercion,[20] could be seen as early forms of the health-diplomatic challenge. Similarly, colonial governments' interventions in the health of the natives also invited these governments to legislate upward, regulating commercial and labor activities when they were harmful to health. These too formed a proto-health-diplomacy as instruments of empire that directly impacted health by way of governance. Political efforts to improve health or legislate health care reforms in this era traveled from metropole to periphery and vice versa as far as the empire(s) reached, but it was not until the colonial era began to see its demise that modern international political treaties regarding health policy were seen.

In sum, one senses a diplomatic imperialism that was built into the era of colonial medicine. With active acquiescence of natives to colonial medical care, natives and their diseases could be studied, counted, tracked, and understood, forming an infrastructure of knowledge about how to control diseases in ways that directly enhanced the government's ability to both govern and protect the colony, which, in turn, served the colonizing nation.[17] Still, the institutions of public health that eventually emerged out of these efforts created a foundation for international health agencies in a postcolonial era. In fact, the colonial period generated insights that are also foundational to health diplomacy today. The more investment that colonial administrations made in the health of the colonized, the more the idea arose that epidemic diseases required surveillance and control measures which exceeded any single nation's capacity to respond. The growth of academic and scholarly research on tropical medicine and hygiene reinforced and deepened an understanding of the links between trade, tourism, and colonialism itself and the spread of diseases. The London School of Hygiene and Tropical Medicine, for example, developed a large database of information about the pathologies, etiologies, and means of controlling the spread of infectious diseases, devoting particular attention to the containment and treatment of numerous tropical and epidemic diseases (malaria, leprosy, yaws and tuberculosis are good examples).

The rise of international campaigns to control infectious diseases was, in many ways, a product of the colonial experience. Most international health exchanges in the European context in the 19th and early 20th century revolved around preventing the spread of infectious diseases,[25-27] accompanied to a lesser extent by efforts to provide medical education, research, or even curative clinical care. This focus had advantages. Colonialism helped pave the way for a global understanding of how the same diseases thrived in different regions of the globe and how they spread through the movement of goods and people related to colonial advancement and commerce.[24] It was not long before this same set of related interests — economic, medical, and political — was pulled into new institutional arrangements that gave rise to the contemporary notions of international health governance that we see today.

For instance, quarantine and restrictions on travel to prevent the spread of diseases first emerged in Europe during the 14th century as a result of various plagues; other, similar forms of restrictions were found in Arabian empires before that.[28] Thus, although hygiene programs aimed at limiting the spread of air- and water-borne diseases were already in place by the time of empire in the 19th century,[26] the colonial era gave rise to contemporary notions of epidemic disease control involving large-scale, cross-national dialogue and cooperation. Conventions declaring quarantine and restrictions on trade and travel because of the fear of spreading diseases emerged before the turn of the century and as a result numerous international conferences were held as public health came to be seen as something that reached far beyond the confines of nation and state. As colonialism itself began to unravel at the turn of the 20th century (although in large parts of Africa it was only beginning), these new conventions also demanded the attention of newly independent governments that could implement and enforce consensus-driven public health policies.

Health as Politics: Postcolonialism and the Rise of Multilateral and Bilateral Health Aid

The First International Sanitary Conference was held in Paris in 1851, in part as a response to the rise and spread of cholera associated with merchant trade in Europe and the Middle East. It had representatives from European countries, and it was followed by more than 10 other conferences in different countries up through 1903, with each conference focusing on a series of epidemic diseases. These conferences — notably the Paris Convention of 1903, which included representatives from 21 countries — resulted in the first international political treaties devoted explicitly to a health outcome.[29] Such efforts exemplify *health politics* in action.

In 1907, the first International Office of Public Hygiene was established;[29] it remained in existence until the beginning of World War II. The Hygiene Section of the League of Nations was formed around 1917 as a result of fear of the typhus epidemic in Europe. Although the Americas and the East Asian nations were not participants in these European conferences, similar efforts in the Americas were already forming by the end of the 19th century, resulting in the First Sanitary Convention of the American Republics in 1902. The Pan American Sanitary Bureau devoted its efforts to promoting cross-national conventions for quarantine, hygiene, and surveillance, and it was the precursor of the Pan American Health Organization.[29]

At the turn of the 20th century, regional representation of nations in these international consortia had roughly followed the contours of former colonial power structures but, by mid-century, nearly all regions of the globe were included in the conversations around what would come to be called "international health." The first postcolonial global health diplomacy efforts were found in the conventions on health and hygiene for the prevention of diseases and in the international infectious disease eradication effort that followed. These organizations emerged as postcolonial, transnational institutions and created the basis for what would later become the World Health Organization. They provided a template for a kind of health politics in which the interests of promoting health might transcend the economic and political interests of specific nations, despite the fact that, for some nation participants, politics continued to be prioritized over global health.

In these precursor organizations, we find a mixture of humanitarian and political objectives. Some nations (Great Britain, for example) participated reluctantly in these late 19th and early 20th century conventions, precisely because they feared that measures such as quarantine would hamper essential trade relations.[29] Contributions to these conventions (and the willingness to enforce their rules) were often influenced by regional and national politics, with some nations supporting health interventions only if they were linked to trade or other development investment policies. Some nations engaged in negotiations around health conventions only because economic trade and commerce had been undermined by the spread of epidemics (in Europe) and because not doing so might have led to further adverse fiscal outcomes. Some nations participated because of their interest in using health measures to restrict or otherwise limit the inflow of immigrants, who were seen (particularly in Europe and the

United States) as "disease carriers." Clearly, these measures were linked to fears about immigrants displacing native populations in jobs, but also to a general sense of xenophobia. Finally, for many of the idealists involved in these efforts, the ultimate goal was quite simply "health," and they were not concerned as to whether their efforts also promoted political or economic goals. In fact, the distinction between these two priorities was, in all likelihood, quite blurry for many and, just as today, a moving target.

Nevertheless, early postcolonial efforts to promote health as a global public good and economic benefit required policy infrastructures for international collaboration that could facilitate the control and eradication of diseases across national borders. These efforts formed a critical nexus that would give rise to the concept of health diplomacy that we see today. In particular, it is important to recognize that such organizations provided a paradigmatic platform for the birth of what was to follow in programs of international health development — the institutional basis for global health governance that accompanied decolonization.

The institutions involved with international health governance that emerged soon after World War II under the United Nations (UN) and the Bretton Woods financial organizations, i.e. the World Bank (WB) and the International Money Fund (IMF), arose in part from the dreams of collaborative health conventions, such as seen in the Paris Convention and the Pan American Sanitary Code. These conventions were based on direct observation of the benefits of cross-national political collaboration for health. In the post-World War II era, the dream for such transnational institutions was put in motion through policies and practices of postcolonial development aid. A more detailed account of the heritage of development aid is given in William Easterly's *The White Man's Burden*.[30]

The World Health Organization (WHO) was established in 1948 as a specialized agency of the UN, in part to continue with the effort begun by the League of Nations Health Organization in the previous decade.[31] The primary focus of the organization, like that of the "conventions" before it, was the eradication of epidemic diseases. In the context of postwar development, however, the WHO had also taken on a much broader mandate. The multilateral institutions of the UN, the WB, and the IMF, were created with funding from all participating governments with the intention of enabling collaborative international programs that could rebuild war-torn Europe and the newly decolonized world, thereby preventing another world war. Consequently, these organizations targeted a wide range of development goals, including infrastructure, education, health, technology, and economy. The role of the WHO was both to focus specifically on health and to provide an institutional resource for ensuring that health was not overlooked in the larger drive toward modernization of what was then considered the "developing" or "third" world. The Third World was, in fact, more of a political concept indicating those countries not aligned with either the capitalist West or the communist Eastern Bloc.[4] Certainly, health would come to play a role in the standoff between the First and Second Worlds that would affect the Third World as well.

The governance that emerged from international health programs and agendas differed markedly from the kinds of governance implemented under colonial regimes. The formal recognition of health as part of the overall development agenda in many ways undermined the notion that health could be used for political purposes. Under organizations such as the WHO, health became a political goal in its own right — a global public good with a mandate for economic and political cooperation among all of the member states of the WHO. Health diplomacy in this era was tied to multilateral development aid, and it ushered in a new sort of health politics that revisited commitment to a politics of health: health was seen as itself a critical political investment. That is to say, health was seen as a critical component of all other development goals, whether economic, infrastructural, educational, or technological. This orientation culminated in the deployment of numerous international health declarations (from the 1978 Alma Ata *Declaration of Health for All by the Year 2000*, to the 1986 Ottowa *Charter for Health Promotion,* to the 1998 revised *Declaration of Health for All by the 21st Century*), which have successively seeded funding for the dispersal of health resources to the poorest and least-developed nations of the world.

Just as decolonization gave rise to multilateral agencies, so too did wealthy nations respond to the new world order by developing their own governmental branches devoted to international aid (e.g. the US Agency for International Aid, the UK Department for International Development, the Swedish International Development Cooperation Agency, the Canadian International Development Agency, and the Japanese International Cooperation Agency). Alongside multilateral agencies, bilateral aid programs began to emerge. However, unlike the multilateral groups, bilateral agencies were often driven by more explicit political interests of the countries they served, because they were accountable to the foreign affairs or state department offices in their own countries more than to their target communities. The notion that development aid could be used as a tool of foreign policy in its own right worked in parallel with or sometimes even in opposition to efforts of multilateral agencies that prioritized "health for all" above all other political goals.

Development Era Health Diplomacy: From Health Politics to Integrated Health

In the half-century since the advent of the development era, global health has undergone several important paradigm shifts. Initially, most of the programs advanced by the WHO and subsidiary health-related programs were focused on attacking the problems of single diseases. Vertical programs that targeted the prevention, eradication, and treatment of tuberculosis, malaria, leprosy, and smallpox, for example, initially involved the training of teams of health workers to be specialized in these activities.[32] Health politics in this era were primarily focused on the idea that technical expertise, if provided with enough political and financial backing, could eliminate most of the most debilitating sources of morbidity and mortality.[32] Using a "silver platter" approach, health development programs deployed massive spraying and clean water campaigns to eliminate pathogens and vectors, vaccination and quarantine strategies to isolate and eradicate diseases, and the building of latrines and in some cases curative hospitals.

By the mid-1970s, health programs began to recognize that, without attacking other infrastructural problems in health development, vertical programs were limited in their ability to effectively eliminate diseases. Along with the rising interest in various socialist programs of health care that prioritized basic health care over single diseases, the WHO began to promote a more integrated basic program of health.[33] The WHO's Alma Ata Conference of 1978 advanced a Primary Health Care Initiative that called for health development programs focusing on a wide range of pre-ventive measures — immunizations, education, hygiene, clean water, and nutrition — instead of only the specialized strategies of eradication of single diseases and the construction of large, specialized hospitals.[34]

Eventually, the notion of "integrated development" grew out of this shift in focus. Under integrated development models, health goals were tied to other development targets so that, for example, new mothers could receive nutritional supplements and small loans if they agreed to simulta-neously receive prenatal and postnatal care and nutritional health educa-tion.[35] In the case of interventions that focused on single targets, those working on the interventions were asked to reconstitute them in ways that attended to multiple health, economic, and educational goals at the same time. Health was no longer one of several tracks for development aid; it was now linked to other development goals as an integral component and outcome measure of the overall development process.[36]

Integrated development programs continued to be promoted through the 1980s and 1990s, even as neoliberal reforms in donor countries rather significantly shifted the priorities and the paradigm of development aid. Growing concerns over debt relief for recipient nations and the depend-ency of recipient nations on donor nations, as well as fears that develop-ment aid could not show sustainability, led to large-scale reforms within international health development. Structural adjustment programs aimed at reducing dependency while growing free-market, fiscally driven solu-tions to ongoing problems of poverty and ill-health sutured many health programs to measures of financial accountability. Increasingly, programs that made better use of market-driven economic models of development or that incorporated economic sustainability into their interventions were seen as more viable and more worthy of support.[37] Thus, programs for "social marketing" of interventions (clinical care), prevention strategies (condoms), health resources (family planning), and technologies (e.g. diagnostic instruments) began to flourish in the 1990s. Microfinance pro-grams that tied aid and relief work to a program of financial incentives were designed to increase local sustainability and fiscal responsibility. Most health development aid given before structural adjustment reforms were initiated by donor nations was less tied to financial sustainability concerns, but, by 1993, even the WB had turned its attention to health development as a part of the "investment" strategy in developing nations.[38] By the turn of the 21st century, nearly all health development aid included "cost-effectiveness" as a measure of success and viability. After these reforms, nearly all aid was seen as problematic if it was not developed within the framework of larger fiscal and economic concerns.

Thus, in the era of postwar development, the relationships between health and politics took on new and layered complexities. The early visions of health for all as a global goal conceived by the WHO, over time often gave way to political concerns that defined health as not the primary goal, but as one of a series of development achievements that could be evaluated by measures in which health metrics were only one concern among many others. In some cases, health was *only* measurable in terms of other fiscal and social metrics. In fact, efforts by the WHO or the US Centers for Disease Control and Prevention to establish international health policies and bring about decentralized and integrated health interventions have led, in many ways, to a new way of thinking about global health governance in general. The more that health interventions are linked to other development priorities (from education to economic opportunities), the more health itself seems achievable. At the same time, health itself becomes redefined in terms of a wide range of impact areas that exceeded bodies and diseases (including the growth of civil society, increases in employment, improvement in infrastructure, etc.). In this conceptualization, health is not a freestanding target of intervention or evaluation but rather a possibility that is contingent on multiple other kinds of achievements.

The health politics of international health and development programs from at least the 1990s return us to some of the same foundational concepts found in the work of Virchow in which political goals become as important as those of health. International public health is conceptualized as bringing together a larger set of social, political, and economic interventions through which health is made possible. Health diplomacy in this context calls for attention to not only questions of how to reduce the disease burden but also how to engage subjects in an active and multidimensional way with living more healthful lives — in essence, to help make them good citizens by way of their commitment to improving health by way of being better farmers, more resourceful entrepreneurs or businesspeople, being more monogamous, and thinking of their bodies in relation to new technologies that make them visible as what Cohen[48] calls "operable" and what Petryna[47] calls "experimental" subjects. Becoming subjects who are willing to undergo surgeries, from sterilization to organ donation, and who are willing to enroll in randomized clinical trials for new drugs, is part of the package of politics embedded within global health today.

Modern health governance involves paying attention to how people live in ways that reach far beyond their immediate health care needs, while also channeling many other societal demands (economic, political, research) through the funnel of health. In international health programs, we can see the working of what Foucault[39] identified as a distinctly modern form of governance called *biopolitics*. Health governance, in this view, is not simply about creating international treaties across sovereign bodies. Rather, it is about how medical knowledge, definitions of health, policies deployed to improve health, and services given in the name of health create a basis for new kinds of subjects and new kinds of governance. The health of the person (in the Latin sense of *bios*) is the site for governance through science, medicine, and social policy, all of which in turn create new kinds of citizens, civil societies, and economic infrastructures through health.

Health as Biopolitics: From International Health to Global Health Science

Comprehensive approaches to global health diplomacy recognize that sometimes health and politics are competing and sometimes they are complementary, but understanding the relationship between health and politics also necessitates recognition of how politics are built into health and health care. One of the primary goals of health diplomacy is to ensure that positive health outcomes are a goal. In this effort, it is impossible to overlook the intertwining of the two poles of the health–politics continuum in programs that target a wide range of social behaviors that collectively form the basis for modern health governance. Health and politics are intertwined today in the same ways that they have been historically, and understanding these relationships in terms of biopolitics helps us to see where and when new kinds of health diplomacy may be necessary for engaging in a global health politics.

Health interventions are already political in the sense that they work through a nexus that ties the "biological subject" to multiple other modern institutions of global health governance in relation to economy, technologies, and sociality.[40,41] Commitments to the "good society" are built into medical messages and treatment regimes that ask patients to participate in one lifestyle rather than another, and these mandates are now more than ever tied to culturally specific notions of what it means to be productive, fiscally responsible, hygienic, and educated according to global aspirations and standards. HIV treatment programs — e.g. the President's Emergency Program for AIDS Relief (PEPFAR), which require unsubstantiated abstinence programs — are an obvious example of this, as are reproductive health programs (which require limiting family size, prenatal exams, and hospital deliveries), and even endemic disease eradication programs (which ask parents to use mosquito nets and include spraying malarial regions, etc.). Today, health citizenship is tied to new kinds of intervention strategies, in which those who are ill or potentially ill are asked to participate in experimental and entrepreneurial activities that help generate knowledge and sustainable systems of delivery. We see this in the emphasis on evidence-based public health, health education, and sustainable intervention strategies.

These emergent trends have arisen over the past few years, as international health programs have been undergoing a shift to being renamed and, in some cases, reshaped as programs in global health, global health science, or global public health. The inspiration for global health diplomacy emerges in part from this recent paradigm shift, which entails, among other things, new ways of including input from both the global North and South to shape intervention policies. With recognition that poverty and wealth play a greater role in health than does national origin, there has emerged a need for new kinds of accountability through evidence-based health development. The conversion of international health programs and agendas to global health sciences and global heath agendas is also accompanied by shifts in financing of health care and changes in the goals of some health programs.

One of the most significant developments in global health programming has been an increase in collaboration between biomedical bench scientists and international health experts, under the rubric of translational

research. Pharmaceutical industries and the basic sciences have been globalizing, as a result of both the need for more drug-naïve populations[42] and
the need to understand the global contours of emerging and re-emerging
viral, bacterial, and other pathogens. Another reason for the merger
between biosciences and international health has been the growing need
for more scientific rigor in international health interventions. Evidence-
based medicine, in particular, has put increasing pressure on international
health programs to generate better evaluation and accountability measures
with regard to their interventions. The shift toward a more scientific
means of accounting for intervention outcomes has led, more generally,
to the adoption of new intervention programs that insist on "experimental-
izing" interventions that use controls, randomization, and statistically
powerful outcome measures, as opposed to simple evaluations based on
operational data such as overall expenditures, clinics built, and number of
patients treated or immunized.[43] In some cases, only projects conceived
this way are now considered worthy of funding, whether from government, NGOs, or private foundations. Similarly, in some of the poorest
regions, target populations find that they are only able to access treatment
by enrolling in clinical trials managed by Contract Research Organizations,[47]
creating new and significant challenges for determining the protection of
human subjects and maintaining a focus on the health goals and priorities
of local populations.

Another significant issue arising with the new global health paradigm
has been that of the proliferating role played by NGOs in health development. Although some large NGOs (e.g. Rockefeller Foundation, Red
Cross, Medecins Sans Frontiers, Save the Children) have always played a
significant role in global health, the last decade has witnessed a proliferation in the scale and number of organizations. From "mom and pop"
foundations that are formed in the wake of personal disasters (e.g. the loss
of family members in disasters or adventure travel), to a growing number
of evangelical Christian missions that operate small-scale projects all over
the world, to the Bill and Melinda Gates Foundation, we see an enormous
proliferation of resources that at one time were funneled primarily through
or managed by governmental institutions.

The infrastructural widening of health care resources that are not
accountable to or working with government, bilateral, or multilateral

institutions has raised questions about effectiveness and efficiency, redundancy, and accountability. These concerns emerge alongside the growing interest in public–private health partnerships, including those in the global pharmaceutical industry, health care delivery structures, insurance schemes, and hospitals.[44] When delivery of health services is interlaced with private sector interests in expanding markets for bio-pharmaceuticals, consumption of new medical technologies and even agricultural resources, questions about whose interests are being served and how to maximize health outcomes are pushed to the center stage.[49]

Understanding what kinds of negotiations are called for in global health today requires a greater sensitivity to the nature of contemporary geopolitics and to the political nature of contemporary health interventions themselves. If, 100 years ago, putting politics in the service of health was seen as a revolutionary idea, then today the idea that all health is inherently political (in relation to the governmental management of lives, productivity and subjectivity) offers yet another cause for reflection. This idea necessitates an international dialogue that is informed by history and an understanding of how politics operate, not just at official bureaucratic levels associated with government, but in and through new institutional resources and interventions that are decentralized through education, science, and industry. In this situation, putting "politics" in the service of "health outcomes" is a call for critical reflection on the best and most appropriate kinds of health interventions, on the systems by which accountability is generated for these interventions, and on the notion that the most politically profitable interventions are not always the right interventions.

Conclusion

Global health diplomacy calls for a recognition that health interventions can be the work of foreign policy, particularly in bilateral development assistance and in multilateral governance. Sometimes, global health governance is openly political — as when it takes to task governments that have failed to prioritize the interests of health over security, economic, or political interests. However, global health diplomacy does not simply involve negotiating political agreements to reduce disease, morbidity, and mortality across national boundaries. It must be used as a platform for new forms of collaborative intervention and refiguring national agendas. Global health diplomacy can identify how global health cooperation is a critical part of national security,[45] but it can also redefine how humanitarian relief and health aid are negotiated in and through deployment of security apparatuses[42,46,47] sometimes overlooking built-in political demands and opportunities already found in the interventions and aid deployed to manage health. The tools for health diplomacy are no longer only found in geopolitical negotiating and treaty-making. They must be aware of how politics penetrate into the very infrastructures of economy, knowledge production, and sociality that impact and produce health.

Both health politics and a politics of health could better serve the interests of global health today if the global health community had a better understanding of all the ways in which health and politics are intertwined. Global conventions on the distribution of health resources, the prevention of disease, or the elimination of toxic exposures, for example, are needed as acts of global health cooperation. However, fully understanding these instruments of diplomacy requires us to trace the history of interactions between health and politics in ways that move beyond the narrow conceptual frameworks of both politics and health.

References

1. Alland A. (1966) Medical anthropology and the study of biological and cultural adaptation. *Am Anthropologist* **68**: 40–51.
2. Armelagos GJ. (1969) Disease in ancient Nubia. *Science* **163**: 255–259.
3. McNeill WH. (1976) *Plagues and Peoples*. Anchor, New York City.
4. Wallerstein I. (1974) *The Modern World-System I: Capitalist Agriculture and the Origins of the European World-Economy in the Sixteenth Century*. Academic, New York City.
5. Jones SG, Hilborne LH, Anthony CR, *et al.* (2006) *Securing Health: Lessons from Nation-Building Missions*. RAND Corporations, Santa Monica, CA. Available from www.rand.org/pubs/monographs/MG321 (accessed May 14, 2011).
6. Taylor R, Rieger A. (1984) Rudolf Virchow on the typhus epidemic in Upper Silesia: An introduction and translation. *Sociol Health Illness* **6(2)**: 201–217.

7. Porter D. (1999) *Health, Civilization and the State: A History of Public Health from Ancient to Modern Times.* Routledge, London.

8. Engels F. (1845 [1969 edition]) *The Condition of the English Working Class in 1844.* Panther, Moscow.

9. Navarro V. (1976) *Medicine Under Capitalism.* Neale Watson, New York City.

10. Adams V. (1998) *Doctors for Democracy: Health Professionals in the Nepal Revolution.* Cambridge University Press.

11. Doyal L. (1979) *The Political Economy of Health.* South End, Boston.

12. Townsend P, Davidson N. (1982) *Inequalities in Health: The Black Report.* Pelican, Harmondsworth, UK.

13. Birn A-E, Pillay Y, Holtz TH. (2009) *Textbook of International Health: Global Health in a Dynamic World*, 3rd edn. Oxford University Press, New York City.

14. Frankel S. Lewis G. (1989) *A Continuing Trial of Treatment: Medical Pluralism in Papua New Guinea.* Kluwer Academic, Boston.

15. Comaroff Jo, Comaroff Je. (1991) *Of Revelation and Revolution: Christianity, Colonialism and Consciousness in South Africa.* University of Chicago Press.

16. Vaughan M. (1991) *Curing Their Ills: Colonial Power and African Illness.* Stanford University Press.

17. Anderson W. (2006) *Colonial Pathologies: American Tropical Medicine, Race and Hygiene in the Philippines.* Duke University Press.

18. Taussig M. (1987) *Shamanism, Colonialism, and the Wildman: A Study in Terror and Healing.* University of Chicago Press.

19. Packard R. (1989) *Black Labor: Tuberculosis and the Political Economy of Health and Disease in South Africa.* University of California Press, Berkeley.

20. Fanon F. (1963) The Wretched of the Earth: Handbook for the Black Revolution That is Changing the Shape of the World. Grove Weidenfeld, New York City.

21. Fanon F. (1978) Medicine and colonialism. In: Ehrenreich J (ed.), *The Cultural Crisis of Modern Medicine.* Monthly Review, New York, pp. 229–251.

22. Brown RE. (1978) Public health and imperialism: Early Rockefeller Programs at home and abroad. In: Ehrenreich J (ed.), *The Cultural Crisis of Modern Medicine*, Monthly Review, New York City, pp. 897–903.

23. Marglin F. (1990) Smallpox in two cultures. In: Marglin SA, Appfel Marglin F (eds.), *Dominating Knowledge: Development, Culture, and Resistance.* Clarendon, Oxford, UK, pp. 120–144.

24. Prakash G. (1999) *Another Reason: Science and the Imagination of Modern India*. Princeton University Press.
25. Morris RJ. (1976) *Cholera 1832*. Holmes and Meier, New York City.
26. Brandt AM. (1985) *No Magic Bullet: A Social History of Venereal Disease in the United States Since 1880*. Oxford University Press.
27. Brandt A. (1976) *No Magic Bullet: A Social History of Venereal Disease in the United States Since 1880*. Oxford University Press.
28. Cipolla CM. (1973) *Cristofano and the Plague: A Study in the History of Public Health in the Age of Galileo*. Collins, London.
29. Cueto M. (2004 [Spanish]; 2006 [English]) *The Value of Health: The History of the Pan American Health Organization*. PAHO, Washington, DC.
30. Easterly W. (2006) *The White Man's Burden*. Penguin, New York City.
31. World Health Organization. (1952) *The World of WHO, 1952*. WHO.
32. Foster G. (1987) World Health Organization behavioral science research problems and prospects. *Soc Sci Med* **24(9)**: 709–717.
33. Justice J. (1989) *Policies, Plans and People: Foreign Aid and Health Development*. University of California Press, Berkeley.
34. World Health Organization. (1978) Declaration of Alma-Ata International Conference on Primary Health Care (Alma-Ata, USSR; September 6–12, 1978). Available from http://www.who.int/hpr/NPH/docs/declaration_almaata.pdf
35. Overholt C, Anderson MB, Cloud K, Austin JE. (1985) *Gender Roles in Development Projects: A Case Book*. Kumerian, Hartford, CT.
36. Pigg SL. (1992) Inventing social categories through place: Social representations and development in Nepal. *J Comp Stud Soc Hist* **34(3)**: 491–513.
37. Farmer P. (1999) *Infections and Inequalities: The Modern Plagues*. University of California Press, Berkeley.
38. World Bank. (1993) *The World Development Report: Investing in Health*. Oxford University Press.
39. Foucault M. (1973) *The Birth of the Clinic: An Archaeology of Medical Perception*. Vintage, New York City.
40. Nguyen V-K. (2010) *The Republic of Therapy: Triage and Sovereignty in West Africa's Time of AIDS*. Duke University Press.
41. Petryna A. (2002) *Life Exposed: Biological Citizens after Chernobyl*. Princeton University Press.

42. Adams V. (2010) Evidence-based global public health and the disappearing subject. Paper presented at the conference "When People Come First: Anthropology and Social Innovation in the Field of Global Health (Princeton University, March 11–13, 2010). Available from http://joaobiehl.net/manu-scripts/when-people-come-first

43. Adams V, Novotny TE, Leslie H. (2008) Global health diplomacy. *Med Anthropol* **27(4)**: 315–323.

44. Lakoff A, Collier SJ. (2008) *Biosecurity Interventions: Global Health and Security in Question.* Columbia University Press, New York City.

45. Katz R, Kornblet S, Arnold G, *et al.* (2011) Defining health diplomacy: Changing demands in the era of globalization. *Milbank Q* **89(3)**: 503–523.

46. Biehl J. (2008) Drugs for all: The future of global AIDS treatment. *Med Anthropol* **27(2)**: 99–105.

47. Petryna A. (2009) *When Experiments Travel: The Global Search for the Clinical Subject.* Princeton University Press.

48. Cohen, L. (2005) Operability, bioavailability and exception. In: Ong A, Collier S (eds.), *Global Assemblages: Politics and Ethics as Anthropological Problems.* Available online at doi:10.1002/9780470696569.ch5

49. Sunder-Rajan, K. (2003) *Biocapital: The Constitution of Postgenomic Life.* Duke University Press.

3

Governance and Actors in Global Health Diplomacy

*Wolfgang Hein**

Introduction

Health diplomacy, as described in other chapters of this volume, reaches back into the 19th century. Although the negotiations leading up to the adoption of the World Health Organization (WHO) Constitution in 1946 can certainly be seen as a masterpiece of this diplomacy, since then there have been profound changes in the field of international health. These changes are far more complicated than the increase in WHO membership from 48 full members in 1948 to 193 in 2010. Instead, we have observed a transition from an international to a global political health environment, with the emergence of a complex web of state and non-state actors. Global health governance is now defined by the interplay of different institutional forms and actors at many different levels. This interplay points to a growing discrepancy between the density of social relations in a rapidly globalizing society and the effective organization of all important actors on a global scale. Indeed, there is a critical need to understand how this complexity affects the political approach to reaching global health targets and to the governance necessary for such progress.

Martin Wight, one of the founders of the English school of international relations, serves as a good starting point for a description of the

---
*German Institute of Global and Area Studies, Hamburg, Germany.
E-mail: hein@giga-hamburg.de

complexity of global health diplomacy and governance (GHG): "Diplomacy is the attempt to adjust conflicting interests by negotiation and compromise; propaganda is the attempt to sway the opinion that underlies and sustains the interests."[1] Although, of course, the defense of political interests and the practice of advocacy by global health actors cannot be reduced to the conventional meaning of "propaganda," these actions might be called a propagation of positions in order to sway political or social processes toward the achievement of an organization's objectives. Concerning global health, this focus can be seen as another way of approaching what has been called an "unstructured plurality of actors"[2,3,a] or "open-source anarchy."[4] Concerning the mobilization of resources and the flexibility needed to tackle specific challenges, the new era of GHG has permitted results beyond those possible within the formal procedures of international organizations. However, this new arrangement has also raised questions about a more effective use of resources through a better adjustment of conflicting interests through negotiation and compromise. These possibilities may include a more effective operational coordination and a higher degree of legitimacy among the growing array of actors, which lead back to questions of diplomacy, but diplomacy within a new global institutional setting that reflects the new diversity of actors in global health.

In recent years, there have been a considerable number of publications on GHG[5-9] and a very good overview of the global health system in a four-part series published in 2010 in *PloS Medicine*.[10-13,b] Concerning the link between GHG and the role of the WHO, one may consider one of the conclusions by Moon and colleagues[13] in that series: "In the present complex global environment, no single actor can or should set the agenda for action.... Broad-based, participatory processes for agenda setting, anchored by WHO's global political legitimacy, will be required to define priorities, avoid unnecessary duplication, and share knowledge."

---

[a] This phrase was introduced by Beck and Lau[2] and first used to characterize global health in Ref. 3.

[b] For an overview of the topic, see: Szlezák NA, Bloom BR, Jamison DT, *et al.* (2010). The global health system: actors, norms, and expectations in transition, *PLoS Med* **7(1):** e1000183. doi:10.1371/journal.pmed.1000183.

In this chapter, a larger vision of governance[c] in global health will be offered through a broad approach to the link between GHG and global social and political dynamics. In addition to the social and political implications of globalization, the work of Fidler[4,16] and the nodal governance discourse of Burris and colleagues[17] will be dealt with. The sections of this chapter will discuss (i) the historical background of GHG; (ii) globalization and its implications for (a) transnational social relations and the changing character of politics beyond the nation-state, (b) new challenges in global health, (c) new types of actors in global health, and (d) the rise of global health governance; (iii) the changing relationships between state and non-state actors focusing on conflicts and norm-building in the field of access to medicines; (iv) critical approaches to GHG; and (v) perspectives, taking into account the new challenges for health diplomacy through negotiation and compromise.

This discussion addresses the complex universe of partners in global public health, which currently exists without a coordinating governance structure. Such a situation calls for what Wiseman has termed "polylateral diplomacy,"[18,d] which links the bilateral, the multilateral, and the non-state actors in negotiations that may help reach binding goals through better forms of GHG.

The Prehistory of Global Health Diplomacy

As long as territorial borders have existed, diseases have been a cross-border phenomenon. In the second half of the 19th century, 14 International Sanitary Conferences were held to discuss the spread of infectious diseases and to agree on coordinated activities to control them without unduly restricting trade and mobility. Since 1900, permanent organizations have been established: the International Sanitary Bureau of the Americas (1902; today the Pan-American Health Organization), the

---

[c] Governance is defined as "the management of the course of events in a social system."[14,15]

[d] Wiseman[18] proposed; "[T]raditional state-centered bilaterial and multilateral diplomatic concepts and practices need to be complemented with explicit awareness of a further layer of diplomatic interaction and relationships. Accordingly, the diplomat of the future will need to operate at the bilateral level, the multilateral level, and, increasingly, the polylateral level (relations between states and other entities)."

Office Internationale d'Hygiène Publique (Paris, 1907), the League of Nations Health Organization (1920), and its 1948 successor, the WHO, a specialized agency of the United Nations (UN).

The extensive participation of non-state organizations is not frequently recognized as part of this history. These organizations have included professional associations, the Red Cross, foundations, and, above all, missionary and philanthropic religious groups. The role of the Rockefeller Foundation was particularly important and, during the 1920s, the Rockefeller Foundation financed between one-third and one-half of the League of Nations' Health Office budget.[19,20] Until the 1970s, the WHO remained unchallenged as the leading international organization in health; financial support by non-state actors played a negligible role, while a small number of nongovernmental organizations (NGOs) had a well-defined role only as observers of the governance process.

The WHO was entrusted with the following tasks: (a) "to act as the directing and co-ordinating authority on international health work, and (b) "to establish and maintain effective collaboration with the United Nations, specialized agencies, governmental health administrations, professional groups, and such other organizations as may be deemed appropriate."[21] From its inception, the WHO had close cooperation with other UN institutions, such as the United Nations Children's Fund (UNICEF) in the field of child health; the Food and Agriculture Organization (FAO), concerning food safety and security; the International Labor Organization (ILO), concerning occupational safety and the health of workers; the UN Educational, Scientific and Cultural Organization (UNESCO), regarding scientific documentation; and the International Civil Aviation Organization (ICAO), regarding transport safety. One of the first tasks of the WHO Executive Board was to appoint the WHO members of the UNICEF/WHO joint committee on health policy.

Since those developments, the growing interdependence of various fields in global health has meant that health is part of the deliberations not only of specialized health organizations but also of those organizations that have more indirect connections with health issues. In addition, other bodies, such as the World Bank, World Trade Organization (WTO), World Intellectual Property Organization (WIPO), UN Development Programme (UNDP), and UN Conference on Trade and Development (UNCTAD), have become increasingly involved in health affairs because of health-related policies in areas including development, trade, and intellectual property rights. Clearly, there is an increasing interdependence in the norm-setting process (e.g., intellectual property and health) and an increase in joint operational activities of several intergovernmental organizations (IGOs), such as the WHO and the FAO, in the case of the Codex Alimentarius. Finally, new UN organizations for health, such as the UN Program on HIV/AIDS (UNAIDS), have been created.

WHO negotiations have always been subject to coalition and bloc-building processes among Member States as well as attempts by powerful states to curtail the WHO's autonomy. These processes have, at times, created near-paralysis. In the 1990s, many UN institutions faced a serious financial crisis because of nonpayment of arrears by key Member States. Much of this crisis resulted from the attempts of some high-income countries (HICs) to impose their views of international relations on UN organizations. In spite of their majorities in the governing assemblies [such as the World Health Assembly (WHA)], states of the global south [low- and middle-income countries (LMICs)] could not prevent the United States or other HICs from withholding financial resources[e] or from establishing new institutional arrangements to circumvent IGOs. In addition, non-state actors intervened more vigorously, through direct or indirect lobbying of both Member States and the WHO Secretariat to push specific policies. Thus, to some extent, it has been the Member States themselves that weakened their IGOs, in particular through the ceiling put on the assessed contributions — specifically, the so-called United Nations Reform Act (Helms–Biden Agreement), a 1999 US law that set a number of conditions for reform of the UN system before the United States would release its total arrears payment to the UN. This intervention introduced the principle of "zero nominal growth" into the WHO budget process and forced the organization to be increasingly dependent on extra-budgetary resources. Such resources invariably come "with strings attached," and it is these strings that may weaken the overall governance of specialized UN agencies by Member States.

---

[e] In 2003, the United States and, to a lesser degree, Japan and Italy were in arrears for their assessed contributions to the WHO.[22]

This scenario further implies that the WHO has to compete for funding with other institutions, NGOs, and even countries. Because resources are linked to specific activities supported by donors, this possibility further implies the risk of undermining the WHO's "...crucial role as trusted neutral brokers between the scientific and the technical communities on the one hand, and governments of developing countries on the other."[23]

Globalization and Health

Globalization, defined as an intensification of cross-border flows of goods, services, finance, people, and ideas, has been facilitated by techno-logical developments and by changes in the institutional and policy regimes at the international and national levels (for example, by the pro-motion of trade liberalization).[24] Globalization has produced further changes in the character of global politics, which extend far beyond eco-nomic activities to political, cultural, environmental, and security issues. It implies an increasing transnational interconnectivity of people and communities, which leads to an increasing density of transnational social relations and the creation of common identities based on characteristics other than nationality. Such interconnectivity has had important conse-quences for the dynamics of global health issues as well as for the archi-tecture of international relations. Today, the transnational discourse on health, magnified through the media, is very important in raising issues, setting agendas, and, in particular, producing the frameworks within which problems are debated in international fora.

Transnational Social Relations and Politics Beyond the Nation-State

In a world of sovereign nation-states, international organizations are based on the aggregation of interests at national levels. IGOs have been estab-lished whenever governments recognize a common interest in coordina-tion, and they are legitimized by the consent of participating sovereign states. Participation in international treaties developed under their bylaws requires signature and subsequent ratification within national government agencies. The agreements are binding only for those states that become parties to them. This traditional system is also called the "Westphalian" system of international relations.[f]

On the one hand, globalization increasingly puts this system of inter-governmental organization under stress, both because of the slowness of decision-making within many IGOs and because of the problems of representation (one country = one vote). On the other hand, the mounting interconnectivity within a globalizing society implies a growing extent, intensity, and velocity of global interactions,[24] and that has strengthened various types of non-state actors, transnational norms, and conflicts extending beyond Member States' sole influence in IGOs.

Thus, transnational corporations (TNCs), foundations, civil society organizations (CSOs), and various other private groups are progressively changing the structure of the global polity. They defend their own interests and also pursue advocacy positions by exerting political pressure from inside national polities as well as on the global level. They also offer resources (financial resources as well as expertise) to achieve public goals. Proactively, they associate with national and international state actors to form hybrid alliances in the pursuit of specific goals. Non-state actors also play a significant role in developing transnational norms among themselves (e.g. *lex mercatoria* and standard-setting instruments such as the International Organization for Standardization) and in building and defending international law (e.g. in the field of human rights). This "new diplomacy" is most clearly exemplified by the Ottawa Process,[26] which led to the treaty banning antipersonnel landmines; by the Rome Statute to establish the International Criminal Court; and by the Access to Medicines Campaign in global health (see the subsection "Global health partnerships" and the section "States and Non-State Actors...").

New Challenges in Global Health

There is now general agreement that the processes of globalization have catapulted health to a more prominent political place on the global agenda.

---

[f] This concept is derived from the 1648 Peace of Westphalia, which is seen as the original of a system of international relations based on interactions between sovereign nation-states.[16,25]

In many parts of the world, there is a "growing consciousness of a global responsibility for global health,"[7] and the complex (two-way) interactions between social and economic development and health have been broadly documented by the reports of the Commission on Macroeconomics and Health[27] and the Commission on the Social Determinants of Health.[28] A wide range of factors have contributed to this increased attention to global health:

- Health threats such as HIV/AIDS, influenza, severe acute respiratory syndrome (SARS), and avian flu threaten each and every country and the global community as a whole, as a result of rapid spread based on global travel and mobility.
- The globalization of lifestyles has led to the rapid growth of chronic disease challenges such as diabetes and is linked to the impact of global industries such as tobacco, alcohol, and food.
- Health systems are critically important for economic stability in all countries, and health care financing is a key political issue for health systems viability.
- The mobility of patients and health care professionals is a global issue that needs global solutions.
- Health is one of the largest industries worldwide, involving several critical issues, such as intellectual property and trade in goods and services related to health. In particular, this issue gained notoriety concerning access to antiretrovirals (ARVs) for treatment of HIV/AIDS and the conflicts related to the production and marketing of generic versions of these and other medicines.
- Inequality of access to preventive and curative health care around the world is gaining more attention and has become a subject of major discourse on human rights and social justice.

Irrespective of whether globalization was perceived as a threat or a challenge, supporters and opponents started to acknowledge the need for international and transnational coordination, which would make it possible to "govern" the process in the absence of a central political authority (see the next major section of this chapter).

New Types of Actors in Global Health and the Rise of Global Health Governance

Today, a large number of different actors interact with each other at various levels, including national governments, IGOs, bilateral agencies, and non-state players, such as public–private partnerships (PPPs). All of these actors have their own agendas, are guided by specific interests, and operate from disparate power bases. Their ability to influence politics on the global level varies according to the actors' properties and the specific interfaces in which they participate with donors, governments, and recipient organizations.

The very flexibility of the organization and cooperation characterizing the evolving system of global governance may offer multiple ways to overcome barriers within UN organizations. The establishment of the Global Fund to Fight AIDS, Tuberculosis, and Malaria (GFATM) illustrates this. The Group of Eight (G-8) proposed making large funds available for the fight against HIV/AIDS; this proposal was supported by then UN General-Secretary Kofi Annan. Because some G-8 members refused to allocate funds via a UN organization (which was seen as not sufficiently "results-oriented"), an independent fund was established, based on the PPP model (state governments, representatives of private enterprise, and civil society organizations as decision-makers; IGOs only as nonvoting members of the Executive Council).

The implementation of the human rights norm of "universal access to essential medicines" can be seen as another example of the role of organizational flexibility in GHG. The intellectual property system, which encourages research- and development-intensive industries to finance product development, is a factor obstructing universal access to essential medicines in an unequal global society. However, the changing norm to ensure universal access to critical medicines has gained strength during the past decade. It has necessarily demanded changes in policies by pharmaceutical companies (supported by some form of financial subsidy) toward *voluntarily* selling medicines at specific places and/or to specific populations at greatly reduced prices. The vehicle of differential pricing is used by PPPs such as the Accelerating Access Initiative.[g]

In this post-Westphalian system of global governance, traditional forms of state regulation through nation states and IGOs are both complemented by and competing with new forms of transnational activities through non-state actors and hybrid organizations such as those mentioned above. Furthermore, global health has become a concern in quite a number of other policy fields, such as foreign policy, geopolitics, security, and marketing. Next, the most important groups of new actors in global health will be characterized.

Global health partnerships

Beyond the fight against HIV/AIDS, PPPs — or global health partnerships (GHPs) — have contributed significantly to the changing approach to global health. Through the integration of a number of different actors (government health departments, multilateral and bilateral organizations, pharmaceutical enterprises, private foundations, and CSOs) in different combinations as required by the specific tasks and social and political environments, flexible forms of cooperation have become possible. These partnerships combine specific needs identified by governments, IGOs, or CSOs with the scientific and technological capacities of private corporations and the financial resources of donor countries, public funds, or private foundations.

A number of such partnerships (e.g. the Medicines for Malaria Venture, the Global Alliance for TB Drug Development, the International AIDS Vaccine Initiative, and the Foundation for Improved Diagnostics) have attempted to address the absence of research and development on neglected diseases and products. A different group of partnerships has been established to address the lack of access to existing medicines. These

---

[g]The Accelerating Access Initiative (AAI) is a cooperative endeavor of UNAIDS, the WHO, UNICEF, the UN Population Fund, the World Bank, and seven research-based pharmaceutical companies (Abbott Laboratories, Boehringer Ingelheim, Bristol-Myers Squibb, GlaxoSmithKline, Gilead Sciences, Merck & Co., Inc., and F. Hoffmann–La Roche). For more information, see www.ifpma.org/health/hiv/health_aai_hiv.aspx

initiatives include drug donation programs by drug manufacturers (e.g. Mectizan for river blindness, Diflucan for the treatment of AIDS-related opportunistic fungal infections, and Malarone for malaria in Africa), as well as programs aiming to reduce the costs of medicines (e.g. the Green Light Committee for TB medicines, and the Accelerating Access Initiative for ARVs). Other alliances catalyze action and improve coordination on a range of issues, from tuberculosis (the Stop TB Partnership) and malaria (the Roll Back Malaria Partnership) to health measurement (the Health Metrics Network), and to the crisis in human resources for health (the Global Health Workforce Alliance).

Some of these partnerships have taken over a broad field of activities, concerning either the fight against a specific disease (e.g. Roll Back Malaria and Stop TB) or a specific area of health services such as the Global Alliance for Vaccines and Immunization (now called the GAVI Alliance). The composition of the GAVI Alliance Board (Fig. 1) points to a broad-based governance structure and linkages to varied actors in global health. These large initiatives have recently also been called Global Health

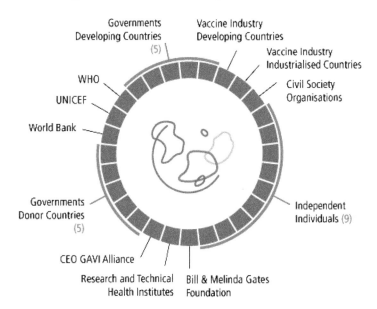

Fig. 1. Composition of the Board of the GAVI Alliance. Reproduced here with permission from the GAVI Alliance website, www.gavialliance.org/about/in_partnership/index.php

Initiatives (GHI) but, because this term is also used for other "initiatives" of IGOs [such as the World Bank's Multicountry HIV/AIDS Program (MAP)] and single states (the new US Government Global Health Initiative), it lacks clarity concerning the types of actors involved. Nevertheless, it is clear that the current situation is beyond the capacity of any one structure to provide coordination, let alone governance.

Advocative CSOs

CSOs have played a role in international health for quite a long time but, in a rather tightly interconnected world, they are particularly important for their advocacy power rather than in a role as service providers (although they are also extending this role). Extremely divergent in form, size, and political position, CSOs mirror the diversity of global civil society.[29] CSO activities often relate to more than one policy field (e.g. trade and health, human rights and health, or, more generally, global welfare and market creation), which also gives them an important advantage over many other actors with regard to knowledge and communicative relations.

One of the most important activities in this context is the representation of interests from civil society that are not mirrored in other types of organizations. CSOs advocate for many marginalized and weak groups through political campaigns (e.g. Access to Essential Medicines), through the dissemination of information and knowledge on specific issues [e.g. the Médecins sans Frontières (MSF) Guide to ARV prices], and through lobbying at decision-making institutions on both the national and international levels. Furthermore, CSOs participate in international conferences, establish consultative relationships with IGOs, and even participate in the decision-making bodies of some IGOs and GHPs as Officially Recognized NGOs. They also play the role of watchdogs (e.g. Global Health Watch) by monitoring other global health actors, UN conferences, specific programs carried out by IGOs, national politics, or the behavior of transnational companies. They may use "naming and shaming" approaches and monitoring of published codes of conduct to sustain their advocacy work. These activities may improve voluntary compliance with existing rules and might also support further legal bases for global policies along with stricter enforcement of them.

Large foundations

The role of large foundations in global health has grown significantly in recent years, and they influence GHG along four main dimensions. The most obvious of these is the financial dimension, with monetary contributions provided directly to existing or new global health programs. In 2006, the Development Assistance Committee[h] countries' bilateral aid to health was US$8.6 billion, and multilateral agencies' aid accounted for US$4 billion; in the same year, the Gates Foundation alone provided health grants of nearly US$1 billion.[30,31] Second, there is the operational dimension, which pertains to the activities of foundations in service delivery, programming, and grant-making. It reflects the priorities which the foundation sets out for its engagement and has direct impact on policy processes at the global, national, and local levels. The third dimension is the institutional setting of GHG. This dimension is influenced by the recent increase in the number of philanthropic organizations, by the preference of most of them for the PPP model, and by their active participation in the decision-making processes of these initiatives. The fourth dimension is the ideational dimension, in which private foundations, through their application of business models and their focus on performance, contribute to the diffusion of market norms and principles that affect both the theory and the practice of global public health.

In conclusion, the evolution of GHG can be summarized by the following points:

- GHG development is closely related to the more extensive integration of global society. In a complex global health arena (see Fig. 2), different types of actors from all over the world are increasingly interactive with one another, which reflects a growing need for global norms and a growing risk of cross-border health threats that have an impact on the lives of people globally.
- GHG responds to the growth of global trade institutions. At the same time, many UN organizations, such as the WHO and the ILO, have

---

[h] The OECD's Development Assistance Committee (DAC) is a forum within which selected member states can discuss issues surrounding aid, development, and poverty reduction in developing countries. For more information, see www.oecd.org/dac/stats/daclist

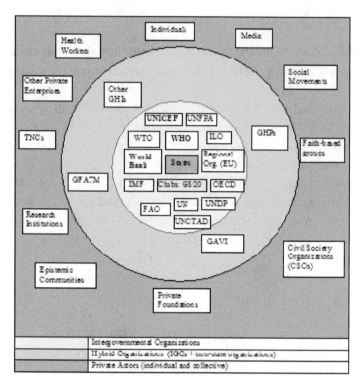

Fig. 2.   The global health arena: Actors in global health. [Reproduced with permission from Hein W (2010); Hein W, Kickbusch I, *Global Health, AID Effectiveness and the Changing Role of the WHO*, GIGA Focus International Edition.]

been weakened through ideological conflicts involving demands for "effectivity" versus "equity." This conflict has been complicated by the nonacceptance of majority decisions among the major national financial contributors to those institutions.

- GHG structures involving hybrid regulations and networks among different actors facilitate integration and compromise at the global level. This structure has permitted formerly weak actors to advance agendas, such as those for human rights, in the face of resistance from traditionally powerful actors.

- GHG has become a product of both ethical values and material interests emerging in an evolving, integrated social system. It accompanies the increased density of social interactions on the global scale and the development of a globalized society.

States and Non-State Actors in Global Health Governance[i]

The fight against HIV/AIDS has raised issues around which many of the new features of GHG have developed. Although this disease is quite specific in its medical as well as social characteristics, the conflicts about prevention versus treatment and about the affordability of and access to ARV therapies have stimulated the development of GHG structures.

The issues involving ARV access have assumed a multidimensional character, involving, in addition to groups of countries defending and opposing strict intellectual property rights (IPRs), a large number of CSOs networked through multiple access campaigns.[j] Through various means, such as domestic production of ARVs, import of generics, and negotiated concessions from pharmaceutical companies, developing countries succeeded in significantly lowering the prices of ARVs.[35] At the same time, developing countries have been able to reach international agreements to assert their rights to use the safeguards of the Trade-Related Aspects of Intellectual Property Rights (TRIPS) Agreement, such as compulsory licensing[k] and parallel importing,[l] to "protect public health," thus decreasing the risk of trade conflicts related to stringent patent rights protection.

Regulations based on international law result from conflictive and cooperative processes, and may also initiate new conflicts about specific health policies. Regulations affect the interfaces between actors with conflicting perceptions, values, and interests.[37] Interfaces are defined as

---

[i] This section of the chapter is based on Ref. 32.

[j] The role of global civil society in this conflict has been analyzed in more detail by Hein *et al.*[14]; see also Refs. 33 and 34.

[k] Under WTO rules, a compulsory license allows governments to produce or to grant a third party authority to produce a drug without the consent of the patent holder in cases of national public health emergency, among other limited circumstances (www.wto.org/English/thewto_e/minist_e/min01_e?mindecl_trips_e.htm). The TRIPS Agreement, as confirmed by the Doha Declaration and adopted on November 14, 2001, affirmed governments' right to use the agreement's flexibilities, in particular to use compulsory licenses in order to avoid any reticence the governments may feel (www.who.org/English/tratop_e/dda_e/dohaexplained_e.htm#trips).

[l] The phrase "parallel importing" refers to the import of goods purchased in a foreign market by an independent third party and later resold in the domestic market, where much lower prices compete with the prices charged by authorized distributors.[36]

"sociopolitical spaces of recurrent interactions of collective actors in the handling of trans-national and international affairs."[34] There are four major types of interfaces that closely relate to the different types of power employed in them: legal, resource-based, organizational, and discursive. This differentiation highlights the changing financial, economic, institutional, political, and social aspects of GHG.

The recurrent interactions between major global health actors manifest themselves in different ways, according to the types of interfaces involved. While the two approaches are closely interconnected, rational (discursive) discussions were more important in shaping the global conflicts around access to treatment for HIV/AIDS than were the seemingly powerful resource-based interfaces. The emerging legal and organizational interfaces reflect that constellation of discourse, and these findings should have significant implications for present and future GHG development.

The fight against AIDS and the confrontation over ARV prices by Brazilian and South African governments (and their supportive local and global CSOs) against transnational pharmaceutical corporations (TNPCs) (and their supportive governments in industrialized countries) reveal two important points for future policy decisions. First, TNPCs were forced to negotiate and, basically, to accept the policies of two large developing countries in the throes of a global health crisis. While the importance of the NGOs' involvement is undeniable (and has been cited here and elsewhere), the emergence of strong national health governance in Brazil and the successful opposition of both Brazil and South Africa to a narrow, TNPC-oriented interpretation of the TRIPS agreement were crucial examples for other LMICs. Second, the successful actions of CSOs against the South African government concerning the provision of access to ARVs illustrated the strength of global civil society in asserting human rights in health issues and attested to the fact that conflicts about access to medicines are not fought along ideologically hardened North–South lines alone.

These accomplishments were made through the artful use of different interfaces, the combination of which made possible a power shift in GHG. Important as it was as a first step, the defense of presumed national interests along legal interfaces, the path which the Brazilian[m] and South African[n] governments followed, was a necessary effort, but it was insufficient to have an impact on the overall rules and regulations governing access to medicines. That step was accomplished by using opportunities and reacting to challenges along resource-based, organizational, and, especially, discursive interfaces in the multi-level global polity. As a consequence, future developments of GHG will depend on policy-makers using the multiplicity of interfaces to achieve comprehensive solutions for global health challenges.

The round of negotiations on funding of health research ongoing at the time of this writing (2008 Global Strategy and Plan of Action on Public Health, Innovation and Intellectual Property) and the evolving norm of "universal access to essential medicines" have called for new institutional forms in GHG.[40] On the one hand, intergovernmental agreements continue to play an important role in establishing binding rules. On the other hand, state actors are also becoming part of a more open field of global politics in which various types of non-state actors are strengthening their positions by using a multitude of interfaces. Private companies and CSOs are playing an important role in pushing for legal agreements, amendments, or authoritative interpretations of existing rules.

The First Five Years of the 21st Century: Stock-Taking in GHG

Since the turn of the millennium, the development of the GHG concept in academics has been closely related to a stock-taking of institutional

---

[m]In patent-rights-related conflicts with the US government and TNPCs, the Brazilian federal government was able to reach price reductions on ARVs; Brazil also successfully negotiated the terms of cooperation with major financial donors and creditors.[38]

[n]The South African government, although for many years having taken a rather idiosyncratic position on HIV/AIDS, fought two rounds of legal conflicts with TNPCs about the right to import generics on the basis of the right to "parallel importation." In both rounds, the TNPCs finally withdrew their lawsuits because of ongoing protests by CSOs and the corporations' fear of image loss.[39]

changes in global health.° Health in developing countries has a newfound and privileged position in the eyes of the general public and for the world's political leadership. During recent years, many actors in global health have in fact made important contributions to research on neglected diseases, to financing of health activities in specific fields, and to improvement in access to medicines in poor regions. Health challenges now play a role in national security strategies, and they appear regularly on the agenda of meetings of leading economic powers. The connections between health and the environment, trade, economic growth, social development, and human rights have been well established, and they are seen as affecting both LMIC and HIC interests. However, the "unstructured plurality of actors" also entails several considerable problems.

(1) From the 1980s until well after the turn of the millennium, there was mainly a focus on vertical global health activities — i.e. controlling and treating specific infectious diseases (some of them of global concern and others seen as "diseases of the poor" in developing countries) — an effort reinforced by the experience with HIV/AIDS. Horizontal activities such as improving national health systems and developing systems of primary health care (PHC) were given less attention. Already in the 1980s, the implementation of the PHC concept was hindered by a variety of factors, among them the politics of the Washington consensus,ᵖ including a lack of long-term political and financial commitment to

---

° Earlier publications introduced the concept of global health governance and the issues at stake, including the health impacts of globalization,[41] the impact of globalization on health policy-making,[42] the growing role of public–private partnerships in health,[43,44] and global public goods for health.[45] Since 2003, a substantial literature has been produced on global health and GHG in general.[46–49] See also the overview by: Walt G, Spicer N, Buse K. (2009) Mapping the global health architecture. In: Buse K, Hein W, Drager N (eds.), *Making Sense of Global Health Governance: A Policy Perspective.* Palgrave Macmillan, London, pp. 47–71.

ᵖ The term "Washington consensus" was coined in 1989 by economist John Williamson to describe neoliberal economic policies involving market fundamentalism in LMICs. These policies were developed by Washington, DC-based institutions, including the International Monetary Fund, the World Bank, and the US Department of the Treasury, and they have been roundly criticized by many other economists.

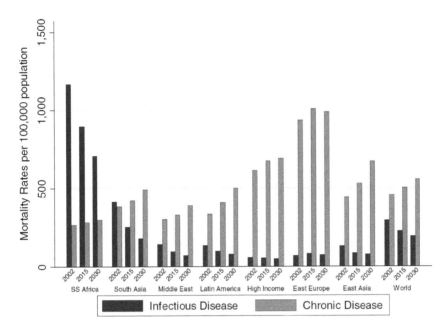

Fig. 3. Evolution of the global burden of disease, 2002–2030. Infectious disease classification is based on the WHO's type 1 infectious disease cluster. Chronic disease classification is based on the cardiovascular disease, cancers, respiratory disease, and diabetes mellitus subcategories of the WHO's type 2 burden-of-disease cluster. Reproduced here with permission from Stuckler D (2008), *Millbank Q* **86**: 492–494.

comprehensive PHC development. Horizontal activities have gained stronger support only during recent years, mostly linked to the Millennium Development Goals (MDGs),[q] even though the World Bank focused on health systems development in the *1993 World Development Report.*[50]

(2) There has been a lack of focus on noncommunicable diseases, although they have been playing a growing role in LMICs during the most

---

[q] The Millennium Development Goals (MDGs) are eight time-bound, comprehensive, and specific development goals for tackling global poverty. They include goals and targets for income, hunger, maternal and child mortality, infectious disease, inadequate shelter, gender inequality, environmental degradation, and economic development. For more information, see www.undp.org/mdg/basics.shtml

recent decades. In 2002, in only two world regions was the burden of disease brought by infectious diseases higher than that brought by chronic diseases and, in 2015, this will be so only in Africa (Fig. 2).

(3) The need for prevention and the need to foster more healthy lifestyles are the basis for preventing noncommunicable diseases, but these needs have been underestimated in most GHG discussions.[52] It should be stressed, however, that the WHO recently refocused on this perspective, as well as on the role of lifestyles and the social determinants of noncommunicable diseases, in the context of the Commission on the Social Determinants of Health (CSDH).

(4) There has been a growing critique concerning a lack of transparency and accountability of most of the new nonstate actors in the GHG field. Large CSOs, GHPs, and financially strong, internationally active foundations (such as the Bill and Melinda Gates Foundation) are having an important impact on the orientation of many global health efforts without being accountable to the people who are affected by their activities. GHG should not be left to the market or to chance, as those options may lead to suboptimal health outcomes. There are grounds for much more proactive approaches to identifying collective governance solutions to collectively identified problems. Past efforts have too readily dismissed the possibility of reinvigorating and reforming existing institutions, and have been overly *ad hoc* and disjointed. Thus, we need to deliberatively assess the relevance and adaptability of existing institutions and, where necessary, develop and refine their organization, authorizing legislation, rules, norms, principles, and decision-making procedures. It is hoped that such a reassessment may bring some order to the disconnected global health enterprise and thus improve health outcomes for all. IGOs might also suffer from a number of legitimacy problems, but they are clearly accountable to governing bodies in which sovereign states are represented (at least formally).

(5) Complexity constitutes a huge challenge to global health. The determinants of health as well as the components of health care systems continue to increase. Hence, an increasingly dense web of actors and initiatives is involved in and has an impact on GHG. Particularly for those countries receiving aid from a large number of different

organizations, international aid has become a burden as much as a necessity. The proliferation of actors has made it difficult for national governments to pursue consistent national strategies for developing their own health systems and controlling the activities in their sovereign territories. These problems have been addressed in the increasing dialogue about aid effectiveness that has accompanied the enormous new financial investments being made in global health. It is still far from clear what impact that dialogue will have (see below). Balancing the demands of sovereignty with those of a shared responsibility for global health, as well as the self-interest of a range of groups and organizations, is a difficult task. Yet, to craft health policy today, governments, international organizations, and NGOs must find mechanisms for managing the health risks and programs that spill into and out of every country.

(6) There is an urgent need "to bring order to the chaos of global health governance."[7] The strong emphasis on some problems (communicable diseases and HIV/AIDS, in particular) and approaches (i.e. care and treatment) deflects attention from other disease burdens and their approaches (e.g. strengthening health systems, preventing disease, and addressing noncommunicable diseases). There is currently no forum to bring order to this chaos. Such a forum is necessary in order to allow the involved parties to set priorities, link them with investment decisions in both the public and private sectors, and add to the legitimacy, credibility, and effectiveness in decision-making among IGOs.

Perspectives of Global Health Governance — Nodal Governance and the Role of the WHO

As indicated above, the question of donor diversity has been at the center of the dialogue on aid effectiveness, and this has a significant influence on GHG. The 2002 International Conference on Financing for Development (in Monterrey, Mexico) paved the way for a negotiation process that led to the 2005 Paris Declaration on Aid Effectiveness. This declaration articulated five target areas of improvement for aid effectiveness: ownership, harmonization, alignment, results, and mutual accountability. Donor countries must coordinate and harmonize their aid in order to effectively support their partners' national development strategies, but those strategies will basically follow internationally-agreed-upon concepts of good governance. The hope is to make these entities reliable partners in a global system. The Paris Declaration thus refers to some of the problems in GHG: the need for both better coordination of actors and a stronger link to the country level that can foster legitimacy and accountability as well as strengthen health systems.

The salience of aid effectiveness in the health sector was stressed during the preparation of the Accra High Level Forum on Aid Effectiveness (monitoring progress on the Paris objectives). The WHO, World Bank, and Organization for Economic Co-operation and Development–Development Assistance Committee (OECD-DAC) proposed using health as a "tracer sector" for tracking progress on the Paris Declaration. At this conference, it was pointed out that "[A]id effectiveness is particularly challenging in health…. [D]ifficulties are the result of inefficiencies in the global aid architecture and of poor country policies; however, problems in health are exacerbated by the inherent complexities of the sector itself."[r]

Health has an important place in the MDGs, but the health-related MDGs (goals 4–6 and target 8E) were oriented to the 1990s foci on infectious diseases, maternal health, and child mortality.[s] Slow progress in MDG indicators necessitated refocusing aid on health systems, and in particular on PHC.[53] In addition, the work of the WHO Commission on the Social Determinants of Health[54] supported the revival of PHC.

The High Level Forum (HLF) on the Health MDGs[55] held three meetings in 2004 and 2005. "Scaling up aid for health" was the HLF's main target, which implied better coordination between GHPs, improved health

---

[r] For more information, see www.oecd.org/dataoecd/14/37/42254322.pdf

[s] Some of the coordination measures are aimed at reducing the problems with parallel activities of different actors in the same field. For example, UNAIDS promoted several coordination activities, of which the concept of the "three ones" is the most important. It aims at the establishment of "one" agreed-upon AIDS action framework that provides the basis for coordinating the work of all partners, "one" National AIDS coordinating authority, and "one" agreed-upon country-level monitoring and evaluation system.[55] In relation to that, in 2007, a Country Harmonization and Alignment Tool (CHAT) developed by UNAIDS and the World Bank, was presented (see http://www.aidstar-two.org/Tools-Database.cfm?action=detail&id=23&language_id=).

fund-ing, and a greater effort to address problems with health systems in poor countries. Participants developed "best practice principles for GHPs," demanding that GHPs adhere to the Paris Declaration's principles, and established an issue-oriented annual forum as well as informal information-sharing plans among the five or six largest GHPs. These meetings also criticized the misalignment of funding with government priorities — 50% of health Official Development Assistance (ODA) is earmarked for specific diseases or programs — and the lack of stable, long-term support for government ministries. The Scaling up for Better Health (IHP+) Initiative was established by a Scaling-up Reference Group (SuRG), which brought together the eight most important agencies or initiatives in global health: WHO, World Bank, GAVI, UNICEF, UN Population Fund, UNAIDS, GFATM, and the Bill and Melinda Gates Foundation. Under a new name, "Health 8," this group has since gained importance beyond IHP+.

Still, the Paris–Accra process is a limited domain of GHG. There is an urgent need for health diplomacy in other fields, which are more directly related to the role of health in the provision of global public goods[t] — as, for example, in the control of infectious diseases, in the production and distribution of health-related knowledge, or in the improvement of global health institutions.

The dynamics of the increasingly dense transnational community are worthy of both research and more dialogue. These dynamics have been transformed from the rather thin and simply structured flows of international communication between governments into a dense web of exchange. In such a dynamic situation, well-informed policy networks and policy coherence become key issues in global health coordination.

In very open forms of organization, networking is the logical complement to a system that "anybody can access, use, modify and improve."[4] In these networking processes, specific actors or institutions emerge as nodes of information and coordination in the pursuit of specific goals. This development creates network power that is described as "nodal governance."[14] Informal and formal meetings in Geneva and other regular

---

[t] The issues of public goods in themselves, of global public goods in particular, and of global public goods in health are too complex to be treated in detail in this chapter. For more information, see Refs. 45 and 56.

global health events, such as the Pacific Health Summit, create flexible links between global health actors. The concept of "interfaces" can then be used to design a power map of the GHG system and describe the characteristics of governing nodes. The interactions taking place may reshape the goals, perceptions, interests, and relationships of the various actors.[37]

The WHO has in recent years succeeded in strengthening its nodal role in global health. This organization has assumed a more active role in global health diplomacy, in particular through the successful negotiations of two important international agreements, the Framework Convention on Tobacco Control (FCTC) and the new International Health Regulations, which played an important role in the approaches to SARS, avian flu, and "swine flu" (pandemic influenza, or H1N1). Furthermore, recent developments suggest that, after a decade of learning how to adjust to the proliferation of actors in global health, the WHO might play a growing role in coordinating GHG. High-level expert commissions, such as the Commission on Macroeconomics and Health (CMH), the Commission on the Social Determinants of Health (CSDH), and the Commission on Intellectual Property Rights, Innovation and Public Health (CIPIH), constitute a valuable forum in which to establish dialogue on significant GHG issues. These commissions are important instruments of policy-making for stakeholders with conflicting interests; they may produce meaningful consensus through debates and the subsequent decision-making processes of participants. They can also refer to the WHA for debate any problems that need multinational deliberations by Member States.

For example, the publication of the report of the CIPIH in 2006[57] stimulated development of a consensus on the need for more general changes in the global system of innovation for medicines and for health research. This step led to the establishment of the Intergovernmental Working Group on Public Health, Innovation and Intellectual Property (IGWG) under the auspices of the WHO. The IGWH was open to all interested Member States and included civil society actors; it was mandated to develop a global strategy and plan of action on innovation. This strategy aims to secure an enhanced and sustainable framework for needs-driven health research and development that is relevant to diseases that disproportionately affect LMICs. This global strategy and parts of the plan of action were adopted in a resolution passed at the WHA in 2008 (WHA

Resolution 61.21). Later negotiations were related to financing for the plan of action. The funding of health research and development proposed by the Taskforce on Innovative International Financing for Health Systems was estimated at (by 2015) US$7.4 billion per year. Whatever the results of these deliberations, they are an indication of the stronger role of the WHO in leading negotiations on global health funding issues. This situation contrasts with the establishment of the GFATM, a process in which the United States and other industrial countries pursued funding strategies outside the UN system.

Nodal governance operates in a landscape of mixed social interactions and a conflict-laden cultural and political economy.[14] A recent survey identified more than 80 organizational actors in the city of Geneva alone, and that number did not include the missions and representations of national governments. However, the WHA provides the interface among Member States that possess disparate goals, perceptions, and interests and between the Member States and the many other global health actors seeking to influence the policy process. Indeed, one could well argue that the political activity associated with the WHA each May in Geneva has become one of the central channels for global health governance — quite independent of what is being discussed in the formal WHA committees.[19] Here, polylateral health diplomacy is conducted: formal and informal meetings take place, agreements are reached, deals are struck, NGOs exert influence, the private sector lobbies, and receptions are organized. In short, a diversity of key global health players participate in these activities, even if they do not enter the formal committee rooms at the Palais des Nations, where the WHA holds its formal meetings.

Because the WHA represents a legitimate international decision-making forum, it permits nations that are not powerful in other governance processes, such as the G-8, to express their interests and to influence the multinational consensus-seeking process. Indeed, HICs strive to see their interests reflected in the decisions taken by the WHA, because it is the only body with such legitimacy in global health governance: powerful countries are compelled to negotiate with less-powerful entities because the latter may reflect the positions of multinational alliances that oppose the HIC positions.

As recognition of the diversity of global health actors, Gostin proposed that the WHO take full advantage of its treaty-making capabilities and establish a Framework Convention on Global Health that ties all major stakeholders together.[58] Effective global health programs require the coordinated political and financial commitment of all the relevant actors,[58] and thus capacity-building, priority-setting, coordinating, and progress-monitoring may benefit from such revised GHG.

Some have recommended that the WHO should make much better use of the nodal governance process currently displayed in the WHA, but with a more continuous interaction among all actors, including non-state actors. It has been recommended by global health scholars[19,59] that a Committee C of the World Health Assembly be established that, in addition to Member State representatives, would include as active participants international agencies, philanthropic organizations, multinational health initiatives, and representatives from major civil society groups, particularly those that legitimately represent the most vulnerable populations. The proposed Committee C would debate major health initiatives and provide an opportunity for many important non-state players involved in health to present their plans and achievements to the Member States and to offer expanded consideration of issues that are of concern to them. Committee C could pass resolutions that are then forwarded to the other committees (e.g. Committee A, dealing with program issues, and Committee B, dealing with administrative issues). The work of Committee C would complement rather than supplant the program focus of Committee A and the budget and managerial responsibilities of Committee B.

Such a reform would link the flexibility of what Fidler called "open source anarchy" to the WHO's role as the "directing authority" in global health and to its global political legitimacy. The more vibrant political framework that it would help to produce would allow negotiation of conflicting interests and a search for compromises among the plurality of actors. The existing density of social relations will continue to generate increased organizational growth in the transnational space, but it will also require an expanded mechanism to address the health conditions of people in all parts of the world and to coordinate the large number of initiatives. These activities might be undertaken directly, as in the case of specific disease programs, or indirectly, by focusing on the social determinants of disease, of which poverty is the leading factor. Nevertheless, powerful actors in GHG will not be inclined to entirely relinquish their hegemony in the pursuit of global health cooperation.

Conclusion

GHG has been characterized since the 1990s by a rapid proliferation of actors reacting to new health challenges that had been insufficiently addressed by the post-World War II international health architecture. Facilitated by globalization, the emergence of new actors added expertise and financial resources to the field of international health and contributed to a higher degree of flexibility in dealing with global health problems. However, it also contributed to new problems:

- An underlying tendency to focus on controlling and treating infectious diseases and, vice versa, a lack of focus on noncommunicable or chronic diseases.
- Underestimation of the need for disease prevention and promoting healthy lifestyles.
- Increasing doubts about the legitimacy and accountability of most of the non-state actors in the GHG field.
- The huge challenge of complexity, with the urgent need "to bring order to the chaos" — but without losing the creativity of multi-actor engagement.

Since the 1990s, a number of activities have been undertaken or proposed to improve coordination in this field while building on the achievements of GHG. These activities include:

- Coordination activities following the Paris Declaration.
- A stronger focus on health systems and primary health care.
- Strengthening the WHO's role as the "directing authority" in global health, particularly by using the nodal role of the WHA (as in the proposal to create a Committee C for the representation of non-state actors).

References

1. Wight M. (1979) *Power Politics.* Penguin, Harmondsworth, UK.
2. Beck U, Lau C. (2004) *Entgrenzung und Entscheidung.* Edition Zweite Moderne, Frankfurt, Germany.
3. Bartlett CLR, Kickbusch I, Coulombier D. (2006) *Cultural and Governance Influence on Detection, Identification and Monitoring of Human Disease.* Foresight Project — Infectious Diseases: Preparing for the Future. Government of the United Kingdom. Available from www.bis.gov.uk/assets/bispartners/foresight/docs/infectious-diseases/d4_3.pdf (accessed May 29, 2011).
4. Fidler D. (2007) Architecture amidst anarchy: Global health's quest for governance. *Global Health Govern* **1:** 1–17.
5. Rosenberg ML, Hayes ES, McIntyre MH, Neil N. (2010). *Real Collaboration: What It Takes for Global Health to Succeed.* University of California Press, Berkeley.
6. MacLean SJ, Fourie PP, Brown S. (2009) *Health for Some: The Political Economy of Global Health Governance.* Palgrave, Basingstoke, UK.
7. Buse K, Hein W, Drager N (eds.). (2009) *Making Sense of Global Health Governance: A Policy Perspective.* Palgrave, Basingstoke, UK.
8. Kay A, Williams O. (2009). *Global Health Governance: Crisis Institutions and Political Economy.* Palgrave, Basingstoke, UK.
9. Cooper AF, Kirton JJ. (2009) *Innovation in Global Health Governance.* Ashgate, Aldershot, UK.
10. Szlezak NA, Bloom BR, Jamison DT, *et al.* (2010) The global health system: Actors, norms and expectations in transition. *PLoS Med* **7(1):** e1000183.
11. Frenck J. (2010) The global health system: Strengthening national health systems as the next step for global progress. *PLoS Med* **7(1):** e100183.
12. Keusch GT, Kilama W, Moon S, *et al.* (2010) Global health system: Linking knowledge with action — Learning from malaria. *PLoS Med* **7(1):** e1000179.
13. Moon S, Szlezak NA, Michaud C, *et al.* (2010) The global health system: Lessons for a stronger institutional framework. *PLoS Med* **7(1):** e1000193.
14. Hein W, Burris S, Shearing C. (2009) Conceptual models for global health governance. In: Buse K, Hein W, Drager N (eds.), *Making Sense of Global Health Governance: A Policy Perspective.* Palgrave, Basingstoke, UK, pp. 72–98.

15. Rosenau J. (1995) Governance in the twenty-first century. In: Farer T, Sisk TD (eds.), *Global Governance: A Review of Multilateralism and International Organizations*. Lynne Rienner, Boulder, CO, pp. 13–43.

16. Fidler D. (2004) *SARS, Governance and the Globalization of Disease*. Palgrave, Basingstoke, UK.

17. Burris S, Drahos P, Shearing C. (2005) Nodal governance. *Austral J Legal Philos* **30:** 30–58.

18. Wiseman G. (2005) "Polylateralism" and new modes of global dialogue. In: Jonsson C, Langhorne R (eds.), *Diplomacy*. Sage, London, Vol. 3, pp. 36–57.

19. Kickbusch I, Hein W. Silberschmidt G. (2010) Addressing global health governance challenges through new mechanism: the proposal for a Committee C of the World Health Assembly. *J Law Med Ethics* **38:** 550–563.

20. Berridge V, Loughlin K, Herring R. (2009) Historical dimensions of global health governance. In: Buse K, Hein W, Drager N (eds.), *Making Sense of Global Health Governance: A Policy Perspective*. Palgrave, Basingstoke, UK, pp. 28–46.

21. World Health Organization. (2006) *Constitution of the World Health Organization*. Available from www.who.int/governance/eb/who_constitution_en.pdf (accessed May 29, 2011).

22. World Health Organization. (2003) *Status of Collection of Assessed Contributions, Including Members in Arrears to an Extent Which Would Justify Invoking Article 7 of the Constitution: Report by the Secretariat*. Available from www.who.int/governance/eb/committees/EBABFC19–2en.pdf (accessed May 20, 2011).

23. Ravishankar N, Gubbins P, Cooley R, *et al.* (2009) Financing of global health: Tracking development assistance from 1990 to 2007. *Lancet* **373:** 2113–2124.

24. Held D, McGrew A, Goldblatt D, Perraton J. (1999) *Global Transformations: Politics, Economics and Culture*. Stanford University Press.

25. Linklater A. (1996) Citizenship and sovereignty in the post-Westphalian state. *Eur J Int Relat* **2(1):** 77–103.

26. Davenport D. (2003) The new diplomacy. *Policy Rev* **116:** 17–31.

27. World Health Organization. (2001) *Macroeconomics and Health: Investing in Health for Economic Development — Report of the Commission on Macroeconomics and Health*. World Health Organization.

28. World Health Organization. (2008) *Closing the Gap in a Generation: Final Report of the Commission on Social Determinants of Health.* World Health Organization.

29. Bartsch S, Kohlmorgen L. (2007) The role of civil society in global health governance. In: Hein W, Bartsch S, Kohlmorgen L (eds.), *Global Health Governance and the Fight Against HIV/AIDS.* Palgrave, Basingstoke, UK, pp. 92–118.

30. Organization for Economic Cooperation and Development–Development Assistance Committee. (2008) Measuring aid to health. Available from www. oecd.org/dataoecd/15/49/42584150.pdf (accessed May 5, 2011).

31. Bill and Melinda Gates Foundation. (2007) *Annual Report 2007.* Gates Foundation.

32. Wogart JP, Calcagnotto G, Hein W, von Soest C. (2009) AIDS and access to medicines: Brazil, South Africa and global health governance. In: Buse K, Hein W, Drager N (eds.), *Making Sense of Global Health Governance: A Policy Perspective,* Palgrave, Basingstoke, UK, pp. 137–163.

33. Sell S, Prakash A. (2004) Using ideas strategically: The contest between business and NGO networks in intellectual property rights. *Int Stud Quart* **48:** 143–175.

34. Hein W, Bartsch S, Kohlmorgen L. (2007) *Global Health Governance and the Fight Against HIV/AIDS.* Palgrave, Basingstoke, UK.

35. Hein W. (2007) Global health governance and WTO/TRIPS: Conflicts between "global market-creation" and "global social rights." In: Hein W, Bartsch S, Kohlmorgen L (eds.), *Global Health Governance and the Fight Against HIV/AIDS.* Palgrave, Basingstoke, UK, pp. 38–66.

36. Kuhl H. (2002) *TRIPS and AIDS in South Africa: New Actors in International Relations — Weighing Patents, Pills and Patients.* Occidental College, Los Angeles.

37. Long N. (1989) *Encounters at the Interface: A Perspective on Social Discontinuities in Rural Development.* Wageningen Agricultural University, Wageningen, Germany.

38. Calcagnotto G. (2007) Consensus-building on Brazilian HIV/AIDS policy: National and global interfaces in health governance. In: Hein W, Bartsch S, Kohlmorgen L (eds.), *Global Health Governance and the Fight Against HIV/ AIDS.* Palgrave, Basingstoke, UK, pp. 172–201.

39. Von Soest C, Weinel M. (2007) The treatment controversy: Global health governance and South Africa's fight against HIV/AIDS. In: Hein W, Bartsch S, Kohlmorgen L (eds.), *Global Health Governance and the Fight Against HIV/AIDS*. Palgrave, Basingstoke, UK, pp. 202–225.

40. Hein W, Moon S. (2013) Informal Norms in Global Governance, Human Rights, Intellectual Property Rules and Access to Medicines, Asgate, Farnham.

41. Lee K. (2003) *Health Impacts of Globalization: Towards Global Governance*. Palgrave, Basingstoke, UK.

42. Lee K, Buse K, Fustukian S. (2002) *Health Policy in a Globalising World*. Cambridge University Press.

43. Buse K, Walt G. (2000) Global public–private partnerships: Part 1 — A new development in health? *Bull World Health Organ* **78(4):** 549–561.

44. Buse K, Walt G. (2000) Global public–private partnerships: Part 2 — What are the health issues for global governance? *Bull World Health Organ* **78(5):** 699–709.

45. Smith R, Beaglehole R, Woodward D, Drager N. (2003) *Global Public Goods for Health: Health, Economic, and Public Health Perspectives*. Oxford University Press.

46. Thomas C, Weber M. (2004) The politics of global health governance: Whatever happened to "health for all by the year 2000"? *Global Govern* **10:** 187–205.

47. Aginam O. (2005) *Global Health Governance: International Law and Public Health in a Divided World*. Toronto University Press.

48. Walt G, Buse K. (2005) Global cooperation in international public health. In: Merson M, Jamison D, Mills A (eds.), *International Public Health*. Jones and Bartlett, Boston, pp. 649–680.

49. Cooper AF, Kirton JJ, Schrecker T. (2007) *Governing Global Health: Challenge, Response, Innovation*. Ashgate, Aldershot, UK.

50. World Bank. (1993) *World Development Report 1993 — Investing in Health*. Oxford University Press.

51. Stuckler D. (2008) Population causes and consequences of leading chronic diseases: A comparative analysis of prevailing explanations. *Millbank Q* **86:** 492–494.

52. McQueen D, Kickbusch I. (2007) *The Role of Theory in Health Promotion*. Springer, Berlin.

53. World Health Organization. (2008) *Primary Health Care. Now More Than Ever. The World Health Report.* World Health Organization.

54. Commission on Social Determinants of Health (2008). Closing the gap in a generation: Health equity through action on the social determinants of health. Final Report of the Commission on Social Determinants of Health. World Health Organization.

55. World Bank and World Health Organization. (2006) *High Level Forum on the Health Millennium Development Goals. Selected Papers 2003–2005.* World Bank and World Health Organization.

56. Kaul I, Conceièção P (eds.), (2006) *The New Public Finance: Responding to Global Challenges.* Oxford University Press, New York City.

57. World Health Organization. (2006) *Public Health, Innovation and Intellectual Property Rights: Report of the Commission on Intellectual Property Rights, Innovation and Public Health.* World Health Organization.

58. Gostin LO. (2007) A proposal for a framework convention on global health. *J Int Econ Law* **10(4):** 998–1008.

59. Silberschmidt G, Matheson D, Kickbusch I. (2008) Creating a Committee C of the World Health Assembly. *Lancet* **371:** 1483–1486.

4

Instruments of Health Diplomacy

Ebony Bertorelli, BA, MA, *
Steven A. Solomon, BA, JD, †
and Nick Drager, BSc, MA, MD, PhD ‡

Introduction

The rapid changes in the global health landscape over the past few decades have led to an increasingly varied and chaotic environment for global health governance (GHG).[a] With recent episodes of infectious disease

*Program Officer, Global Health Diplomacy, McGill World Platform for Health and Economic Convergence.

†Principal Legal Advisor, World Health Organization.

‡Former Director of the Department of Ethics, Equity, Trade and Human Rights and Senior Adviser in the Strategy Unit, Office of the Director-General at the World Health Organization; Honorary Professor, Global Health Policy, London School of Hygiene & Tropical Medicine; Professor of Public Policy and Global Health Diplomacy, McGill University; Adjunct Research Professor, Norman Paterson School of International Affairs and Senior Fellow, Global Health Programme, The Graduate Institute, Geneva.

[a]Global governance has been defined as "not only the formal institutions and organizations through which the rules and norms governing world order are (or are not) made and sustained, the institutions of the state, intergovernmental cooperation and so on — but also those organizations and pressure groups — from multinational corporations and transnational social movements to the plethora of nongovernmental organizations — which pursue goals and objectives which have a bearing on transnational rule and authority systems"[1] Accordingly, global health governance can be understood as the entities, movements, and organizations (at subnational, international, and supranational levels) that pursue public health goals and objectives that impact international systems of authority.

97

outbreaks, such as severe acute respiratory syndrome (SARS) and influenza A subtype H1N1, the mounting interest in issues involving trade and health, negotiations over virus sharing, the concern over intellectual property rights, the renewed funding for neglected diseases, and the growing concern about chronic diseases, there are more issues than ever that demand attention to GHG.[2-7] At the same time, in addition to the traditional leadership of the World Health Organization in dealing with global health issues, there has been a proliferation of new nongovernmental actors and entities, including global public–private partnerships (GPPPs), nongovernmental organizations (NGOs), private industries and foundations, and multinational institutions. This proliferation has created an increasingly interconnected and confusing global "forum" of public health actors. The construction of meaningful and broadly supported guidelines, norms, standards, rules, and legislation for GHG is, consequently, extraordinarily challenging.[2,8,9] Indeed, many current global health initiatives are characterized by fragmented and uncoordinated efforts that lack transparency, leadership, and normative clarity, which can undermine both the scope and the effectiveness of global health programs.[7,8]

As part of an effort to better understand this environment and with a view to building a more effective architecture for GHG, interest in the structures and practice of global health diplomacy (GHD) has grown.[3,4,10] GHD refers to the policy elaboration processes through which "[s]tates, intergovernmental organizations, and [non-state] actors negotiate responses to health challenges or utilize health concepts or instruments in policy-shaping and negotiation strategies to achieve other political, economic, or social objectives."[3] Within this arena, the instruments of GHD may be considered as a critical tool kit that assists the various actors in achieving workable solutions for the most pressing health challenges. Because of the myriad actors and enterprises now in play, effective GHD instruments are vital to ensuring cooperation among them. Thus, understanding the operation, range, strengths, and weaknesses of these instruments is crucial to successful GHD in the 21st century.

This chapter offers a typology of instruments currently used in GHD. We use the word "instrument" in the sense of mechanisms or vehicles of public health action. Even though that term may suggest tools such as resolutions and treaties, other mechanisms are also used to address global health problems. Firstly, the instruments or tools are divided into four categories: advisory, operative, collaborative, and normative. Within each of these categories, the instruments are further characterized by where they fit on a scale from "less formal" to "more formal" in terms of their structural and normative nature. An explanatory framework for each of these subsections will then be presented, along with historical and current examples. Next will be an assessment of each instrument's strengths and weaknesses. Finally, we will conclude with reflections on the paths forward in addressing gaps in GHD practice.

Instruments Used in GHD

Rather than presenting strict groupings of instruments, it is perhaps more useful ontologically to think of GHD instruments as falling within a dynamic matrix (Fig. 1). Within this matrix, various instruments can be characterized as "softer" or "harder" as well as more or less structurally

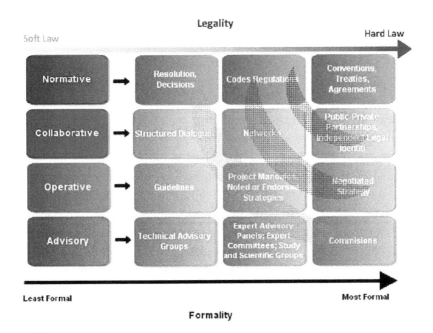

Fig. 1. Matrix of global health diplomacy instruments.

"formal." GHD strategies or actions may be made up of a number of different instruments from multiple categories.

This matrix encompasses the four previously mentioned GHD instrument categories. It is important to note that this typology is heavily influenced by the WHO's framework of governance. Although, as discussed above, the landscape of GHG is changing because of the appearance of many new actors, the WHO has been, since its creation in 1948, the central multinational institution within which global health practice and negotiation takes place.[8,11,12] As Taylor has noted, "[A]s the specialized agency with the primary constitutional directive to act as the 'directing and coordinating authority' on international health work, WHO has the cardinal responsibility to implement the aims of the [United Nations (UN)] Charter with respect to health."[12] Due to this mandate, many of the central instruments used in GHD, within and outside of the WHO, are those that fit within the categories shown in Fig. 1.

Advisory Instruments

Research on the science that is the base for global health practice is critical to setting the global health agenda. When crises or challenges emerge, there is often very little basic research upon which program development can be based, particularly in regions of the world where there is little capacity to address new health crises.[13,14] For example, non communicable or chronic diseases (NCDs) have gained attention as major contributors to the global burden of disease. Such diseases (cardiovascular diseases, cancers, and diabetes) often are linked to human behaviors (alcohol consumption, high-calorie diets, and lack of exercise), but there is little evidence in the developing world on, for example, trans-fat consumption and the linkage of these substances to health outcomes. Such information is necessary for securing international attention and generating subsequent action to restrict these substances.[13] Conversely, tobacco use has gained enormous attention as a developing-world problem, through the science-based negotiations behind the Framework Convention on Tobacco Control (FCTC), which is sponsored by the WHO and which involves nearly all Member States.

Advisory instruments may play a role in translating science into action. These efforts require research, problem identification, database development, and strategic analyses to address global health problems. Collaborative actions based on advisory instruments include the development of disease surveillance systems, program evaluation, and monitoring systems for a given health issue. They may be used by a wide range of actors, including policy-makers, NGOs, governments, and researchers, to support actions on health issues in relevant fora.

Less-formal advisory instruments

Less-formal ("softer") instruments may include recommendations from technical advisory groups and processes such as the WHO's Health Impact Assessments (HIAs). In general, these instruments review existing research and data to build a clearer picture of a particular health issue and to create linkages explaining the depth and breadth of the issue's global health impact. To stimulate further action, research findings are interpreted by advisory and expert groups for the relevant actors and the public.

Advisory instruments are frequently used by the WHO, where reports are presented formally to the Director-General, to the World Health Assembly (WHA) or the WHO Executive Board (EB), and, often, to the general public through WHO communication channels. A recent example can be seen in the deliberations surrounding innovations in financing for neglected diseases of the poor. Recognizing that the issue lacked a sufficient evidence base, the WHO, mandated by the WHA, created an Expert Working Group on Research and Development Financing to address the issue.[15–17] Interestingly, the Working Group was created as part of the previous Public Health Innovation and Intellectual Property Strategy, itself a "harder" (see the next section for the definition) operative instrument, which demonstrates the interconnected nature of GHD instruments.[18] Data for the Expert Working Group report were obtained from several background papers, gleaned during three meetings with scientific presentations, and provided in response to electronic solicitation of public commentary.[17] After one year, the Expert Working Group submitted its report, "Public Health, Innovation and Intellectual Property: Report of the Expert Working Group on Research and Development Financing," to the EB of the WHO. This deliberative body considered the report and arranged for a consultation on it among WHO Member States.[17]

HIAs are a slightly different type of advisory instrument. They are used specifically in scenarios in which a potential initiative is planned and concerned parties are interested in evaluating whether the action may be harmful to the health of a population.[14] Moreover, like advisory groups, HIAs can make recommendations as to how to shape a future initiative to ensure greater operative success. HIAs can be especially useful for clarifying the health aspects of ostensibly non-health-related concerns, such as foreign policy and trade, by highlighting the potentially negative impact that activities in these arenas might have on public health. As Lee *et al.* have noted, "HIAs are intended to improve the quality of decision-making so that policies, projects and programs in all areas lead to improved public health or minimize harm to the health of the particular population."[14] For example, before the negotiation of the FCTC, the World Bank undertook a major study of the global economic impact of tobacco use.[14] The resulting information was extremely effective in illustrating the importance of tobacco control to such diverse agendas as economic development, illegal trade, and pharmaceutical policy.[14]

More-formal advisory instruments

Advisory instruments in the more formal range of the matrix shown in Fig. 1 are generally more structured and may have a higher impact. An example of this type of "harder" advisory instrument is the Commission. Within an international organization such as the WHO, a commission is generally established after preliminary research and policy work has been conducted (usually through the softer advisory instruments mentioned above). The core product of a commission is a set of firm recommendations as to further action that should be taken.

For the 2008 WHO Commission on the Social Determinants of Health, the WHO Secretariat provided administrative support from its Department of Ethics, Equity, Trade and Human Rights.[19] Three work streams were identified to help implement the Commission's recommendations: a policy implementation stream, a policy coherence stream, and a health equity and analysis research stream. These streams provided a structural interface for Member States in the development of and advocacy for new policies dealing with social determinants of health.[15]

Limitations of Advisory Instruments

The central limitation of an advisory instrument is the inability to force actors to conform or to act on the instrument's recommendations. Advisory instruments are simply not constituted as instruments of binding obligation. Therefore, regardless of the degree of "hardness" of the instrument, there is no legal mechanism for translating recommendations into governance. However, sometimes such a translation actually does occur, which underscores the interconnectedness of the GHD instrument matrix. For example, the Codex Alimentarius Commission is an advisory instrument that produces standards for food safety. These standards provide benchmarks against which restrictive national measures on food importation may be evaluated within World Trade Organization (WTO) agreements.

Second, advisory instruments do not always benefit from a clear set of supporters. In many cases the basic research is undertaken by individuals, institutes, or a group of self-appointed experts who may not have the support or the official authorization of Member States. Thus, advisory instruments must assimilate this research and then present an unbiased technical overview of the issues so that appropriate policies may be deliberated on by the governing institutions. However, without policy champions, issues and evidence might not see the light of day in multinational fora. Recently, the work of NGOs and scientific think tanks has been important in pushing evidence to the fore at the WHO and in other GHG bodies.

In summary, the use of advisory instruments is a first step in identifying solutions or instrumentation for global public health practice. However, they generally do not, in and of themselves, provide the initiative to tackle the specific health challenge. The use of other instruments is necessary for bringing about action by policy-makers or GHG bodies.

Operative Instruments

Advisory instruments identify and frame the technical aspects and evidence necessary for addressing health issues, but they do not describe procedures or codes of conduct. Operative instruments, on the other hand, can bring about more rigorous and targeted actions, which operationalize norms through plans of action and strategies. Fundamentally, operative instruments prescribe specific guidelines and procedures for tackling global health challenges.

International organizations, whose governing bodies are made up of Member States, generally produce these operative instruments on behalf of the membership. However, for softer forms of operational instruments, non-state actors such as NGOs can, and often do, disseminate formal advice on various public health issues. Unless these operational activities receive more formal recognition and endorsement, they will have less of an impact on the various actors. Operative instruments generally target governments in terms of action and accountability; however, many of these instruments also offer guidelines for civil society and the private sector.

Less-formal operative instruments

Operative instruments that fall into the less-formal range include guidelines and standards — developed by WHO expert bodies or by the WHO Secretariat itself — which are published by the WHO but not formally endorsed by the WHA. Such guidance may be put forth by the Secretariat on the basis of an explicit authorization of the WHA or the EB or as part of the Secretariat's ordinary function within areas of its regular mandate. Because this less-formal guidance does not require Member States to approve or implement any actions, it can be easier to set in motion, thus facilitating operational programs and agendas. This guidance may also provide reference points for various actors that are looking to influence Member State behavior.

Such guidance or protocols (the word "protocol" is used in this context to mean "a procedure to follow," rather than in its meaning in treaty law, which is "a binding international obligation") are usually based on existing standards and national, regional, and global norms. For example, the WHO Interim Protocol on Rapid Operations to Contain the Initial Emergence of Pandemic Influenza (2007) was based on an earlier version of the same document that was updated with expert input.[20] In the case of the Interim Protocol, the guidelines were formulated without Member State input, and they relied largely on technical expertise from relevant WHO staff.[20] The Interim Protocol, although a formal document, serves as a technical guideline for Member States to use in developing national policy, rather than as a binding international legal agreement.[20]

Importantly, operational instruments, at a purely technical level, can be flexible and responsive to emerging issues. They also can be used to distribute critical technical information without being impeded by legal and negotiation processes.

More-formal operative instruments

Mid-range operative instruments are produced through more formal methods and are frequently referred to as "strategies," a word that in WHO practice usually indicates the involvement, at some level, of governmental representatives or intergovernmental processes. Such strategies are a fairly regular feature of the WHO's work; the WHA has agreed upon more than 20 strategies, on matters ranging from medicines to sanitation to immunization.[b]

---

[b]WHA strategies include the following:

WHA 60.25: Global strategy on public health, innovation, and intellectual property

WHA 58.15: Global immunization strategy

WHA 57.12: Reproductive health: strategy to accelerate progress toward the attainment of international development goals and targets

WHA 57.17: Global strategy on diet, physical activity, and health

WHA 56.21: Strategy for child and adolescent health and development

WHA 56.30: Global health-sector strategy for HIV/AIDS

WHA 55.25: Infant and young nutrition (drafted on the basis of the draft global strategy for infant and young child feeding)

WHA 54.11: WHO medicines strategy

WHA 52.19: Revised drug strategy

WHA 51.28: Strategy on sanitation for high-risk communities

WHA 51.18: Noncommunicable disease prevention and control (urges states to cooperate with the WHO in developing a global strategy)

WHA 51.11: SAFE strategy

WHA 51.10: Revised drug strategy

WHA 49.14: Revised drug strategy

WHA 49.12: WHO global strategy for occupational health for all

WHA 48.11: International strategy for tobacco control

WHA 46.20: WHO global strategy for health and environment

WHA 45.35/WAH42.33/WHA40.26: Global strategy for the prevention and control of AIDS

WHA 34.36: Global strategy for health for all by the year 2000

WHA 33.16/WHA31.45: Malaria control strategy

WHA 24.49: Strategy for health during the Second United Nations Development Decade

WHA 22.39: Re-examination of the global strategy for malaria eradication

Strategies fall into two broad categories: those that are elaborated by the Secretariat through expert and technical processes and then endorsed or otherwise approved by the WHA, and those that involve direct inter-governmental processes before approval by the WHA. Both types of strategies involve input from relevant non-state actors as well. The former may be softer instruments than the latter, but both have substantial weight, owing to the fact that they are products of the WHA. However, there is not always a clear line between the two types. The 2004 WHO Global Strategy on Diet, Physical Activity and Health (GSDPAH) is an example of an instrument with a more active Secretariat role; the 2008 Global Strategy and Plan of Action on Public Health, Innovation and Intellectual Property is an example of a more active intergovernmental process.

The GSDPAH was created through a consultation spanning 18 months that addressed guidelines on the role of unhealthy diet and physical inactivity in NCDs.[21] During this period, the WHO conducted formal meetings with Member States at the regional level, with UN agencies outside of the WHO, with organizations of civil society, and with independent experts and private sector actors in a variety of disciplines from both developed and developing countries.[21] Each consultation produced a report that addressed recommendations for the creation of a global strategy. After being formally endorsed at the WHA, the strategy became a set of recommendations for behavior change, targeting not only Member States but also civil society and NGOs, the private sector, and international partners. The global strategy approach, along with the FCTC, forms the principal WHO contributions to the prevention of NCDs.[22]

The process of multi-actor consultation and endorsement by the WHA is considerably lengthier and more structured than that used to establish the Interim Protocol described above. Intergovernmental endorsement, often expressed through a resolution adopting or welcoming such plans, also denotes a level of attention from Member States that raises both the profile and the status of the final recommendations. Thus, operative instruments created in this manner may have greater advocacy effect in leading Member States themselves to adjust policy in response to the guidelines in the instrument.

The harder range of operative instruments are strategies that are, as noted above, more fully elaborated by governments (as opposed to those that are formulated technically and presented as more or less a complete package for intergovernmental consideration) and then adopted by the WHA. Paralleling many of the features of harder normative instruments, operative instruments in this range articulate even more precisely a code of conduct dealing with more controversial issues. Such strategies involve formal Member State negotiation and often include input from non-state actors before formal adoption.

The highly formalized Global Strategy and Plan of Action on Public Health, Innovation and Intellectual Property (GSPAPHIIP) is the first comprehensive plan supporting national strategies for pharmaceutical innovation. Member States and intergovernmental institutions came together in a forum to produce this plan. In addition to formal consultation with Member States, the GSPAPIIP involved formal negotiations with other intergovernmental organizations — specifically, the WTO and the World Intellectual Property Organization (WIPO).[23] A series of discussions concluded with an exchange of formal letters between the Director-General of the WHO and the directors-general of the WIPO and the WTO, as well as the establishment of regular coordination meetings. These processes aim to build a sustainable partnership that delivers effective outcomes for issues related to public health and intellectual property.[23]

In contrast to the time required for negotiations on softer operative instruments, the negotiations behind the Global Strategy and Plan of Action required a larger time investment and a broader consensus from stakeholders. Accordingly, negotiated strategies tend to be more influential and have a greater impact than softer forms, and they are generally supported by more-structured mechanisms (through the Secretariat and other means of support) to help carry out the specific aims and codes of conduct.

Another set of harder operative instruments comprises the country-specific strategies relating to GHG. Recently, national global health strategies have proliferated, and they have responded to calls from the international community and at the WHO to integrate foreign policy more closely with global health policy. The sentiment for making such a change is represented by the Oslo Ministerial Declaration (2007) and the UN General Assembly Resolution on Global Health and Foreign Policy (A/RES/63/33, 2009). Several jurisdictions are developing national global health strategies to better tackle global health challenges through coordinated foreign policy, by utilizing the rubrics of health equity, international coordination, and national security.[c]

The first country to formally adopt a national global health strategy was Switzerland (in 2006), with the document "Swiss Health Foreign Policy: Agreement on Health Foreign Policy Objectives."[28] The agreement was a collaborative effort between the Federal Office of Public Health and the Swiss Department of Foreign Affairs. The United Kingdom and the European Union have followed suit, with the British strategy entitled "Health Is Global: A UK Government Strategy 2008–13" (2008) and the EU White Paper entitled "Together for Health: A Strategic Approach for the EU 2008–2013" (2007).[29] The United States has now joined these countries, with its release of President Obama's Global Health Initiative in 2010.[30]

As "harder" operative instruments, national global health strategies offer opportunities for coordinated intergovernmental communication and cooperation to ensure that national global health priorities are transparent and explicit, that they focus on health security, and that they are equitable on a global scale. In the United Kingdom, "Health Is Global" outlines 41 commitments for various departments of the government, including changes to trade policy and the recruitment of foreign workers, and mandates the government to work more closely with multilateral institutions on global health issues.[29]

A critical strength of an instrument such as a national global health strategy is that, because it is tied to domestic priorities, issues of impingement on national sovereignty are obviated. In this context, sovereign governments recognize that global health is key to domestic health, and international agreements that support global health then are consistent with national priorities — especially national security.

---

[c] All of these declarations and resolutions are directed toward urging Member States to place health issues within their domestic foreign policy domains, along with traditional foreign policy issues such as security and trade.[24]

Limitations of Operative Instruments

The drawback of operative instruments is that they contain few if any provisions for review and monitoring. There is no legal force obliging actors to follow their mandates — rather, these mandates are understood to fall within the WHO's authority to make "recommendations" under Article 23 of its constitution. The effectiveness and enforcement of the instrument's mandates depend, most immediately, on political will and institutional credibility.

Operative instruments, like those found in the normative category, also face weaknesses in terms of financial and technical capacity in targeted actors.[8,31,32] These limitations are widely recognized. Indeed, while discussing the creation of the GSDPAH, the Assistant Director-General of the WHO noted that, although steps were taken to facilitate implementation at the global level, "The next step for WHO is to respond to the requests of the Member States — and we know many will ask us — to support them to facilitate implementation at the national level."[33] Therefore, the overall effectiveness of operative instruments depends on support at the local, national, and regional levels, and thus the plausibility of success for mandates and guidelines is in many countries a major concern.

Collaborative Instruments

As mentioned throughout this chapter, a central feature of the changing global health landscape has been the proliferation and shifting of roles among GHG actors. The recognition on the part of traditional actors, such as governments and intergovernmental institutions, of the private sector, NGOs, and other civil society groups has motivated discussions on GHD.[2,3,7,8,11] Nontraditional actors have expressed a need to be more explicitly integrated into formal policy-making and negotiations, and traditional actors have recognized the need to understand, incorporate, and influence actions of emerging actors.[2,3,7,8,11] As cross-border health issues and new players in global health proliferate, the need for instruments to facilitate global cooperation is becoming more urgent.

New instruments must focus on creating multilevel partnerships and mechanisms for global health decision-making. They can then be accessed

by all actors, and they can offer important channels for effective implementation of complex health progsrams and policies. Moreover, they
present an opportunity to work outside traditional constrained government
channels and to find innovative models and sources of action, additional
resources, and new policy tools.

Less-formal collaborative instruments

The collaborative instrument category includes a newer breed of GHD
instruments. In general, this category has involved more soft tools and
less-formal tools and an emphasis on communication and collaboration in
a flexible and practical framework. One of the longer-standing examples
of these instruments has been the participation of non-state actors in intergovernmental forums where policy negotiations occur. NGOs in particular
have participated in WHO fora for decades and, increasingly, intergovernmental bodies invite nonstate actors to provide recommendations and
enter into consultations on GHG.

By 1998, 188 NGOs from disciplines as varied as medicine, education,
and law were in an official relation with the WHO, and in recent initiatives such as the GSDPAH and the WHO Global Strategy to Reduce the
Harmful Use of Alcohol, a wide range of actors were invited to formally
participate in consultations.[7] Routine participation of these actors also
occurs at the WHA, where recognized NGOs may act as observers during
the plenary sessions and regional committee meetings.[7]

Private sector entities have been formally involved with the WHO
since 1998, when leading pharmaceutical research firms were included
in roundtable discussions on access to medicines for the world's poor, on
research and development for neglected diseases plaguing developing
countries, and on security threats from counterfeit and poor-quality
medicines.[34] Such discussions led to the elaboration of "WHO Guidelines
on Working with the Private Sector to Achieve Health Outcomes (EB
107/20)" and, more recently, to the GSPAPHIIP. The International
Labour Organization has taken the formal participation of non-state
actors one step further: industry and labor unions are included as voting
members of state delegations to the Organization on Health and Safety
Labour issues.[5]

Networks make up another less-formal collaborative mechanism, providing ongoing platforms for cooperation and dialogue on global-health-related issues at the international, regional, and country levels. Collaborative networks may be largely technical in nature, providing services or resources on a specific global health issue. For example, the WHO Global Outbreak Alert and Response Network (GOARN), created in April 2000 to facilitate responses to disease outbreaks of international importance, is a technical collaboration of existing institutions and networks. GOARN pools information from multiple sources to identify and monitor global disease outbreaks, and helps to coordinate the response to these.[35,36] Another network of this type is the WHO Multicenter Collaborative Laboratory Network, which is made up of laboratories that have the capacity to identify samples of suspected outbreak organisms from countries that lack such technical capacity. By utilizing the unique resources and expertise of various nonstate actors, networks such as these are able to effectively and efficiently bridge and fill gaps in global health challenges.

Networks can also support dialogue and advocacy and thus connect groups of varied actors working on various global health issues. One of the longest-surviving networks of this kind, the International Baby Food Action Network (IBFAN), rose to prominence during the global campaign against the marketing of breast milk substitutes in the early 1980s. Composed of NGOs, IBFAN worked collaboratively with the United Nations Children's Fund, the WHO, and several individual countries to emphasize the importance of breast-feeding. This collaboration was critical to the creation of the International Code of Marketing on Breast-Milk Substitutes. A similar advocacy network supports global tobacco control efforts, and this network formed the Framework Convention Alliance (FCA). The FCA played an important role in the WHO FCTC, supporting Member States in efforts to ensure a strong and equitable tobacco treaty and to enable further actions at the national level in support of the FCTC.

A third set of prominent collaborative instruments is made up of GPPPs, which are collaborative organizations that are identified as emerging actors in their own right.[2,7,11,37,38] Buse and Walt have defined GPPPs as "a collaborative relationship [that] transcends national boundaries and brings together at least three parties, among them a corporation (and/or industry association) and [an] intergovernmental organization, so as to achieve a shared health-creating goal on the basis of a mutually agreed division of labour."[39] Although existing as an instrument in GHG for quite some time, GPPPs grew in prominence during the 1990s in relation to the many global health issues of those years.[40] Current domains for some of the largest GPPPs include HIV/AIDS, tuberculosis, NCDs, malaria, innovations and research and development for neglected diseases, and financing for global health.[7,41]

GPPPs such as the Global Alliance for Vaccines and Immunizations (GAVI), the Global Fund to Fight AIDS, Tuberculosis and Malaria (Global Fund), the International AIDS Vaccine Initiative (IAVI), the International Drug Purchase Facility (IDPF), and the International Finance Facility for Immunization (IFFIm) are frameworks that bring together private finance, technical expertise, governments of affected and donor countries, NGOs, and intergovernmental organizations. Together, these entities build resources, create advocacy, expand knowledge, stimulate research and development, improve access to and delivery of care, and provide an effective structure within which stakeholders can address specific global health challenges in a collaborative manner.[7,8]

Importantly, GPPPs can come in a variety of forms and can operate at the international, regional, and country-specific levels — sometimes simultaneously, depending on the given partnership or project. Although primarily a private philanthropic endeavor, the Bill and Melinda Gates Foundation, one of the largest private funders of global health issues, does much of its work through GPPPs involving academic institutions, intergovernmental forums, countries, and NGOs.[42] Other actors, including international financial institutions such as the World Bank and intergovernmental groups such as UNAIDS, also work through GPPPs.[22,43] Considered by many to be the "path of the future" in terms of GHG, GPPPs have at the very least provided a critical pathway for nongovernmental forms of GHG.

More-formal collaborative instruments

Although a large majority of collaborative instruments reside in the softer range of the GHD matrix, there are a few examples that lean toward more-institutionalized and even legal forms. Currently, leading international institutions in the field of health are making strides toward creating and promoting permanent formal collaborative mechanisms and structures to encourage partnership and discussion with nongovernmental actors. One example of new collaborative structures is the Partners Forum on Chronic Disease in the Americas (part of the Pan-American Health Organization), which spans the range of health stakeholders and focuses on developing awareness and consensus across sectors, as well as developing support for international initiatives on chronic disease and lifestyle issues.[44] The Forum thus ensures the participation and incorporation of non-state actors in consultation and dialogue.

There are GPPPs that may be characterized as even harder in terms of their structure and legality. Such partnerships are constituted as distinct legal identities under national law. Examples of such entities are the Global Fund, GAVI, and the Medicines for Malaria Venture (MMV), all of which operate under a highly formal governance and administrative structure. These GPPPs, incorporated as nonprofit foundations under national law (in all three cases, under Swiss law), are also examples of the rapid changes taking place in the GHG environment. The oldest among them, the MMV, was established in 1999.[40]

Limitations of Collaborative Instruments

Although they represent one of the more progressive and inclusive categories of GHD instruments, collaborative instruments face significant limitations in their effectiveness and legitimacy as governance mechanisms. The majority of collaborative instruments are softer and less formal and, thus, they are often very impermanent and limited in their integration within governing institutions. In these instruments, NGOs and the private sector have access to various intergovernmental fora, but they are not systematically consulted or able to formally participate in policy formation.[7,45] Formalizing the participation of these actors in GHG polices would be fraught with complications. Because intergovernmental forums control the participation of non-state actors, these collaborative mechanisms can become excessively one-sided; this leaves little scope for new actors to fully participate in the more-formal arenas of GHG.

There are concerns about accountability and transparency in the governance of GPPPs. Many GPPPs are nongovernmental, and thus there is no government oversight of the actions of these organizations. Furthermore, transparency in terms of where and how funds accrued by the less-structured GPPPs are allocated and spent has not yet been fully attained. As Buse and Walt have pointed out, there is little accessible information as to which parties benefit from actions of GPPPs — those most in need because of health burdens or those that receive more public recognition of their efforts?[39] The private sector makes up 23% of GPPP membership but only 5% are NGOs; the market-based interests of private sector actors may not always align with the global health needs recognized by NGOs, and thus dissonance in objectives may result.[7,34] In addition, GPPPs can often accrue excessive transaction costs related to the conduct of their initiatives, and those costs create extra obstacles or burdens for recipient countries.

Finally, the involvement of multiple GPPPs in a specific global health issue can lead to fragmented policies and duplicative funding efforts. Although some GPPPs, such as IAVI, work to unify and focus efforts among various actors, in many instances GPPPs take a narrow interest in specific aspects of a given challenge, leaving gaps in the overall approach to the problem.[8,38] This piecemeal or issue-specific approach can result in disorganization and may inhibit coordinated approaches that support greater structural change rather than focusing on niche projects.[8,38] Moreover, because resources for global health are already severely constrained, the involvement of multiple GPPPs in a given issue may divert funding from other deserving issues and thus reduce the reach of limited available resources.

Normative Instruments

Often referred to as legal instruments, normative tools are among the most familiar elements in GHG. Beginning in 1851, normative instruments were used by the International Sanitary Conferences to create several health treaties, which many recognize as the first instances of GHG.[5] Fundamentally, normative instruments define the duties, responsibilities, rights, and obligations that actors authorize and enforce by using both binding and nonbinding legal structures. Many normative instruments, such as resolutions of the WHA, often require the creation of a working group or commission. Normative instruments also encourage or commit actors to comply with the recommendations highlighted within various less-formal instruments. Without these legal documentary structures, it would be difficult to control the actions of the various actors. As prominent legal scholar David Fidler has noted, "[I]nternational law is structurally and practically unavoidable as an instrument of GHG."[11]

Notwithstanding the role of legally binding agreements in GHG, the emphasis within most global health negotiations, and especially at the WHO, has been on soft, nonbinding forms of commitment.[8,11] Although the WHO has the constitutional power to create binding international law, throughout its history it has preferred to enact recommendations, resolutions, and other nonbinding forms of normative instrumentation. Indeed, in its 62 years of existence, the WHO has used its constitutional powers to create binding instruments a mere handful of times.[11] In contrast, the use of binding normative instruments has been growing in use for issues affecting global health at the WTO, International Labour Organization, and UN General Assembly. In terms of the actors that are utilizing normative instruments (besides the special constitutional mandate of the WHO), those that are able to invoke them are also those that are constrained by their mandates — namely, Member States.

Less-formal normative instruments

As briefly discussed above, softer normative instruments are those that are often characterized by their nonbinding nature and that include resolutions, decisions, and codes.[8,32] The legal basis within the WHO for such instruments is Article 23 of the WHO's constitution, which provides to the WHA the authority to make recommendations and to adopt annexed codes, strategies, plans of action, or frameworks on all matters within the competence of the WHO. Such recommendations are normally constituted as or approved through resolutions of the WHA. Resolutions that urge or call upon Member States to act or refrain from acting in certain ways are not considered binding obligations in an international legal sense. However, they often have considerable force as a diplomatic agreement, as well as specific implementation requirements. Such instruments become effective immediately upon adoption by a simple majority of the WHA. Very often, however, specific votes are not taken on such resolutions, but rather agreed on as a "consensus" among the Member States. Such a consensus is developed both in formal negotiations on the floor of the Assembly and in informal communications among representative delegations or official foreign office missions.

It is important that these instruments, although often lacking the power to constrain the sovereignty of nation states or some nonstate actor behavior, generally are easier to enact than treaties and can be useful for framing goals, creating consensus, and establishing priorities. Among the most prominent of such formalized instruments are codes adopted by the WHA, only two of which have been agreed upon. The first of these codes was the International Code of Marketing of Breast-Milk Substitutes, adopted in 1981.[d] The second, the Global Code of Practice on the International Recruitment of Health Personnel, was adopted 29 years later.[e] The International Code — created in response to the rising understanding that poor infant-feeding practices were having a damaging impact on the health and development of children, as well as causing a significant proportion of deaths among infants and young children — has been heralded as a "key milestone in global efforts to improve breastfeeding."[8,11,32] It has resulted in actions taken by countries throughout the world to implement and monitor its provisions through national measures and binding domestic legislation, as well as through further relevant WHA resolutions on the issue.[f,g]

Moreover, the creation of soft law in its various forms provides a touchstone by which nonstate actors such as NGOs, institutions, and individuals can hold states and other actors accountable with regard to the issues. Through numerous tactics, such as "naming and shaming," that

---

[d] WHA Resolution 34.22 of May 21, 1981.

[e] WHA Resolution 63.16 of May 21, 2010.

[f] By 1995, 60 countries had implemented aspects of the code into various forms of international law.[63]

[g] WHA Resolutions 33.32, 34.22, 35.26, 37.30, 39.28, 41.11, 43.3, 45.34, 46.7, 47.5, 49.15, 54.2, and 55.25 have further clarified or extended certain provisions of the code.

have been made popular by civil society groups, the existence of international norms and formal expectations can help change government behavior.[46,47] As Keck and Sikkink have noted, non-state actors, especially transnational advocacy groups, "promote norm implementation by pressuring target actors to adopt new policies and by monitoring compliance with international standards… [I]n doing so, they contribute to changing the perceptions that both state and societal actors may have of their identities, interests, and preferences; to transforming their discursive positions; and ultimately to changing procedures, policies, and behavior."[47] For example, the UN Millennium Development Declaration has become an important lobbying tool for both nonstate actors and governments. These actors have used the MDGs to pressure countries around the world to support commitments and to ensure that future action is focused on the core MDG issues.[h]

More-formal normative instruments

Harder normative instruments are those tools that, because of their binding nature, have the ability to regulate state behavior in more formal and concrete terms. They include conventions, treaties, agreements, binding regulations, and other forms of legislation, both international and national. Under its constitution, the WHA, as the supreme governing body of the WHO, may take two types of binding normative actions: the adoption of regulations under Article 21 of the WHO Constitution, on the one hand, and the adoption of conventions under Article 19, on the other. Both actions establish legally binding obligations among the Member States.

Article 21 of the WHO Constitution provides to the WHA the authority to adopt regulations in a number of areas, including "procedures designed to prevent the international spread of disease." Such regulations, unlike recommendations adopted under Article 23, establish obligations under international law for Member States. The International Health Regulations

---

[h] The UK Gender and Development Network, a consortium of leading UK-based practitioners, consultants, and academics working on gender, development, and women's rights issues, highlights the use of the MDGs specifically pertaining to gender as a lobbying tool to pressure governments for pointed policy change.[48]

2005 (IHR) are the most recent example of these regulations; they were adopted by resolution WHA58.3, to which the text of the IHR is annexed. Regulations can be distinguished from recommendations under Article 23 by their terms (for example, the use of prescriptive language such as the verb "shall"), by the understanding and intention of Member States in adopting them, and by the compliance of those instruments with Article 22 as to their entry into force for individual Member States.

Article 19 provides to the WHA the authority to adopt international conventions and agreements on any matter within the competence of the WHO. Like regulations under Article 21, such international agreements are legally binding. The WHO FCTC is the first international agreement to be concluded under Article 19. As in the case of a regulation, a convention is adopted by the WHA through a resolution. The FCTC was adopted by resolution WHA56.1, to which the text of the Convention is annexed. Conventions adopted by the WHA can be distinguished from recommendations under Article 23 by the intention of Member States to adopt a legally binding instrument, as well as by the provision of a process through which individual states agree to be bound by the instrument (typically, the adding of signatures, followed by ratification and governance by a Conference of the Parties).

First created in 1969 and revised most recently in 2005, the IHR has the objectives of directing the international management of public health emergencies and preventing the unnecessary obstruction of global commerce.[49] The extensive 2005 revisions have considerably strengthened these regulations to empower information-gathering and to improve the WHO's coordinating and directing functions, especially during international public health emergencies.[31,32,50–52] Included among the changes are the establishment of requirements for Member States to report potential public health emergencies within 24 hours; the assertion of the WHO's authority to utilize nongovernmental information in disease detection and surveillance; and the recognition of the WHO's ability to issue recommendations, such as travel restrictions, without the authorization of the implicated governments.[51] Lastly, the new regulations also obligate all 194 Member States to improve their national management of public health threats through strengthened detection, reporting, and responding mechanisms.[51] The changes in the IHR make this instrument the most comprehensive international health legal instrument to date and, as Fidler and Gostin have pointed out, "[T]he revised Regulations promise to become a centerpiece for GHG in the 21st century."[50]

A feeling of unprecedented change also surrounded the creation of the FCTC in 2005, as it marked the first international treaty to be adopted under the auspices of the WHO's constitution.[50] The FCTC was created to foster multilateral collaboration that would deter the global tobacco epidemic through science-based strategies for demand reduction and control of smuggling.[32] The negotiation process actually started in 1999, and it required sustained effort on the part of its original backers within the WHO and nongovernmental communities. The process was criticized by some as "ambitious to a fault"[53] and it was not until direct support was received from WHO Director-General Gro Harlem Brundtland that the negotiation process became a reality.[53,54] Although the IHR was executed as a consensus agreement, the FCTC has now been signed by 168 countries and constitutes binding international law for them by a Conference of the Parties.[53] This first use of the framework-convention approach under the WHO's constitution has sent a signal that the WHO may in the future use its political power to prevent or manage global health crises through the use of hard normative instruments.[32]

Other multinational organizations have also used hard normative instruments to tackle global health challenges. In the area of trade and health, some of the most important instruments are found at the WTO in the form the General Agreement on Tariffs and Trade (GATT), the General Agreement in Trade in Services (GATS), the Agreement on Trade-Related Aspects of Intellectual Property Rights (TRIPS), the Agreement on the Application of Sanitary and Phytosanitary Measures (SPS Agreement), and the Agreement on Technical Barriers to Trade (TBT Agreement).[11,55-58] These normative instruments provide the Member States with the legal basis on which to regulate imports of international or domestic goods that are based on dangerous additives, contaminants, toxins, or disease-causing organisms that might threaten human health (SPS); to ensure that technical regulations are not more trade-restrictive than necessary when seeking protection of human health or safety (TBT); to provide a framework for the liberalization of trade in services, including health services (GATS); and to harmonize the intellectual property protections of WTO Member

States, including pharmaceutical patents (TRIPS).[11,55–59] Importantly, unlike the WHO, if disputes concerning violations of these instruments arise, the WTO — unlike the WHO — offers a dispute settlement mechanism, the rulings of which are enforced by the Conference of the Parties.[60] Such an advanced legal framework allows legislation enacted by the WTO to be far more powerful than that enacted by the WHO.

Finally, domestic legislation is also an important subset of hard normative instruments. For both soft and hard international law to have a strong impact in signatory states, Member States must convert international mandates into national law.[8,31,32] Beyond national ratification and implementation of signed agreements, countries often formulate their own legislation that directly affects global health, such as UK regulations on the hiring and recruiting of foreign medical personnel. Therefore, individual countries' direct legislation within the area of public health or legislation within parallel areas is crucial to the success of international law as well as, more generally, to the improvement of global health.

Limitations of Normative Instruments

Although normative instruments are often considered to be the bedrock of GHG instruments, there are significant limitations on and systemic issues with their use. The issue of sovereignty remains a fundamental concern. Although there are clear merits to the use of soft law, such as the greater ease of achieving consensus on instrument introduction and the demonstrated success in influencing state behavior, the fact that soft law is fundamentally nonbinding and thus is a weaker form of instrumentation carries heavy implications for the strength of global health regimes in overcoming issues of individual state sovereignty — especially considering soft law's traditional acceptance.

Indeed, the ability of states to ignore the mandates of declarations, decisions, and regulations in soft law is generally without recourse and has been highlighted by many in the field as a major shortcoming of GHG.[8,11,31,32,61] These observations become even more salient when it is noted that hard law, although binding, still faces significant obstacles in terms of ensuring the compliance of Member States with national laws. This reliance on soft law leaves normative instruments vulnerable to individual state preferences and often results in states withholding their support from a piece of legislation until its rules follow those preferences or are watered down to be vague and merely rhetorical agreements.[8]

In both the FCTC and the IHR negotiations, the resistance of states to restrictions on their sovereignty was observable. Within the FCTC process, it was not until WHO Secretary-General Gro Harlem Brundtland turned her concerted support and efforts to the task that serious negotiations were jump-started.[53,54] Furthermore, a significant number of the FCTC's major provisions contain clauses with wording such as "consistent with domestic law" and "as appropriate" that allows each state to harmonize the Convention's provisions with its own domestic law. This is accomplished through the liberal use throughout the FCTC of phrases such as "consistent with domestic law" and "as appropriate."[62]

There are certain soft aspects to the IHR as well. Mandates to provide technical and financial resources were watered down and made to be nonbinding (Article 13.5 and Article 44.1).[50,51] Moreover, the entire document is subject to the preferences of individual states; as Fidler *et al.* have pointed out, "[S]tates can reject the new IHR (Article 61) or formulate reservations to provisions to which they refuse to be bound (Article 62)."[50] Thus, states may legalistically reduce a critical piece of this legislation to having the same weak impact as soft law.[50,51,89] A last significant example is found in the definition of a "temporary recommendation." Such recommendations are rightly regarded as among the key strengths of the regulations, as they in effect authorize the Director-General to directly issue such recommendations (for example, travel restrictions as in the case of SARS). However, the IHR takes pains to clarify that such "recommendations" are "nonbinding advice issued...on a time-limited, risk-specific basis...."[51,63] Government negotiators clearly felt compelled to clarify the soft nature of such temporary recommendations and, in so doing, highlighted the ways in which concerns about sovereignty continue to be part of normative instrument negotiations.

Still, such soft law elements arguably cleared the way for the overall adoption of both the FCTC and the IHR. The former is fast approaching universalization, and the latter is already a universal instrument. It is doubtful that such broad acceptance would have been possible in the absence of the flexibilities negotiated into the instruments.

Indeed, the terms *soft law* and *hard law* can obscure important aspects of international agreements — aspects that are critical in describing the tradeoffs involved in international negotiations. It is fair to say that those who reflexively place hard agreements at the top of the international normative order often underestimate the benefits of such factors as softer language in binding agreements or harder language in nonbinding arrangements, as paths toward consensus. A clearer understanding of the dynamics of normative instruments may help stakeholders in shaping them to accommodate the variety of agendas and objectives expressed in GHD.

Finally, within binding legislation, there are few means of supporting states in the implementation of their new obligations. Within the IHR, the mandate for states to monitor and report on their national public health conditions requires a substantial amount of regional and local resources.[31,50] In addition, without meaningful compliance mechanisms, such as the dispute resolution tribunal found at the WTO, the WHO as the central body for GHG is disadvantaged in normative compliance. For both the IHR and the FCTC, there are no mandatory third-party dispute resolution procedures.[8] As Gostin and Taylor have noted, "[I]nternational law is largely voluntary: there is generally no supranational authority to develop and enforce law against sovereign states."[8]

Besides their effect on the critical issues of state sovereignty and compliance, the incorporation of nonstate actors in international agreements may create limitations. The proliferation of global health actors continues to affect and shape public health priorities.[2,3,7] The concurrent increases in nonstate funding mechanisms and contributors in the global health field have also shifted the focus of decision-making and GHG to actors outside of the traditional nation-state.[2,8] Lastly, the importance of the private sector as the marketers, producers, and innovators of a range of products that are integral to either global health or health risks — including pharmaceuticals, vaccines, diagnostics, food, health care, tobacco, and alcohol — is also an element of concern in GHG.[8,34] Thus, there is a growing critical need for useful and effective negotiation fora and strategies among these varied actors. Despite the traditional and continued primacy of Member States in GHG, there are now new forces and financing that should motivate Member States to reach outside their domestic political spheres and make a strong case for multi-tiered, complex negotiations in achieving their national health and security objectives and meeting their obligations.

It is important that, at the international level, the participation of non-state actors has been increasing in the formation of both soft and hard law, as can be seen in the role played by NGOs in the negotiation and implementation of the FCTC. In addition, there have been robust efforts on the part of NGOs to enter into official relations with the WHO and, indeed, to participate in many of its normative initiatives.[64] Increased NGO participation is observed at the national level as well. For example, in 2005, Canada passed the Canadian Access to Medicines Regime (CAMR), a piece of national legislation that allows Canada, on the basis of the TRIPS, to issue licenses for the manufacture of generic versions of patented drugs and medical devices and their export to developing countries that do not have the capacity to produce the products themselves.[65] During the creation of this legislation, representatives of Canada's generic and brand name drug companies and various NGOs played a large role in the formulation of the legislation through consultation as well as through lobbying and petitioning the state.[65]

Yet, although international law is now being utilized more widely and flexibly than in the past, there are still issues that must be resolved to allow the involvement of actors outside of the nation state. As Gostin and Taylor have argued, "[W]hile the WHO and other international organizations do interact with non-state actors and incorporate them within GHG through such means as public–private partnerships and participation in global health forums, international law does not provide a sufficient basis [from which] to fully realize the potential synergies of collaboration among stakeholders."[8]

Where Do We Go from Here? The Need for Future Modification and Coordination of Instruments

The world of GHD instruments is diverse. Some are relatively new, especially the collaborative instruments; others, such as the normative tools, have existed since the beginning of GHG and have played a substantial role in constructing today's global health governance environment. However, as this chapter has highlighted, the use of these instruments, especially with the rapidly changing set of global health actors, in a manner that is transparent and accountable, continue to pose challenges.

For GHG to be more effective, there is a need for greater understanding, innovation, and flexibility with respect to the instruments of GHD. Progress will mean clearer and more effective "rules of the game," more research, clearer and more expansive communications, and greater transparency. Even in some of the well-established areas of international law, overcoming the lasting impacts of the Westphalian system, with its almost-total focus on state sovereignty and governance mechanisms, is still a challenge. In addition, finding ways to improve capacity and increase resources for the poorest Member States, many of which are facing the largest health burdens with the least capacity to meet them, is critical to ensuring the success of GHG in the 21st century.

With all of the changes that have occurred because of globalization, it is virtually impossible for actors involved in GHG, including states, to address global health challenges alone. Thus, the time for achieving transformations and innovation in GHD is ripe, as many of the changes that have occurred have involved greater input from non-state actors, access to greater funding through private interests, and linkages between health and traditional state concerns of trade, security, and economic development. Indeed, more than ever, the traditional structures of power and influence that currently exist in GHG are open to change and redefinition for the future.[2–4,7]

GHG is much more than creating and passing binding legislation and using that legislation to guide the actions of national governments.[2–5,7] Critically, it entails producing opportunities for all stakeholders involved in health-related fields to become engaged in the process of change and cooperation. It also entails creating incentives to ensure cohesion, technical skills, and the financial capacity to implement collaborative actions. As Fidler has noted, "[T]he challenge for global health governance in the 21st century is not to generate more international law, even though new treaties may be needed and old regimes modernized. The challenge is to embed public health as a value and interest in (1) sovereign states; (2) their interactions in the international system; and (3) their relationships with global civil society groups."[11]

In conclusion, there is a need to expand and deepen scholarly interest in and evaluation of GHD instruments as the field continues to change and progress. Fundamentally, the nature of these challenges is well known. However, as this chapter has shown, the pathways of action and the instruments required to achieve successful global health outcomes remain to be fully explored, understood, evaluated, and, finally, adopted. Therefore, continued research in GHD is critical.

Key questions for further research include the following:

- Do binding or nonbinding instruments promote deeper commitment and adherence to global health norms? Evidence as to which type of instrumentation is more successful in influencing the actions of governments and the ways in which this success occurs is an important area of study.
- What criteria may be used to assess the effectiveness of different forms of international instruments? Such a system of evaluation would be essential in informing the decisions of various actors as to which GHD instrument may be the most effective to use when targeting specific global health challenges.

References

1. Held D, McGrew A, Goldblat D, Perraton J. (1999) *Global Transformations: Politics, Economics and Cultures.* Policy, Cambridge.
2. Buse K, Hein W, Drager N (eds.). (2009) *Making Sense of Global Health Governance: A Policy Perspective.* Palgrave Macmillan, London.
3. Smith R, Fidler D, Lee K. (2009) Global health diplomacy research, trade, WHO trade, foreign policy, diplomacy and health. In: *Draft Working Paper Series.* World Health Organization.
4. Kickbush I, Silberschmidt G. (2007) Global health diplomacy: The need for new perpectives, strategic approaches, and skills in global health. *Bull World Health Organ* **85:** 3.
5. Fidler D. (2001) The globalization of public health: The first 100 years of international health governance. *Bull World Health Organ* **79:** 8.
6. Fidler D. (2007) Architecture amidst anarchy: Global health's quest for governance. *Global Health Governance* **1:** 17.

7. Dodgson R, Lee K, Drager N. (2002) Global health governance: A conceptual review. In: *Key Issues in Global Health Governance*. World Health Organization and Center on Global Change and Health, London School of Hygiene and Tropical Medicine.
8. Gostin L, Taylor A. (2008) Global health law: A definition and grand challenges. *Public Health Ethics* **1**: 10.
9. Sridhar D. (2009) Introduction in health and foreign policy: Country strategies. WHO Working Paper, World Health Organization.
10. Fidler D. (2008) Navigating the global health terrain: Preliminary considerations on mapping global health diplomacy. In: *Globalization, Trade, and Health Series*. World Health Organization.
11. Fidler D. (2002) Global health governance: Overview of the role of international law in protecting and promoting global public health. Discussion Paper No. 3. In: *Key Issues in Global Health Governance*. World Health Organization and Center on Global Change and Health, London School of Hygiene and Tropical Medicine.
12. Taylor A. (2004) Governing the globalization of public health. *J Law, Med Ethics* **32**: 8.
13. L'Abbe M. (2009) Global and regional collaboration for chronic disease prevention and control — Trans-fat and sodium. Presentation given at McGill World Platform 2008 Think Tank, Convergence Workshop: Harnessing the Power of Business for Better Global Health Diplomacy in Non-communicable Disease Prevention and Control, Experts Meeting, November 16, 2009.
14. Lee K, Ingram A, Lock K, McInnes C. (2007) Bridging health and foreign policy: The role of health impact assessments. *Bull World Health Organ* **85**: 5.
15. World Health Organization. (2010) WHO implementation. Available at http://www.who.int/social_determinants/implementation/en (accessed on December 12, 2011).
16. World Health Organization. (2009) Public health, innovation, and intellectual property. In: *Report of the Expert Working Group on Research and Development Financing*. World Health Organization.
17. World Health Organization. (2008) Resoluton 61.21 on global strategy and plan of action on public health, innovation, and intellectual property. WHO Expert Working Group on R&D and Financing. World Health Organization. Available at http://apps.who.int/gb/ebwha/pdf_files/A61/A61_R21-en.pdf (accessed on December 12, 2011).

18. World Health Assembly. (2008) WHO Expert Working Group on R&D and Financing. Available at http://www.who.int/phi/R_Dfinancing/en/index.html (accessed on February 2, 2010).

19. Commission on Social Determinants of Health. (2008) Closing the gap in a generation: Health equity through action on the social determinants of health. In: *Final Report of the Commision on Social Determinants of Health*. World Health Organization.

20. World Healths Organization. (2007) WHO Interim Protocol: Rapid operations to contain the initial emergence of pandemic influenza. World Health Organization. Available at http://www.who.int/influenza/resources/documents/RapidContProtOct15.pdf (accessed on December 12, 2011).

21. World Health Organization. (2003) World Health Organization process for a global strategy on diet, physical activity and health. WHO/NMH/EXR.02.2 Rev.1. Available at http://whqlibdoc.who.int/hq/2003/WHO_NMH_EXR.02.2_Rev.1.pdf (accessed on December 12, 2011).

22. Magnusson RS. (2007) Non-communicable diseases and global health governance: Enhancing global processes to improve health development. *Globalization Health* **3**: 16.

23. World Health Organization. (2010) Public health and intellectual property. World Health Organization in collaboration with WIPO and WTO. Available at http://www.who.int/phi/documents/CollaborationwithWIPOandWTO.pdf (accessed on December 12, 2011).

24. Ministers of Foreign Affairs of Brazil France, Indonesia, Norway, Senegal, South Africa and Thailand. Oslo Ministerial Declaration. (2007) Global health: A pressing foreign policy issue of our time. *Lancet* **369**.

25. United Nations General Assembly. (2009) Resolution on *Global Health and Foreign Policy*. A/RES/63/33.

26. Chan M, Støre J, Kouchner B. (2008) Foreign policy and global public health: Working together towards common goals. *Bull World Health Organ* **86**.

27. Fidler D, Drager N. (2006) Health and Foreign Policy. *Bull World Health Organ* **84**.

28. Federal Department of Home Affairs and Federal Department of Foreign Affairs. (2006) Swiss health foreign policy: Agreement on health foreign Policy objectives. Government of Switzerland.

29. HM Government. (2008) Health is global: A UK government strategy 2008–13. Available at http://www.dh.gov.uk/prod_consum_dh/groups/dh_digitalassets/@dh/@en/documents/digitalasset/dh_088753.pdf (accessed on October 2009).

30. Government of the United States of America. (2010) Implementation of the Global Health Initiative: Consultation document. Available at http://www.usaid.gov/our_work/global_health/home/Publications/docs/ghi_consultation_document.pdf (accessed on February 2010).

31. Wilson K, McDougall C, Fider D, Lazar H. (2008) *Bull World Health Organ* **86:** 5.

32. Gostin L. (2007) A proposal for a framework convention on global health. *J Int Econ Law* **10:** 18.

33. Zaracostas J. (2004) WHA adopts landmark global strategy on diet and health. *Lancet* **363**.

34. Freymond J. (2009) Global health diplomacy and the private sector: A European perspective — A report. Working text, draft.

35. World Health Organization. (2010) Global outbreak alert and response network — GOARN: partnership in outbreak response. World Health Organization. Available at http://www.who.int/csr/outbreaknetwork/goarnenglish.pdf (accessed on February 15, 2010).

36. World Health Organiztaion. (2010) Global Alert and Response (GAR). Available at http://www.who.int/csr/outbreaknetwork/en (accessed on February 15, 2010).

37. Buse K, Walt G. (2000), Global public–private health partnerships: Part I — A new development in health? *Bull World Health Organ* **78:** 50.

38. Buse K, Harmer AM. (2007) Seven habits of highly effective global public–private health partnerships: Practice and potential. *Soc Sci Med* **64:** 12.

39. Buse K, Walt G. (2000) Global public–private health partnerships: Part I — A new development in health? *Bull World Health Organ* **78:** 10.

40. Burci GL. (2009) Public/private partnerships in the public health sector. *Int Organizations Law Rev* **6:** 23.

41. Fidler D. (2003) Emerging trends in international law concerning global infectious disease control. *Emerg Infect Dis* **9:** 5.

42. Bill and Melinda Gates Foundation. (2010) Programs and parnerships. Available at http://www.gatesfoundation.org/programs/Pages/overview.aspx (accessed on February 16, 2010).

43. World Bank. (2010) Public–private partnership in infrastructure. Available at http://web.worldbank.org/WBSITE/EXTERNAL/WBI/WBIPROGRAMS/PPPILP/0,menuPK:461142~pagePK:64156143~piPK:64154155~theSitePK:461102,00.html (accessed on February 15, 2010).
44. Pan American Health Organization. (2010) Chronic disease prevention. Available at http://www.paho.org/english/ad/dpc/nc/partners-forum.htm (accessed on February 17, 2010).
45. Hulme D, Edwards M. (1997) *NGO's, States, and Donors: Too Close for Comfort?* Macmillan, London.
46. Johnstone AI. (2001) Treating international institutions as social environments. *Int Stud Quart* **45:** 28.
47. Keck M, Sikkink K. (1998) *Activists Beyond Borders: Advocacy Networks in International Politics.* Cornell University Press.
48. Painter G. (2004) *Gender, the Millennium Development Goals, and Human Rights in the Context of the 2005 Review Processes.* Gender and Development Network.
49. World Health Organization. (1969) International health regulations.
50. Fidler D, Gostin L. (2006) The new international health regulations: An historic development for international law and public health. *J Law, Med Ethics* **33:** 9.
51. World Health Organization. (2006) International health regulations. World Health Organization.
52. Kamoie B, Pestronk R, Baldridge P, *et al.* (2008) Assessing laws and legal authorities for public health emergency legal preparedness. *J Law, Med Ethics* **36:** 4.
53. Roemer R, Allyn T. (2005) Origins of the WHO Framework Convention on Tobacco Control. *Am J Public Health* **95:** 2.
54. Mackay J. (2003) The making of a convention on tobacco control. *Bull World Health Organ* **81**.
55. World Trade Organization. (1995) Marrakesh Declaration of 15 April 1994: Agreement on the Application of Sanitary and Phytosanitary Measures. World Trade Organization.
56. World Trade Organization. (1995) Marrakesh Declaration of 15 April 1994: Annex 1B: General Agreement on Trade and Services. World Trade Organization.

57. World Trade Organization. (1995) Marrakesh Declaration of 15 April 1994 Agreement on Barriers to Trade. World Trade Organization.

58. World Trade Organization. (1995) Marrakesh Declaration of 15 April 1994: Annex 1C: Agreement on Trade-Related Aspects of Intellectual Property Rights. World Trade Organization.

59. World Trade Organization, World Health Organization. (2002) WTO agreements and public health: A joint study by the WHO and WTO Secretariat. World Health Organization, World Trade Organization.

60. World Trade Organization. (1995) Marrakesh Declaration of 15 April 1994: Annex 2, Dispute Settlement Understanding. World Trade Organization.

61. Fidler D. (2008) Influenza virus samples, international law and global health diplomacy. *Emerg Infect Dis* **14:** 6.

62. World Health Organization. (2003) WHO Framework Convention on Tobacco Control. World Health Organizaiton.

63. World Health Organization. (2005) Resolution on Revision of the International Health Regulations. WHA58.3.

64. World Health Organiation. (1946) Constitution of the World Health Organization. World Health Organization.

65. Government of Canada. (2010) Canada's Access to medicines regime. Available at http://www.camr-rcam.gc.ca/index_e.html (accessed on January 14, 2010).

5

Global Health in International Politics

*Harley Feldbaum, PhD**

Introduction

In the past two decades, global health issues have undergone a remarkable rise in political priority. For much of the 20th century, global health issues were considered low-priority political issues of a technical nature and largely irrelevant to powerful state interests or to international politics.[1] Now, global health issues such as pandemic influenza, severe acute respiratory syndrome (SARS), HIV/AIDS, and bioterrorism are major issues within international politics. Fidler deemed this change a "revolution" in the political status of global health issues, saying "[N]othing in the prior history of national and international efforts on public health compares to the political status public health has reached today."[2]

There is little recent precedent for understanding the impact of international politics and national interests on the practice of global health. The strong relevance of global health to international politics and, by extension, to the foreign policy interests of nation-states has not been seen since the colonial era, when public health played a key role in supporting colonial expansion and trade.[3,a] The scientific basis of public health and the history of mutual neglect between the fields of global health and international relations

*Director of the Global Health and Foreign Policy Initiative at Johns Hopkins SAIS.
E-mail: harley.feldbaum@gmail.com
[a] See also the chapter by Adams in this volume.

have limited the examination of the role of global health in international politics to a small number of practitioners and scholars.

The study of national interests and international politics is, however, increasingly relevant to an understanding of the prioritization of select global health issues and the enacting of successful global health interventions. To be sure, there are other critical actors in global health that are not nation-states, including nongovernmental organizations (NGOs), transnational companies, and international organizations such as the World Health Organization (WHO). However, nation-states remain a (if not "the") "main actor in international relations," and thus it is critical to understand their interests and interactions on global health issues.[4]

This chapter examines the state (national) interests, international politics, and relationship of science and politics, which increasingly affect global health efforts and demand greater understanding and collaboration between the practitioners of global health and foreign policy.

Global Health and State Interests

Tension will always exist between the pursuit of global health and state interests. It is inherent in this relationship because the goals of global health and the goals that states seek to achieve are different. The pursuit of global health "places a priority on improving health and achieving equity in health for all people worldwide,"[5] whereas states place a priority on the interests and well-being of their political community. These abstract goals result in real tensions: while the goals of global health are cosmopolitan and transnational, efforts to achieve global health are predominantly funded by and implemented through the governments of nation-states. Thus, nations filter global health through the lens of their own interests, a process that creates both synergies and conflicts between global health and states' interests.

How National Interests Prioritize Global Health Issues

A hierarchy of foreign policy issues informs the ways in which nation-states pursue their interests.[6] National security has traditionally been pursued as the number-one priority of governments because "[o]nly if survival is assured can states safely seek such other goals as tranquility, profit, and power."[7] States also pursue economic, political, and humanitarian interests, historically placing a higher priority upon security and economic issues than on humanitarian or public health concerns.[6] This hierarchy of foreign policy issues has an enormous impact on the determination of the level of a state's engagement on particular global health issues.

The US Institute of Medicine (IOM) was one of the earliest entities to recognize and expound on the linkages between global health and national security, arguing in a 1992 report, "[I]n the context of infectious diseases, there is nowhere in the world from which we are remote and no one from whom we are disconnected."[8] That report was, in the words of King, the "centerpiece of a major public health campaign"[3] to link infectious diseases with US economic and security interests. This linkage was an important development that brought increased high-level political attention and funding to the field. A more recent IOM report continued these arguments, stating that the US President should "highlight health as a pillar of US foreign policy,"[9] because saving lives both reflects America's values and supports national strategic objectives.

The powerful impact on funding and political attention of linking health to national security is perhaps most exemplified by the United States' response to the national security threat of bioterrorism. This response to the anthrax attacks of 2001 and the continuing threat of bioterrorism generated the expenditure on biodefense of US$6.3 billion per year from 2004 through 2008, far exceeding investments in any other area of global health.[10] Similarly, US investments to respond to the threat of avian flu were $3 billion per year in 2006 and 2007.[11] These major investments occurred because the United States perceived these select global health issues to threaten its security and economic interests.[12] In Fidler's words, "[w]hen diseases threaten, or show the potential to threaten, national security, military capabilities, geopolitical or regional stability, national populations, economic power, and trade interests, foreign policy-makers take notice."[13]

An understanding of the hierarchy of foreign policy issues can also clarify why some global health issues languish without state attention or funding. Important global health burdens of disease, including road traffic injuries and chronic conditions, and the social determinants of health have yet to be persuasively linked to the foreign policy interests of states. Despite the quantity of scientific evidence mustered to illustrate the importance of these issues, state engagement has been lacking because these major disease burdens are not perceived to be relevant to powerful state interests.

State interests of course do not always impede global health goals. The threat that SARS posed to the interests of powerful states was critical to passage of the revised International Health Regulations (IHR) in 2005.[14] SARS's threat to state interests actually resulted in states ceding sovereignty to the WHO in order to better enhance surveillance of and response to infectious disease epidemics. In this case, "the WHO's authority in infectious disease control [was] strengthened partly because it suited the interests of Western states to allow this to happen."[15]

Divergent State Interests with Regard to Global Health Issues

State interests can determine the political priority of global health issues, but states engage differently with global health issues, depending upon each state's interests. Such divergent state interests with regard to global health issues were clearly shown in the controversy over Indonesia's refusal to share influenza A (H1N1) virus samples with the WHO. Many Western countries sought Indonesia's cooperation in sharing viral samples to prevent delays in virus detection or vaccine production that might have allowed an influenza pandemic that would harm citizens, as well as national and economic interests. It has been argued that Indonesia's actions constituted viral blackmail, which "could [have led] to a devastating health crisis anywhere, at any time."[16] Indonesia, however, objected to the WHO's sharing its virus samples with pharmaceutical companies, because the vaccines produced from these samples would likely be unaffordable to Indonesia if a pandemic occurred.[17] Indonesia, supported by India, Brazil, Thailand, and other countries, sought to protect its own national interests by trying to ensure its access to vaccines for a potentially pandemic strain of influenza. Indonesia used the leverage it had, in the form of withholding influenza virus samples, to pursue its national interests and, it argued, to remedy the "unfairness and inequities of the global system."[17] It is interesting that these divergent state interests were replicated within the global health community, with some countries supporting Indonesia's position to create a more equitable framework for sharing vaccines and pharmaceutical products, and others lamenting Indonesia's undermining of previously uncontroversial global infectious-disease-surveillance activities.

Divergent interests also were implicated in the weakening of the final language of the Framework Convention on Tobacco Control (FCTC). In this case of health diplomacy, tobacco- and tobacco-product-producing countries, including the United States, Japan, China, and Germany,[18] successfully introduced flexibilities and optional language into the final text of the treaty, which "offers an ostensible excuse for... [p]arties to the Convention to avoid development of robust, comprehensive tobacco control policies."[19] These flexibilities were opposed by many of the other state parties to the Convention, which illustrates the impact of divergent state interests on global health priorities.

Domestic Politics and Global Health

It is also worth considering the role that domestic political interests can play in influencing state preferences on global health issues. Despite the principle expounded during the Truman Administration — that politics stops at the water's edge — there is clear evidence that domestic politics affects state actions on global health. The international politics of Indonesia's position on the sharing of H1N1 influenza virus samples was discussed above, but this position should be understood as also containing a domestic political component. Former health minister Supari's championing of this issue was popular domestically, as she was seen as standing up to Western interests, and her statements were tailored to address internal Indonesian dynamics between nationalism and the role of Islam in government.[20] Domestic political calculations were also at play in the recent offering, and then postponement, of US donations of influenza A (H1N1) vaccines to poor countries. Domestic shortages of the vaccine in the United States made donations to other countries politically infeasible; US citizens had to remain at the front of the vaccine line as long as there was domestic demand for the vaccine. The areas of reproductive health, family planning, and HIV/AIDS have frequently been subjected to such domestic political preferences. Successive conservative administrations in the United States have implemented policies banning the funding of NGOs in other countries that perform abortions.[21] Domestic Christian religious advocacy for addressing HIV/AIDS was critical to the passage in 2003 of the President's Emergency Plan for AIDS Relief (PEPFAR). This advocacy usefully supported the incorporation of treatment for AIDS into the program, as well as a focus on sex trafficking; less helpfully from a public health perspective, it also resulted in the incorporation into PEPFAR of abstinence education and an anti-prostitution pledge.[22] The important role that domestic political interests can play in shaping state interests on global health, in both supportive and obstructive ways, indicates that state interests are malleable, a fact that opens the door for activists, NGOs, companies, academics, and other actors to influence state actions on global health.

Health Interventions for Foreign Policy

Not only is the pursuit of global health subjected to state interests, but states increasingly are using health interventions to support non-health foreign policy objectives.[12] The missions of the US Navy's hospital ships *Comfort* and *Mercy* in Latin America and West Africa are described as health diplomacy missions that are "winning hearts and minds through the use of health interventions."[23,b] However, these health interventions are "critical elements of policy" and are undertaken to improve the image of and goodwill toward the United States, and are also useful training missions for future disaster relief activities.[23] The US military offers short-term medical and veterinary clinics in Iraq and Afghanistan as a part of "supporting pacification, gathering local intelligence, or rewarding locals for their cooperation,"[24] and Thompson argued: "Medical interventions are an important component of a diplomatic strategy to regain moral authority for US actions, regain the trust of moderate Muslims, and deny terrorists and religious extremists unencumbered access to safe harbor in ungoverned spaces."[25] Such activities have been criticized for undermining the principle of humanitarian neutrality, politicizing health interventions, and

---

[b]See also the chapter by Bonventre and Denux in this volume.

being ineffective at supporting either health or strategic goals, but they continue, partly because of their relevance to US interests and what Brown calls the "chronic under-investment by the United States in non-military instruments of state-building."[26]

The United States' use of health interventions to support ulterior foreign policy objectives is also driven by the actions of other states in this arena. The US hospital ship missions, in particular, represent a response to long-standing Cuban programs that support Cuban medical teams working abroad, free medical education, and disaster relief activities. The Cuban program has "garnered symbolic capital (prestige, goodwill, and influence)... way beyond what would otherwise have been possible and has helped cement Cuba's role as a player on the world stage."[27] Cuba's health diplomacy programs have also been materially beneficial, as Cuba's "oil for doctors" agreement with Venezuela has shown. In another example, Brazil has used its successful HIV/AIDS programs to build South–South collaborations that have won it "sway with Southern allies that Brazil relies upon to push for bigger goals, such as winning a seat on the UN Security Council or having a stronger voice in the international monetary system."[28] Similarly, China's pursuit of natural resources in Africa is increasingly linked with Chinese health diplomacy efforts, including hospital building and grants for malaria drugs (produced by China), which "not only [help] China gain favorable trading terms and access to necessary resources, but also [support] the government's attempts to portray itself as a good international citizen."[29] These activities show that states often consider support for health interventions within the broader context of their foreign policy objectives and that they increasingly perceive health interventions to be an effective "soft power" tool of diplomacy.

Global Health and Characteristics of World Politics

Examination of state interests is critical to an understanding of states' engagement on global health issues. However, state interests are also affected by larger trends and characteristics of world politics. This section examines the impact of major paradigms, weak states, and divisions between rich and poor states on the actions of states and the implementation of global health programs.

Major Paradigms

Global health efforts occur with the context of world politics. As such, major paradigms in world affairs can affect state interests in relation to their engagement in global health efforts. For example, Cold War politics were integral to both the origin and the obstruction of the campaign to eradicate smallpox — a campaign that is widely regarded as one the greatest success stories in public health.[30]

A substantive proposal to eradicate smallpox was first made by the USSR (Soviet Union) at the 1958 World Health Assembly meeting. The USSR's interest in supporting the eradication of smallpox was threefold. First, the USSR had successfully eliminated smallpox in the 1930s with a low-quality vaccine and thus believed that global eradication was feasible with an improved vaccine. Second, the USSR was forced to respond to frequent smallpox epidemics originating in neighboring Central Asian countries, which gave it a self-interested reason for engaging in improving health outside its borders. Third, support for smallpox eradication "represented a potential counterbalance" to well-publicized but ultimately doomed US-supported malaria eradication efforts.[31]

Cold War and WHO politics prevented the Soviet proposal from being funded, until the United States unexpectedly announced a joint smallpox eradication and measles control program in West Africa in 1965. The reason for the sudden US support was the need for President Johnson to announce a program for the UN's International Cooperation Year.[31] With both Soviet and US support, the smallpox eradication program began to receive the trickle of funding that would eventually result in the eradication of the disease. D.A. Henderson, who was director of the WHO's smallpox eradication campaign, wrote that Cold War politics continued to influence aspects of the eradication campaign, but that the program also facilitated "cooperation across political and cultural barriers."[31]

The US-led wars in Afghanistan and Iraq and the "global war on terrorism" also represent a paradigm that has affected attempts to eradicate polio. In 2003, three northern Nigerian states began a boycott of polio vaccination that would spawn an outbreak of polio that traveled to 20 Nigerian states and severely set back efforts to eradicate the disease.

The boycott was based on rumors that the polio vaccine was "contaminated with antifertility drugs intended to sterilize young Muslim girls."[32] While the context for the boycott implicated internal Nigerian politics, the US-led war on terrorism was a key precipitant of Nigeria's lack of trust in the polio vaccine campaign. The governor of one of the northern Nigerian states said: "Since September 11, the Muslim world is beginning to be suspicious of any move from the Western world.... Our people have become really concerned about [the] polio vaccine."[33] Further reports suggested that the war in Iraq strongly affected Muslim perceptions of the United States: a doctor from the WHO reported, "What is happening in the Middle East has aggravated the situation. If America is fighting people in the Middle East, the conclusion is that they are fighting Muslims."[33] US perceptions of this paradigm also prevented President Bush from directly contacting Nigerian President Obasanjo about the vaccine boycott, because it was felt that "too overt an intervention by the United States could exacerbate the problem in Northern Nigeria."[32] In such examples from the Cold War and the global war on terrorism, these major paradigms in world politics have had strong relevance to the success or failure of certain global health efforts, and they should be considered when implementing global health programs.

Weak States

The existence of weak and failing states, defined as those with weakness or absence of "physical security, legitimate political institutions, economic management, and social welfare," is a characteristic of world politics that affects both health and global disease eradication campaigns.[34] Eradication campaigns in particular show the impact of weak and failing states, because eradication is the "weakest link" as a global public good, which, while having enormous benefits for health and development, depends for global success upon the countries that are the least able to control and eliminate disease.[35]

In addition to Northern Nigeria as described above, the border area between Afghanistan and Pakistan is one of the remaining strongholds of the polio virus. Lack of security, military campaigns, attacks on polio vaccinators, and areas that are "variously ungoverned or under the control of antigovernment, Taliban, Al-Qaeda, or tribal groups" have to date prevented the successful control of polio in this region.[36] The weakness of the states in the border areas of both Afghanistan and Pakistan is a major barrier to the successful global eradication of polio.

Similarly, the GWEP has faced tremendous barriers because of years of conflict and insecurity in Sudan. Despite the availability of inexpensive interventions to prevent Guinea worm transmission and the successful elimination of the parasite across most of the globe, Sudan has "long been the main obstacle to completing the global campaign."[37] The Comprehensive Peace Agreement was signed in 2005, ending the country's second civil war, and strong progress has been made against the Guinea worm, but a 2011 referendum on the independence of Southern Sudan could portend future conflict and therefore imperil efforts to eradicate the parasite. Efforts to eliminate rinderpest — a viral disease of cattle with major implications for food security — from Africa are also impeded by conflict and ungoverned spaces in Somalia.[38] Health measures suffer in these weak nation-states, which present a major barrier to the success of global campaigns to eradicate disease.

Divisions between Rich and Poor States

The existence of inequalities in wealth between states is clearly one driver of global health inequalities, and differences in wealth between states also contribute to divergent interests with regard to global health issues. These differences are most apparent in debates on the protection of intellectual property and access to pharmaceuticals. Continuing conflict arises between largely wealthy states which support stronger intellectual property protections, known as Trade-Related Aspects of Intellectual Property Rights (TRIPS)-plus measures, in service of their economic interests, and poorer states which seek "to interpret and implement [the] TRIPS [Agreement] in a manner supporting the protection of public health and, in particular, access to medicines."[39] Whereas the Declaration on the TRIPS Agreement and Public Health (known as the Doha Declaration) affirms the right of countries to interpret the TRIPS Agreement in a manner that is supportive of public health and access to medicines, developing countries have faced strong barriers to implementing that flexibility.[40]

Similarly, the Doha Development Round of World Trade Organization negotiations is stalled because of conflicts between poorer countries and the United States and the European Union over barriers to trade and subsidies for agricultural products.[41] Finally, economic interests and the desire to attract direct foreign investment for development often undermine occupational health and safety regulations.[42] The differences in economic interests and in exposure to global health threats between rich and poor states cause divisions on these trade issues that affect global health, with economic interests traditionally predominating over public health concerns.

Other cases of divisions between rich and poor countries on global health issues include infectious disease surveillance, the influenza virus sample-sharing controversy, and the IHRs. A flashpoint in these debates has been the concept of "health security." Wealthy states have promoted this concept as a response to the perceived increasing threat of infectious disease epidemics and bioterrorism. The WHO described health security in politically neutral terms, as "activities required… to minimize vulnerability to acute public health events that endanger the collective health of populations living across geographic regions and international boundaries."[43] Developing countries are, however, "increasingly suspicious of global health initiatives justified on the grounds of 'global health security,'"[44] because they perceive that "the harvest of outbreak intelligence overseas is essentially geared to benefit wealthy nations."[45] It has been argued that such surveillance systems do little to address the vast current burdens of disease in poor countries. Many developing countries are increasingly unlikely to support or cooperate with global infectious disease surveillance, capacity building, and reporting unless these efforts also benefit health in their countries. As Aldis wrote, it remains to be seen whether wealthy countries "are prepared to make the technical and financial commitments for development of health systems [that] are necessary to ensure that poor countries benefit from timely and open sharing of information in accordance with the global health security concept."[44] Divisions with regard to global health security and surveillance will likely persist, because they are based upon inequalities in health and wealth that are long-standing characteristics of world politics.

Science and State Interests

National interests and international politics have strong impacts on global health efforts. However, public health's production of scientific and epidemiological insights into the functioning of the natural world also affects the progress of global health issues and does not respond to the politics of state interests. As Fidler wrote, there exist "scientific principles and imperatives that foreign policy cannot overlook," as well as foreign policy "considerations that health cannot ignore."[13] For instance, Chinese attempts to cover up the SARS epidemic for economic and political reasons failed when the disease (abetted by Chinese inaction) spread out of China to Hong Kong and Vietnam.[46] The spread of SARS was based upon its attack rate and human movements, not on Chinese state interests.

A different example is the 2002 US National Intelligence Council estimate of the "next wave of HIV/AIDS."[47] This estimate by the US intelligence community predicted that "five countries of strategic importance to the United States — Nigeria, Ethiopia, Russia, India, and China — collectively will have the largest number of HIV/AIDS cases on earth" and that this next wave of HIV/AIDS was likely "to have significant economic, social, political, and military implications."[47] However, the estimate was based upon erroneous assumptions about the transmission dynamics of HIV, which were quite different in those five countries than in sub-Saharan Africa.[48] In this case, a failure to understand the epidemiology of HIV/AIDS resulted in a failure of the United States to accurately predict the national security implications of the pandemic. Both this case and the SARS case are reminders that scientific inquiry and knowledge stands apart from national interests and international politics.

Conclusion

The rising moral, economic, and strategic impacts of global health issues have brought the field into a prominent role in international politics. Whereas a vast variety of actors are involved in or have an impact on global health, nation-states remain the critical actors in international politics. Thus, state interests play a powerful role in prioritizing and shaping engagement on global health issues. Major characteristics of current world politics, such as the war on terrorism, weak states, and inequities in wealth, also inform national interests and can directly affect the pursuit of health interventions.

In this arena of "high politics," it is no longer enough for global health practitioners to research and present evidence on public health interventions. Epidemiology and biostatistics remain key tools of public health research, but global health practitioners will increasingly be called upon to navigate international politics and national interests to enact and protect global health. Knowledge of the national interests that drive action on global health, understanding the impact of international politics on global health efforts, and maintaining rigorous science in support of global health efforts are critical tools for global health and global health diplomacy in this arena.

References

1. Fidler DP. (2001) The return of microbialpolitik. *Foreign Pol*: Jan./Feb., pp. 80–81.
2. Fidler DP. (2004) Caught between paradise and power: Public health, pathogenic threats, and the axis of illness. *McGeorge Law Rev* **35**: 45–104.
3. King NB. (2002) Security, disease, commerce: Ideologies of postcolonial global health. *Soc Stud Sci* **35**: 763–789.
4. Evans G, Newnham J. (1998) *The Penguin Dictionary of International Relations*. Penguin, London.
5. Koplan JP, Bond TC, Merson MH, *et al.* (2009) Towards a common definition of global health. *Lancet* **373**: 1993–1995.
6. Fidler DP. (2006) Health as foreign policy: Harnessing globalization for health. *Health Promot Int* **21(Suppl 1)**: 51–58.
7. Waltz KN. (1979) *Theory of International Politics*. Addison-Wesley, Reading, MA.
8. Lederberg J, Shope RE, Oaks SC. Institute of Medicine (US Committee on Emerging Microbial Threats to Health. (1992) *Emerging Infection: Microbial Threats to Health in the United States*. National Academies Press, Washington, DC.
9. US Institute of Medicine Committee on the US Commitment to Global Health and National Academies Press. (2009) *The US Commitment to Global*

Health: Recommendations for the Public and Private Sectors. National Academies Press, Washington, DC.

10. Franco C. (2008) Billions for biodefense: Federal agency biodefense funding, FY2008–FY2009. *Biosecur Bioterror* **6(2):** 131–146.

11. Lister S. (2007) *Congressional Research Service Report for Congress. Pandemic Influenza: Appropriations for Public Health Preparedness and Response.* Available from www.fas.org/sgp/crs/misc/RS22576.pdf (accessed May 12, 2011).

12. Feldbaum H, Michaud J. (2010) Health diplomacy and the enduring relevance of foreign policy interests. *PLoS Med* **7(4):** e1000226.

13. Fidler DP. (2005) Health as foreign policy: Between principle and power. *Whitehead J Diplom Int Relats* **6:** 179–194.

14. Fidler DP, Gostin LO. (2006) The new International Health Regulations: An historic development for international law and public health. *J Law Med Ethics* **34:** 85–94.

15. Davies SE. (2008) Securitizing infectious disease. *Int Aff* **84:** 295–313.

16. Holbrooke R, Garrett L. (2008) "Sovereignty" that risks global health. *The Washington Post.* August 2008. Available from www.washingtonpost.com/wp-dyn/content/article/2008/08/08/AR2008080802919.htm (accessed May 28, 2011).

17. Sedyaningsih ER, Isfandari S, Soendoro T, *et al.* (2008) Towards mutual trust, transparency and equity in virus sharing mechanism: The avian influenza case of Indonesia. *Ann Acad Med Singapore* **37:** 482–488.

18. Warner KE. (2008) The Framework Convention on Tobacco Control: Opportunities and issues. *Salud Publica Mex* **50(Suppl 3):** S283–S291.

19. Assunta M, Chapman S. (2006) Health treaty dilution: A case study of Japan's influence on the language of the WHO Framework Convention on Tobacco Control. *J Epidemiol Community Health* **60:** 751–756.

20. Forster P. (2009) *The Political Economy of Avian Influenza in Indonesia.* STEPS Working Paper 17. STEPS Centre, Brighton, UK. Available from www.steps-centre.org/PDFs/Indonesia.pdf (accessed May 12, 2011).

21. Perlman D, Roy A. (2009) Health and development. In: Perlman D, Roy A (eds.), *The Practtice of International Health: A Case-Based Orientation.* Oxford University Press, pp. 9–18.

22. Burkhalter H. (2004) The politics of AIDS: Engaging the conservative activist. *Foreign Aff* **83:** 8–14.

23. Vanderwagen W. (2006) Health diplomacy: Winning hearts and minds through the use of health interventions. *Mil Med* **171:** 3–4.
24. Baker J. (2007) Medical diplomacy in full-spectrum operations. *Mil Rev,* Sep.–Oct., pp. 67–73.
25. Thompson DF. (2008) *The Role of Medical Diplomacy in Stabilizing Afghanistan.* Defense Horizons No. 63. National Defense University, Washington, DC. Available from www.ndu.edu.CTNSP/index.cfm? type=section&secid=16&pageid=4 (accessed May 25, 2011).
26. Patrick S, Brown K. (2007) *The Pentagon and Global Development: Making Sense of the DoDs' Expanding Role.* Center for Global Development Working Paper No. 13. Available from www.cgdev.org/files/14815_file_ PentagonandDevelopment.pdf (accessed May 22, 2011).
27. Feinsilver JM. (2008) Cuba's medical diplomacy. In: Font MA (ed.), *Changing Cuba/Changing World.* Bildner Center for Western Hemisphere Studies, New York City. pp. 273–286. Available from http://web.gc.cuny.edu/dept/bildn/ publications/documents/Feinsilver15_002.pdf (accessed May 15, 2011).
28. Gomez EJ. (2009) Brazil's blessing in disguise: How Lula turned an HIV crisis into a geopolitical opportunity. *Foreign Pol,* July 2. Available from www.foreignpolicy.com/articles/2009/07/22/brazils_blessing_in_disguise (accessed May 28, 2011).
29. Youde JR. (2010) China's health diplomacy in Africa. *China Int J* **8(1):** 151–163.
30. Levine R and "What Works?" Working Group. (2007) *Case Studies in Global Health: Millions Saved.* Jones and Bartlett, Sudbury, MA.
31. Henderson DA. (2009) *Smallpox: The Death of a Disease — The Inside Story of Eradicating a Worldwide Killer.* Prometheus, Amherst, NY.
32. Kaufmann JR, Feldbaum H. (2009) Diplomacy and the polio immunization boycott in Northern Nigeria. *Health Aff* (Millwood) **28:** 1091–1101.
33. Jegede AS. (2007) What led to the Nigerian boycott of the polio vaccination campaign? *PLoS Med* **4:** e73.
34. Patrick S. (2006) Weak state and global threats: Fact or fiction. *Washington Q* **29:** 27–53.
35. Barrett S. (2007) *Why Cooperate? The Incentive to Supply Global Public Goods.* Oxford University Press.
36. Barrett S. (2009) Polio eradication: Strengthening the weakest links. *Health Aff* (Millwood) **28:** 1079–1090.

37. Hopkins DR, Ruiz-Tiben E, Downs P, *et al.* (2005) Dracunculiasis eradication: The final inch. *Am J Trop Med Hyg* **73:** 669–675.

38. Diop BA, Bastiaensen P. (2005) Achieving full eradication of rinderpest in Africa. *Vet Rec* **157:** 239–240.

39. Kerry VB, Lee K. (2007) TRIPS, the Doha declaration and paragraph 6 decisions: What are the remaining steps for protecting access to medicine? *Global Health* **3:** 3.

40. Feldbaum H, Lee K, Michaud J. (2010) Global health and foreign policy. *Epidemiol Rev* **32(1):** 82–92.

41. Elliott KA. (2006) *Delivering on Doha: Farm Trade and the Poor.* Center for Global Development Institute for International Economics, Washington, DC.

42. Shaffer ER, Waitzkin H, Brenner J, Jasso-Agilar R. (2005) Global trade and public health. *Am J Pub Health* **95(1):** 23–34.

43. World Health Organization. (2007) *The World Health Report 2007: A Safer Future, Global Public Health Security in the 21st Century.* WHO Press.

44. Aldis W. (2008) Health security as a public health concept: A critical analysis. *Health Policy Plann* **23:** 369–375.

45. Calain P. (2007) From the field side of the binoculars: A different view on global public health surveillance. *Health Policy Plann* **22:** 13–20.

46. Huang Y. (2004) The SARS epidemic and its aftermath in China: A political perspective. In: Knobler S, Mahmoud A, Lemon A, *et al* (eds.), *Learning from SARS: Preparing for the Next Disease Outbreak.* National Academies Press, Washington, DC, pp. 116–136.

47. National Intelligence Council. (2002) *The Next Wave of HIV/AIDS: Nigeria, Ethiopia, Russia, India, and China.* National Intelligence Council, Langley, VA.

48. Chin J, Bennett A. (2007) Heterosexual HIV transmission dynamics: Implications for prevention and control. *Int J STD AIDS* **18:** 509–513.

6

Health is an Integral Part of Foreign Policy

Santiago Alcázar* and Paulo Buss, MD, MPH†

Introduction

National interests are the main focus of foreign policy, but do they include health? One may identify a wide range of issues and policies that are included in foreign policy activities: human security and political stability; economic prosperity through trade and development; the promotion of ideological goals and cultural values; and the need for preparedness against natural disasters and emergencies. This chapter will discuss the relationship between health and foreign policy and will make the case that health is an integral part of the foreign policy agenda.

The expression "health diplomacy" was used by former US Secretary of Health and Human Services Tommy Thompson in referring to integration of foreign policy and global health.[1] However, it was defined differently in a seminar entitled "Colonizing Societies Through Medical Diplomacy: The Practice and Ideology of Colonialism in International Health and Development Projects," sponsored by the Socialist Caucus during the 128th Meeting of the American Public Health Association.[2]

---

*Mr. Alcázar, formerly the Chief of the International Division of the Brazilian Ministry of Health, is the Brazilian Ambassador to Azerbaijan.

†Mr. Buss is the Director of the Oswald Cruz Foundation (FIOCRUZ) Center for Global Health and a member of the Brazilian National Academy of Medicine.

Here, international public health efforts and development projects were related to colonial history (see also the chapter by V. Adams in this volume). Speakers at the symposium asserted that these processes continue to embody the "ideology of colonialism" by displacing or undermining local organizations and indigenous knowledge, by presenting Europe and the United States as models to emulate, by discouraging progressive social change, and by facilitating the foreign political domination of countries in Latin America, the Caribbean, Africa, and Asia. The term *"health diplomacy"* was also used in 2002 by David Byrne, European Commissioner for Health and Consumer Protection, at the VII European Health Forum in Gastein, Austria, to describe how addressing "hunger, squalor, ignorance, and disease, wherever they arise" may reduce international conflict.[3] The emphasis made by Mr. Byrne, however, was on conflict resolution and not on health issues or their social determinants *per se*.

Whereas health concerns may be germane to conflict resolution, not until recently has health been identified as a specific objective of foreign policy that is on a par with security or trade. It may be argued that the international instruments developed over the past 160 years to control the spread of infectious diseases and narcotic drugs, or to address occupational safety and health,[4] testify to the historical importance of global health diplomacy in foreign policy. These international instruments were designed specifically to protect international commerce, support political stability, and promote economic security; health was not a distinct foreign policy objective in the negotiations leading to these agreements.

Health has had a changing relationship to other sectors as well. During the 2008 financial crisis, the Director-General of the World Health Organization (WHO), Dr. Margaret Chan, expressed her concerns at a meeting convened to examine the possible health consequences of that crisis: "We meet at a time of crisis. We face a fuel crisis, a food crisis, a severe financial crisis, and a climate that has begun to change in ominous ways. All of these crises have global causes and global consequences. All have profound and profoundly unfair consequences for health. Let me be very clear at the start. The health sector had no say when the policies responsible for these crises were made. But health bears the brunt."[5] This important perspective emphasizes that health must be a major consideration in foreign policies that address global environmental, economic, and development issues.

The diplomacy involved in the 19th century sanitary conferences demanded public health approaches to mitigating the potential economic consequences of epidemics. By 2008, however, the health sector demanded action from national and multinational polities to specifically address issues adversely affecting the human condition. This shift in emphasis started to put health forward as a unique foreign policy priority, and not just as an add-on to other issues, for both developed and developing countries. The health focus is not limited to the prevention and treatment of specific diseases; it involves a larger view of the social determinants of health as well as the economic, commercial, and security implications related to public health.[6] Neoliberal economic policies and systemic reforms imposed by international economic institutions in the 1990s swept away entire public health systems in developing countries; "health" in this process was considered more as a market commodity needing fiscal restraint and not a "public good." Such reforms were not beneficial to public health and human development,[7] and they stimulated an alternative approach to health development led by multinational health agencies — the WHO and the United Nations Children's Fund (UNICEF) — on behalf of poor countries. For example, Burkina Faso, one of the poorest countries in the world, participated in the Bamako Initiative,[8] a formal political process. This initiative was adopted in 1987 by numerous African health ministers and called for providing a basic package of integrated services through revitalized health centers, user fees, and community co-managed funds. However, it grew from the multinational economic reforms promoted at that time and not from the specific, identifiable health needs of the participating countries. The Bamako Initiative supported decentralizing health decision-making to local levels and establishing realistic national drug policies to enhance the provision of essential drugs for sub-Saharan Africans.

Another lens through which global health has been viewed is that of security. The extensive negotiations that preceded the adoption of the International Health Regulations (IHR) are a case in point.[9] Public health officials involved with this process emphasized that the goals of the IHR were to prevent and control infectious disease and to define public health responses to new global infectious disease threats. They invoked a global governance approach to potential multinational health crises. The debates shifted discussions about the "risks to health" to an emphasis on the "threats to health." *Risk* is a public health concept, and it expresses the *possibility* of harm, whereas *threat* implies intentionality, which is not part of the traditional public health discourse. As an instrument of health collaboration developed under the convening authority of the WHO, the IHR concentrated on the possibility of harm and not on the intentionality to do harm. As an instrument of security, however, the IHR would also address issues that are a *threat* to population health rather than just a *risk* to individual health. Issues such as pandemic influenza virus A, subtype H1N1, and severe acute respiratory syndrome (SARS) might be considered to be both threats, in terms of the severe disruption of commerce and movement of peoples, and risks, in terms of the specific health consequences of these illnesses, especially for vulnerable persons.

The Health Lens and Foreign Policy: A Copernican Shift

As seen in the above examples, the perception of global health varies according to the lens through which it is viewed. For our discussion, we will consider the question as to whether global health, independent of other policy concerns, could itself be a lens through which foreign policy should be viewed.

In 2007, a group of ministers of foreign affairs took an unprecedented step, stating flatly that health must stand on its own as an objective of foreign policy.[10] In this landmark statement, known as the Oslo Declaration, these ministers agreed to make health a point of departure for foreign policy — and thus a functional lens through which to examine international relations and development strategies. This declaration amounted to a "Copernican shift" in foreign policy, in which concerns about health take center stage and thus demand that foreign and economic policies be evaluated for their impact on global health.[a] It was through this refocused lens that the UN General Assembly adopted, in 2009, Resolution 63/33, entitled "Global Health and Foreign Policy."[11] This consensus statement

---

[a] The term "Copernican revolution" and the related term "Copernican shift" refer to the effects of Copernicus' 16th century publication of astronomic findings that did away with the long-established Ptolemaic model of the heavens, which had postulated that the Earth was at the center of the solar system. This shift moved scientific thinking toward the heliocentric model, with the Sun at the center of the solar system.

recognized the interdependence of these two pursuits. By urging Member States to consider health issues in the formulation of foreign policy, the UN General Assembly validated the Oslo Declaration at the multinational political level.

Orders of Change

What moved health from the subordinate position it has had to the significance it now commands in foreign policy? We shall highlight three orders of change that help to explain this shift.

The first order of change was enabled by the human immunodeficiency virus/acquired immune deficiency syndrome (HIV/AIDS) epidemic. In contrast to the public response to any previous infectious disease crisis, HIV/AIDS-affected communities took matters into their own hands and demanded action from governments, multinational organizations, and the pharmaceutical industry. Before HIV/AIDS, infectious diseases were regarded as issues confined to marginalized populations; they could be taken care of by administering curative measures and not necessarily by addressing upstream causes and social determinants of these infections. Containing the HIV/AIDS epidemic, on the other hand, required that attention be paid to both causes and effects (prevention and treatment).[b] What this horrendous epidemic stimulated was the notion that health policies cannot be limited to the treatment of "effects," but must include efforts to address the entire spectrum of disease.[c] In fact, the many failures of cooperation on health between the "global north" (developed countries)

---

[b] During the early years of the HIV/AIDS epidemic, it was commonly held in many industrialized countries and international institutions that developing countries should focus only on the prevention of the disease, because they would not have the necessary resources to provide antiviral treatment. It is interesting to recall the dialogue on access to highly active anti-retroviral drugs introduced by the Brazilian delegation at the WHO Executive Board session in January 2001. As a result of that dialogue, the World Health Assembly (WHA) adopted Resolution WHA 54.10, the sixth paragraph of whose preamble states that "…prevention and care are inextricably linked, and… their effectiveness is increased when they are used together."

[c] We are not referring to the biological causes of disease, but more broadly to the background of history, economy, political, social, and cultural issues that determine health risks, access to treatment, and priority-setting by decision-makers.

and the "global south" (developing countries) have had to do with an over-emphasis on the effects side, without sufficient attention to the much more complex upstream, social determinants of the diseases, especially for the poor. Curative medicine within global epidemics cannot possibly provide treatment for all those who need it, especially with complex, difficult-to-treat diseases such as HIV/AIDS. This is the medical model that the global north still mainly supports, yet it does not address the social, political, ethical, and cultural complexities of dealing with global health challenges in the global south. Far greater understanding of these complexities is necessary in order to fully engage science-based health diplomacy.

Although WHO defines health as "a state of complete physical, mental, and social well-being and not merely the absence of disease or infirmity,"[12] the second part of this definition was the basis for health development strategies until the 1990s. Once the global focus among WHO member states changed to include the first part of the definition, engaging upstream determinants of health became necessary for multi-level action against specific global health challenges. For example, regarding global tobacco control, critical issues include health inequity, national economics and international trade, information asymmetry between the north and the south, and concern for environmental issues related to tobacco-growing. These issues became part of the key negotiations on the WHO Framework Convention on Tobacco Control (FCTC) in 2000.[13] As another example, access to essential medicines in developing countries required negotiations within the World Trade Organization (WTO) related to the 2001 Doha Declaration on the Trade-Related Aspects of International Property Rights (TRIPS) Agreement and Public Health.[14] This declaration reaffirmed the flexibility of TRIPS so that WTO signatories could circumvent patent protections to ensure affordable access to essential medicines, including those needed to address HIV/AIDS in poor countries. However, it should be noted that there is no official health presence within the WTO; the WTO is a multinational regime concerned only with maintenance of fair trade. Nevertheless, the Doha Declaration asserted the primacy of health over trade and patent protections for countries experiencing public health emergencies such as HIV/AIDS.

In 2008, developing countries were able to put this issue to a test of health diplomacy within the WHO environment — Executive Board

Meetings and the World Health Assembly (WHA). Dramatic negotiations culminated in adoption of the Global Strategy on Public Health, Innovation and Intellectual Property (GSPHIIP) by the 61st WHA.[15] This new strategy and plan of action encourages needs-driven, rather than purely market-driven, research to target diseases that disproportionately affect people in developing countries. Health diplomacy was utilized by Member States to level the playing field for health research, moving global cooperation toward resolving the 10/90 global health research gap.[d]

The second order of change is related to the growing concerns about the legitimacy and representativeness of formal and informal international organizations. A decision taken in an international structure is legitimate if it is in accord with established legal agreements and requirements, and it is representative if it expresses the general will of those entities bound together by the structure of these international organizations. To be effective, a decision has to be both legitimate and representative. Thus, decisions taken at the inception of an international structure are both legitimate and representative, because they reflect a common agreement that brought countries together as an organization. However, if the governance structure of the organization loses representativeness, its legitimacy may be questioned. The growing influence of the Group of Twenty (G-20) countries and the waning power of the Group of Eight (G-8) countries illustrate how changing times and economic conditions may warrant new rules and representation in global negotiations.[e] Because many emerging economies (now part of the G-20) may feel disadvantaged in various international negotiations (dominated until now by the G-8), the legitimacy of the decisions made within the UN agencies and other political/economic alliances is increasingly called into question. This phenomenon has led to a *power*

---

[d] The 10/90 gap refers to assertion by the Global Forum for Health Research that only 10% of worldwide expenditure on health research and development is devoted to the problems that primarily affect the poorest 90% of the world's population. See http://www.globalforumhealth.org/?s=10%2F90+gap

[e] The ongoing debate on reform of the UN Security Council with regard to categories of membership and regional representation may also be seen as a reaction to the sense of an institutional "disconnect" among global south countries that are part of the organization (see http://www.un.org/apps/news/story.asp?NewsID=38390&Cr=security+council&Cr1=reform).

shift in global health negotiations involving countries such as Brazil, Russia, India, China, and South Africa (BRICS).

This power shift suggests the third order of change in international politics. The negotiations and the adoption of resolutions cited above regarding TRIPS would never have been possible if participants from these countries had not asserted that health takes precedence over trade, especially in response to the global crisis of HIV/AIDS. Determined diplomats from these emerging economies invoked moral arguments for improving access to essential medicines; they negotiated the maze of norms and procedural rules within the multilateral organizations so that health-focused trade agreements with the dominant powers of the north became possible. The disconnection from decision-making experienced by the global south and the failure of agreements proposed by developed countries signaled the need for new types of negotiations on global health issues. Diplomacy outside of purely economic and trade concerns allowed health to be raised as a central objective of foreign policy for several emerging economies. It is this third order of change that ultimately moved health into focus as a key element of 21st century foreign policy. This then suggests that there truly has been a Copernican shift in global diplomacy.

The health priority in foreign policy is, arguably, more conspicuous in countries that led the negotiations and adoption of the FCTC, the Doha Declaration, and the GSPHIIP. This same group of countries witnessed the failure of the Seattle WTO Ministerial Conference in 1999 to include the legitimate interests of the global south with regard to access to affordable medicines, attention to poverty alleviation, and human rights, and they thus created the G-20. This new political grouping attempts to expand the influence of the global south in trade, agriculture, and other economic negotiations. A change in the emphasis of national interests — from mainly economic and security *raisons d'état* to include health, poverty, social exclusion, empowerment of women, human rights, and sustainable development[f] — compels a change in foreign policy practices that are also at the heart of the Doha Declaration and the formation of the G-20.

---

[f] Even efforts to change the multinational banking and financial systems signal a departure from business as usual in global governance.

Health as an objective of foreign policy requires new notions of global solidarity to change or transform "the conditions in which people are born, grow, live, work, and age."[6] These notions are in turn "shaped by the distribution of money, power, and resources at global, national, and local levels,"[6] and they may radically transform the nature of foreign policy. For many, public health, with its ethical basis in social justice and human rights, has actually been perceived as a barrier to rather than as a basis for the making of foreign policy; it could be tolerated as a component of foreign policy only if it were attached to an economic or security issue. For example, in 2000, the US National Intelligence Council linked security concerns to emerging infectious diseases, thus implying that foreign policy priorities should include this concern.[16]

There is, nevertheless, room for optimism. The UN Economic and Social Council adopted at its high-level meeting in July 2009 a Ministerial Declaration that reiterates the WHO definition of health and links it firmly to the social determinants of health.[17] This declaration may be considered a landmark, in that its adoption was universal and not restricted to a group of countries or to a specialized UN agency. It clearly recognized the centrality of health in all policies — domestic or foreign — in order to accomplish the UN Millennium Development Goals. These goals, then, require serious foreign policy agreements to resolve global poverty and social inequalities, eliminate discrimination and alienation, empower women, and support human rights overall. As such, they are a radical departure from business as usual in foreign policy.

The focus of health within foreign policy further requires a change in the way the global south is represented in multilateral health organizations, international financial institutions, and informal groups (such as working groups on specific issues and groups of common-language countries). The segregation of those countries that dominate international decision-making from those that may suffer from these decisions, as demonstrated in the 2008 financial crisis, is no longer viable in our globalized world. When decisions that broadly affect the world are made behind closed doors by a small group of countries, it is necessary to ask: How is such decision-making legitimate within today's global governance regime? Governance requires that those who are governed acquiesce to being governed; historically, there has not been equitable representation of the global south in global governance regimes. For example, in the 1980s, a group of trade ministers created the Quadrilateral Group,[g] which involved the world's largest trading partners at the time; this group could in fact influence world trade without representation from any other entity. Similarly, wealthy countries also function within the G-8 and the UN Security Council as independent national groupings that do not seek representation from the low-income countries. However, according to the GSPHIIP background documents, "Currently, 4.8 billion people live in developing countries, representing 80% of the world population, [and of] this number, 2700 million, representing 43% of the world population, live on less than US$2 a day."[15] Thus, a closed grouping of wealthy national decision-makers today seems outdated with regard to global health and development in a globalized, interdependent world. Global health problems affect both rich and poor and require cooperative decision-making, as those problems do not adhere to geographic borders. Such closed-door diplomacy is now dysfunctional in addressing persistent and emerging global health problems and, in particular, this model is dysfunctional in resolving the historical inequities in health development, the 10/90 global health research gap, and the disparities in income that create overwhelming suffering from poverty-related diseases.

Public Health and Foreign Policy: The Case of Brazil

Only a handful of countries have included health issues in their foreign policy priorities, and it may be helpful to examine how Brazil has demonstrated this recent shift in emphasis. Brazil's Constitution guarantees that health is a universal right and that its provision is a duty of the state. Health shall be guaranteed by social and economic policies aimed at reducing the risk factors for illness and also by assuring universal and equal access to services for health promotion, protection, and rehabilitation. There are two parts to that constitutional guarantee. The first part confers the right to health on all Brazilians. It is important to note that the right to health does not discriminate between different levels of health care and that it includes everything from low-complexity interventions,

---

[g] Canada, Japan, the United States, and the European Union.

such as those found in primary health care, to medium-complexity treatments, such as elective surgeries, and to high-complexity treatments, such as those necessary for HIV/AIDS. All of these levels of health care are guaranteed by the public health system.[h] Privately insured persons in Brazil (22% of the population) may also make use of the public health care system, especially when their insurance does not cover high-complexity treatment and emergency surgery. In a country such as Brazil, which historically suffered extreme social exclusions and inequities, guaranteeing universal health care for the entire population is an historic accomplishment.

The second part of the Brazilian constitutional principle frames health as official state policy throughout government and not just as a health care program. What this means is that national interests should include health in all policies and that health is not subordinated to any other national interest. These principles are not necessarily specified *a priori* as to economic development, trade, or security programs, but these sectors must prioritize health issues when they arise; this was not the case before the adoption of the 1988 constitution.

To better understand the transformation of the Brazilian health system, it may be helpful to review the history of the Brazilian MoH. Until 1930, health issues were the remit of the Ministry of Justice, an arrangement that then associated health with policing. From 1930 to the early 1950s, health was placed within the Ministry of Education and constituted the majority programmatic emphasis of that ministry. It was only in 1954 that a separate MoH was created, and it remained a rather small institution until the adoption of the 1988 constitution. Today, the MoH has the largest budget of all of the Brazilian ministries. With the political changes brought about

---

[h] The Brazilian Unified Health System (the acronym for the name in Portuguese is SUS) was established by the Brazilian Constitution and further developed by Acts 8080 and 8142. It is driven by principles of universality, equity, integrity, decentralization, and community participation. SUS is nationally coordinated by the Ministry of Health (MoH) and is present in all 27 states and about 5700 municipalities. Although the entire population has a right to free health care services within SUS, around 22% of the population uses private services through health maintenance organizations. However, public health activities, such as immunizations, health surveillance (both epidemiologic and sanitary), and health promotion, are supported by SUS nationally.

by the 1988 constitution and with the development of institutional arrangements necessary for complying with the constitution, it is clear that health would also become a priority for Brazilian foreign policy.

Brazil's public health system is far from perfect, but it is, perhaps, the greatest transformational social force in Brazil. The experience of Brazil may be informative for other developing countries. In fact, Brazil has engaged in South–South health cooperation with several African nations — through the Community of Lusophone Countries (CPLP)[i] — and in South America — through the Union of South American Nations (UNASUR).[j] The CPLP is a political locus for coordination of policies and cooperation among the Portuguese-speaking countries. It is a structured and hierarchical body composed of a Conference of Heads of State, a Council of Foreign Affairs Ministers, a Permanent Steering Committee, a group of Co-operation Focal Points, and an Executive Secretariat.

Overwhelmed by underdevelopment and general poverty, the African Portuguese-Speaking Countries (the Portuguese acronym is PALOPs) have deficient population health indicators (infant mortality, attended childbirth, maternal mortality, etc.) and weak health systems. Using the Millennium Development Goals to guide cooperation among PALOPs, the CPLP conducted a lengthy negotiation process to define the 2009 Strategic Health Cooperation Plan (the Portuguese acronym is PECS; the combined entity is the PECS/CPLP).[18] This document recognizes the link between health and development, the universal right to health, and the duty of the state to support population health programs. The PECS/CPLP incorporates the following seven thematic areas: (1) development of the health workforce; (2) information and communication in health issues; (3) research for health; (4) reduction of dependency on imported medicines and other health products; (5) epidemiologic surveillance and monitoring; (6) response to emergencies and natural disasters; and (7) health promotion and protection.[19–21]

---

[i] The Community of Lusophone Countries includes Angola, Brazil, Cape Verde, East Timor, Guinea-Bissau, Mozambique, Portugal, and Sao Tomé and Principe. For further information, see www.cplp.org

[j] UNASUR is an intergovernmental union involving two existing trade organizations: Mercosur and the Andean Community. It is part of an ongoing process of South American integration. Its Constitutive Treaty was signed in 2008 in Brasilia, Brazil, by the heads of state of 12 South American nations. It is modeled on the European Union. For further information, see www.unasur.org

Each of the thematic areas is quite complex. The first thematic area, for example, aims to strengthen national health institutes, national schools of public health, schools of health policy, and schools for health technicians. The second thematic area has as one of its objectives the creation of a network of virtual health libraries, as well as electronic connections among health policy-makers, practitioners, and researchers. The third thematic area aims to produce autochthonous, evidence-based knowledge in health. The fourth aims to reduce external dependence on products and equipment, as well as to create networks for service and maintenance of medical equipment. The fifth aims to improve epidemiologic surveillance systems for communicable and noncommunicable diseases, external causes of morbidity and death, and behavioral risk factors. The sixth thematic area aims to build response and coordination capacities in natural disasters. The seventh thematic area specifically addresses the social determinants of health, such as sanitation, education, employment, and a fairer distribution of income. In substance, the PECS/CPLP is a result of the focus on health within Brazilian foreign policy; it is also a consequence of a foreign policy based on the principle of solidarity, because it is the health resource surpluses in Brazil and Portugal that are utilized to implement the strategy with the PALOPs.

UNASUR has a complex structure similar to that of the CPLP. It should be emphasized that these two institutions were developed by foreign affairs officials, and thus they emphasize health as an integral part of the involved countries' foreign policy. In negotiations involving these partners, the participants report to the ministers of foreign affairs, who report, in turn, to the heads of state. UNASUR's first meeting of heads of state, in Brazil, resulted in many political declarations and in the development of the constitution of the South American Health Council,[k] which estab-

---

[k] The South American Health Council is composed of the ministers of health of the 12 member states. UNASUR Salud consolidates South American health interests through policies based on mutual agreements, coordinated activities, and cooperation among countries. The Council includes a Coordinating Committee, constituted of representatives from the ministries of all countries; a Technical Secretariat, based at the country currently holding UNASUR's *pro tempore* presidency, plus the country that previously held that position and the country that will hold it immediately after; and Technical Groups, composed of representatives from all countries, established to develop the components of the South American Health Agenda to be approved by the Council.

lishes health priorities for South American political leaders. These priorities are currently under development within the South American Health Quinquennial Plan 2011–2015, and they include the following thematic foci: (1) development of the South American network of epidemiologic surveillance and control in accordance with the IHR; (2) development of health systems that ensure the universal right to health; (3) establishment of policy on medicines and other health commodities to attain self-sufficiency through development of a South American health-industrial complex; (4) development of a common health promotion policy and a common approach to the social determinants of health; (5) development of the health workforce, including the creation of the South American Institute on Health Governance, which will prepare professionals to manage health systems and to conduct health diplomacy.[22]

The second, third, and fourth thematic foci of this strategy represent an unprecedented regional process. The second focus, for example, cannot be developed unless health holds a prominent place in domestic and foreign policy-making for the collaborating nations. The third focus ensures that essential medicines and commodities are economically accessible, thus preventing serious public health crises that impact all the partners. It captures the essence of the WTO's concerns for developing countries: nothing in trade agreements can interfere with signatory countries taking measures to protect public health. The fourth focus, emphasizing the social determinants of health, is revolutionary, in the sense that it represents the Copernican shift to include global health within foreign policy processes. Further, health has to be considered with every other policy-making enterprise, such as with employment and income redistribution.[1] The profound changes observed in UNASUR are without precedence and signal the shift to make foreign policy more relevant to human rights issues; in so doing, it will re-emphasize the Copernican shift in national priorities on health.

---

[1] In Brazil, the Bolsa Familia Program, or Family Allowance, is the largest conditional cash transfer program in the world. Families enrolled in the program have to comply with educational and health objectives and are closely monitored by the state. Income redistribution through the Program moved 11 million families, or roughly 44 million people, out of poverty; this led to subsequent improvement in several health indicators in that target population.

It is interesting to note that the South American Council of Ministers has a mandate to coordinate positions among Member States in the WHO, the Pan American Health Organization, and other international fora. This coordination is another example of the South-to-South process.

Conclusions

Both the PECS/CPLP and the South American Health Council are consequences of the Copernican shift in these countries that moved health from a subordinate policy position within various national priorities to become a central objective across government. Related to this shift is the profound change in the way foreign affairs are conducted, as can be seen from the institutional structures built by ministers of foreign affairs to deal with health through South-to-South cooperation. Substance changes form, as form changes substance. We now have new forms of health cooperation, more focused health diplomacy for both the global north and south, and new directions in the conduct of foreign affairs for all nations. We have also presented some examples of how the attachment of health issues to non-health priorities can distort health programs; this is the case of the neoliberal economic policies that disrupted public health systems in the name of economic and health system reform in the 1990s.

The adoption of UN General Assembly of Resolution 63/33 on health and foreign policy and the UN Economic and Social Council's Ministerial Declaration emphasizing the social determinants of health have actually codified the Copernican shift described above. The Copernican shift concept allows us to understand how health is now a point of departure and a defining lens through which to practice foreign policy and implement development strategies in the 21st century.

We have described three orders of change underlying the Copernican shift: (1) the fundamental change in perception of health as a foreign policy priority; (2) the redress for deficiencies in legitimacy and representativeness for low-income countries in international organizations; and (3) the emergence of a grouping of countries (the G-20) that seek more transparent international decision-making processes and health cooperation models.

The insertion of health into foreign policy is possible only if actions to ensure international solidarity toward health, reduce poverty, eliminate social exclusion and discrimination, and empower women are embraced by cooperating nations. It is through health that foreign policy must acquire an expanded ethical dimension, which may be counter to traditional political realism. At the same time, transformed foreign policy toward health may help alleviate international power asymmetries and improve the representation of developing countries in global governance. The case of Brazil and the examples of South-to-South cooperation through the CPLP and UNASUR deserve careful scholarly attention for future research. In this chapter, we have presented our own personal examples from our work in foreign policy and health, in the hope that they may contribute to the growing field of global health diplomacy.

References

1. Thompson TG. (2011) Health diplomacy is critical to US foreign policy. *Huffpost World* (posted February 11, 2011). Available at http://www.huffingtonpost.com/tommy-g-thompson/the-case-for-health-diplo_b_823382.html (accessed July 18, 2011).
2. Brechwald JE, Birn A-E, Avilés LA, *et al.* (2002) Colonizing societies through medical diplomacy: The practice and ideology of colonialism in international health and development projects. Presented at the 128th Annual Meeting of the American Public Health Association (Boston, MA) Available at http://apha.confex.com/apha/128am/techprogram/session_969.htm (accessed July 18, 2011).
3. Byrne D. (2002) Future priorities in EU health policies. Presented at the VII European Health Forum, "Common Challenges for Health and Care" (Gastein, Austria, September 26, 2002). Available at http://europa.eu/rapid/pressReleasesAction.do?reference=SPEECH/02/462&format=HTML&aged=0&language=EN&guiLanguage=en (accessed July 18, 2011).
4. Fidler DP. (2001) The globalization of public health: The first 100 years of international health diplomacy. *Bull World Health Organ* **79(9)**: 842–849.
5. Chan M. (2008) Remarks at the United Nations General Assembly panel discussion on globalization and health, New York, NY, October 24, 2008. Available at http://www.who.int/dg/speeches/2008/20081024/en/index.html

6. World Health Organization. (2008) Closing the gap in a generation: Health equity through action on the social determinants of health. Commission on Social Determinants of Health — final report. World Health Organization. Available at http://www.who.int/social_determinants/final_report.en (accessed October 29, 2011).
7. World Bank. (1993) World development report 1993: Investing in health. World Bank. Available at http://econ.worldbank.org/external/default/main?pagePK=64165259&theSitePK=469728&piPK=64165421&menuPK=64166093&entityIK=000009265_3970716142319 (accessed October 29, 2011).
8. United Nations Children's Fund. (1987) The Bamako initiative. Available at http://www.unicef.org/sowc08/docs/sowc08_panel_2_5.pdf (accessed October 29, 2011).
9. World Health Organization. (2005) International health regulations. Available at http://www.who.int/ihr/en/ (accessed October 29, 2011).
10. Ministers of Foreign Affairs of Brazil, France, Indonesia, Norway, Senegal, South Africa, and Thailand. (2007) Oslo Ministerial Declaration — Global health: A pressing foreign policy issue of our time. *Lancet* **396(9570)**: 1373–1378. doi:10.1016/S0140–6736(07)60498-X.
11. United Nations General Assembly. (2009) Resolution adopted by the General Assembly: 63/33. Global health and foreign policy. Available at http://www.who.int/trade/events/UNGA_RESOLUTION_GHFP_63_33.pdf (accessed October 29, 2011).
12. World Health Organization. (1946) WHO definition of health. Preamble to the Constitution of the World Health Organization as adopted by the International Health Conference, New York, June 19–July 22, 1946; signed on July 22, 1946 by the representative of 61 states (Official Records of the World Health Organization, No. 2, p. 100) and entered into force on April 7, 1948. Available at www.who.int/suggestions/faq/en (accessed on October 29, 2011).
13. Conference of the Parties to the WHO FCTC. (2003) WHO Framework Convention on Tobacco Control. Available at http://www.who.int/fctc/text_download/en/index.html# (accessed October 29, 2011).
14. World Trade Organization. (2001) The Doha Declaration on the TRIPS Agreement and Public Health. Available at http://www.who.int/medicines/areas/policy/doha_declaration/en/index.html (accessed October 29, 2011).

15. World Health Assembly. (2008) The global strategy and plan of action on public health, innovation and intellectual property. Resolution WHA61:21. Available at http://www.who.int/phi/implementation/phi_globstat_action/en/index.html (accessed October 29, 2011).

16. Gordon D. (2000) National Intelligence Estimate 99–17D: The global infectious disease threat and its implications for the United States. The National Intelligence Council, Washington, DC. Available at http://www.fas.org/irp/threat/nie99–17d.htm (accessed October 29, 2011).

17. United Nations Economic and Social Council (ECOSOC). (2009) *Ministerial Declaration — 2009 High-Level Segment: Implementing the internationally agreed goals and commitments in regard to global public health.* Available at http://www.un.org/en/ecosoc/julyhls/pdf09/ministerial_declaration-2009.pdf

18. PECS/CPLP. (2008) *Plan Estratígico de Cooperacão em Saúde da CPLP* ("Strategic Health Cooperation Plan") (in Portuguese). Available at www.cplp.org/Default.aspx&ID=1787 (accessed October 29, 2011).

19. Almeida C, de Campos RP, Buss P, *et al.* (2010) Brazil's conception of South–South "structural cooperation in health." *RECIIS* **4(1)**: 23–32. doi:10.3395/reciis.v4i1.343en. Available at http://www.reciis.cict.fiocruz.br/index.php/reciis (accessed October 29, 2011).

20. Buss P, Ferreira JR. (2010) Critical essay on international cooperation in health. *RECIIS* **4(1)**: 43–53. doi:10.3395/reciis.v4i1.350en. Available at http://www.reciis.cict.fiocruz.br/index.php.reciis (accessed October 29, 2011).

21. Buss PM, Ferreira JR. (2010) Health diplomacy and South–South cooperation: The experiences of UNASUR Salud and the CPLP's Strategic Plan for Cooperation in Health. *RECIIS*. doi:10.2295/reciis.v4i1.351en. Available at http://www.reciis.cict.fiocruz.br/index.php/reciis (accessed October 29, 2011).

22. Kickbusch I, Silberschmidt G, Buss PM. (2007) Global health diplomacy: The need for new perspectives, strategic approaches and skills in global health. *Bull World Health Organ* **85(3)**: 230–232.

7

Global Health and Security

Kristofer Bergh* and Bates Gill, PhD†

Introduction

During the past couple of decades, our understanding of international security has changed greatly. Major events such as the fall of the Berlin Wall in 1989 and the terrorist attacks against the United States in September 2001 have forced us to redefine the very concept of security by asking "security for whom?" and "security from what?" What is becoming clear is that we are not isolated from the developments around us. In an increasingly global world, threats to the security of the state or its citizens can take many forms. Poverty and instability in a seemingly remote part of the world may have serious security implications closer to home. After the September 2001 attacks, the President of the United States said; "America is now threatened less by conquering states than we are by failing ones."[1] Similarly, we have become acutely aware of the fact that diseases have little respect for national borders, and potentially grave infectious disease may be merely an airplane ride away. The possible outbreak of a global pandemic or the intentional release of lethal pathogens has further raised concerns at the nexus of health and security.

Yet, despite increasing attention to the relationship between health and security, more work is needed to analyze and define this relationship

*Researcher, Stockholm International Peace Research Institute, Sweden.
†Chief Executive Officer of the United States Studies Center at the University of Sydney, Australia.

165

and to translate that understanding for the benefit of local, regional, and international society. A number of experts examining the nexus of health and security have noted the lack of analytical agreement within this emerging field. Some are concerned that conceptual confusion may have negative implications for public policy.[2–5] References to security are routinely attached to discussions on global health issues, often without further explanation of how, precisely, health affects security or even what, exactly, the term *security* means. The terms *health security*, *public health security*, and *global public health security* are used interchangeably and will have different significance to different actors in the field.[a]

To advance the intellectual and policy agenda at the nexus of health diplomacy and security, this chapter presents and assesses three analytical approaches to this linkage: normative, subjective, and objective. The chapter then looks at high-profile real-world policy challenges in which security and health diplomacy intersect: conflicts and catastrophes; sanctions; infectious diseases; and biological threats. Risks and opportunities of the health–security nexus are also discussed. The chapter concludes by briefly considering the pluses and minuses in linking health diplomacy and security and by noting that far more work is needed in the research and policy community to define that linkage and to build a more coherent field that draws from and pulls together the diverse experience and insights of public health, foreign policy, bioscience, development, and security expertise.

The Normative Approach — Human Security

In his 1941 State of the Union address, US President Franklin D. Roosevelt outlined four universal freedoms that people everywhere should enjoy.[6] The first two, freedom of speech and expression and freedom of religion, had already been addressed in the US Constitution. But

---

[a]Global public health security is defined by the WHO as the activities, both proactive and reactive, required to minimize vulnerability to acute public health events that endanger the collective health of populations living across geographical regions and international boundaries. The title of this chapter refers to the relationship between global health and security, rather than trying to define a new field.

the other two freedoms, freedom from want and freedom from fear, spoke to a new vision. "Freedom from fear" suggests that people should be able to live their lives without concern that violence may be perpetrated against them. Given his times, Roosevelt was thinking of avoiding the horrors of the war that then wracked Europe and Asia. "Freedom from want" speaks to the aim of all people to have healthy and ample lives. Roosevelt called for this new "moral order" to overcome the "order of tyranny" that he saw emerging from fascism in Europe and Japan. After World War II, the four freedoms partly inspired the Universal Declaration of Human Rights adopted by the General Assembly of the United Nations (UN) in 1948. The idea of freedom from want put forward by Roosevelt, however, became marginalized in the bipolar world of the Cold War, and emphasis was put on national security and freedom from fear.

The seminal 1994 UN Development Programme (UNDP) Report argued that a shift toward freedom from want is necessary if we are to address the source of inequities and instabilities in the world. The report suggested a shift from a focus on state-centric national security to a focus on human security — the well-being of the individual and attention to the threats he or she faces in day-to-day life.[7] A human security approach is more concerned with the question of whose security is being threatened and less concerned with what exactly constitutes the threat. Human security is difficult to define; yet, proponents of the concept embrace its breadth and argue that, whereas human security is not academically "neat," it nonetheless offers an appealing framework within which policymakers can aim to reach more discerning decisions.[8] Human security focuses above all on the well-being and survival of the individual, and, therefore, health is essential to the core of the concept. Health is also instrumental to human security, because poor health limits life choices and reduces the potential for individual fulfillment. From a human security perspective, health is not only constituted of the absence of disease but is a "state of complete physical, mental, and social well-being."[9] Health security, as described by the UNDP, makes little distinction between suffering caused by a preventable disease and that caused by a stray bullet.

From this perspective, the human security approach to health will encompass a wide variety of challenges, given the diversity of potential threats to health in different parts of the world. The spread of infectious diseases such as HIV, malaria, and tuberculosis and poor access to fundamental health care constitute the largest threats to people's security in many developing countries and areas. However, in more-developed parts of the world, lifestyle-related diseases, such as diseases of the circulatory system and diseases related to the use of tobacco and drugs, are a far greater threat to the security of the individual. In both the developing and the developed worlds threats to health security are greatest within the poorest part of the population. Children and women are also particularly vulnerable to and affected by poor health infrastructure and distribution. The 2003 report by the Commission on Human Security accorded much importance to the relationship between health and human security, and underscored the unevenness in the distribution of health resources. According to the report, poor health equity and uneven development, in both the developed and the developing world, are the most apparent obstacles to achieving health security.[9] As a concept, human security is intrinsically linked to development, and strategies for achieving human security should overwhelmingly rely on sustainable human development, rather than resort to arms.

Yet, even though poverty-related health threats constitute one of the heavier burdens of human security and, by extension, foreign policy, other factors related to health seem to garner the most attention. For example, the malign use of biological agents, the destabilization of societies by disease, and health crises arising during and after conflicts and humanitarian emergencies are health problems easily accepted as security concerns by the global security community, especially in the developed world. These problems may or may not enter into diplomatic discourse as security issues, however. Other diseases, such as malaria, tuberculosis, and cholera, pose little or no direct threat to the wealthy part of the world and are often given a lower priority by those who set global agendas. A great challenge to the human security approach is to move the alleviation of health problems that are induced and exacerbated by poverty and uneven development higher on the global agenda, not only as a worthy humanitarian end in itself but also, more broadly, as a critically important component of multilateral foreign and security policy cooperation.

Critics of human security discourse have argued that the approach is too comprehensive and all-encompassing to be useful to researchers and policy-makers. In other words, "[I]f human security means almost every-thing, then it effectively means nothing."[10] In this view, the human security concept is too broad to offer much analytical value, and any attempt to narrow the concept will result in arbitrariness that can undermine the aims of the concept's comprehensive approach. However, proponents of the approach embrace the inclusiveness of the concept and maintain that what human security lacks in analytical rigor, it makes up for in normative power and utility.

The UNDP is one of the international institutions in which the human security approach has been most influential. It is instrumental in promot-ing the achievement of the Millennium Development Goals (MDGs), which are aimed at reducing poverty and advancing development. The MDGs have the same normative point of departure as the human security approach, and they share several of the assumptions of the links among development, human rights, and security for the individual. Three of the MDGs are directly related to health, which places health firmly at the center of this important global development agenda.[b]

The Subjective Approach — Securitization

It is important to distinguish between what might be termed the "deepen-ing" of security that flows from the question "security for whom?" and the "widening" of security that comes with the question "security from what?" The narrow approach of the traditional security concept in interna-tional relations limited the focus to military threats to the integrity of the territory and regime of a given state by external enemies — most notably, other states. Several processes have driven analytical thinking toward broader conceptions of security, not least the end of the Cold War and the attacks on the United States in September 2001. These processes under-score that the most important threats to national security do not neces-sarily come from other states. New actors and circumstances make up a plethora of nontraditional security challenges that threaten the security and stability of states, in both the developed and the developing world.

---

[b]The MDGs directly related to health are: Goal 4 — reduce child mortality; Goal 5 — improve maternal health; and Goal 6 — combat HIV, malaria, and other diseases.

Scholars of security studies and international relations and members of the intelligence community have been forced to think more innovatively to identify and prepare for new, often non-state-driven threats. Where the practicalities of health diplomacy will fit into this new development is still an open question.

In this context, several health issues have been elevated to national security concerns. As opposed to the human security approach that has defined health as a general security concern for individuals, the health issues that are considered national security threats have been elevated through a process of what has been termed "securitization." In their seminal work, *Security: A New Framework for Analysis*, Buzan and colleagues explored the construction of threats and established the case for a broader security concept.[11] Security, for these scholars from the Copenhagen School, becomes a concern when a certain issue is described as an existential threat to a referent object — most often the state, but not necessarily so. One of the more important concepts developed by the Copenhagen School is the act of securitization. A securitizing actor that frames an issue within the context of security can move it from traditional politics into the area of security concern and may thus legitimize measures that would not otherwise be possible or acceptable. The process of securitization involves neither objective threats nor subjective perceptions; rather, the successful securitization of an issue is contingent on a receptive audience that accepts the securitization terminology.[11] Securitization is thus "the move that takes politics beyond the established rules of the game and frames the issue either as a special kind of politics or as above politics."[11]

According to David Fidler, the securitization of health has already occurred, and we currently exist in a "post-securitizing phase."[12] He uses this term to mean that framing a public health issue in a security context is widely considered within the public health community as an effective way to influence policy.[12] To claim that health in general has been securitized, however, seems premature: most events with negative health impacts are never mentioned within a security context. In the populations of the European Union, for example, circulatory disease and cancer are without a doubt the biggest killers, yet these diseases are practically never linked to national security concerns. That fact does not mean that there are no health issues that are being securitized or regarded as security threats. Several health-related challenges have in recent years been elevated to the level of the "high politics" of national security concerns, such as bioterrorism and the spread of pandemic diseases. Following a report by the US National Security Council, the Clinton Administration declared HIV/AIDS a threat to US national security interests in 2000.[13] Whether there might be utility in a similar declaration concerning the looming epidemics of noncommunicable diseases, which threaten economic development and health systems across the board, is worthy of further analysis. Until now, noncommunicable diseases have largely been absent from this kind of security discussion.[c]

It is interesting that the securitization of a particular health issue does not necessarily correspond to its objective threat to the state or individual. Rather, the securitization of some issues, but not others, has to do with other values, such as the level of fear that a certain issue may impose upon a population or the ability for advocates to publicly link the specific issue to security. The fear that may be induced by an infectious disease or by the malevolent use of biological agents will be more instrumental to the securitization of an issue than will concern about the long-term health impact of an unhealthy lifestyle. As opposed to the more inclusive approach of human security, in which health is, in itself, an indication of security, the various issues that have been securitized can become so in a relatively ad hoc manner, and the securitzation process may appear arbitrary and even controversial to many observers. Issues that may pose less of an actual threat receive more attention simply because they are deemed more newsworthy or because of successful human agency in promoting the issue as a security concern. In this sense, the securitization of health issues is a subjective process.

The Objective Approach — Criteria-Based Frameworks

In an attempt to bridge the gap between the normative (human security) and the subjective (securitization) approach, Feldbaum and Lee constructed

---

[c]A notable exception to this silence has come from high-ranking US military leaders, who link obesity to the country's ability to defend itself. See Shalikashvili JM, Shelton H. (2010) The latest national security threat: Obesity. *The Washington Post*, April 30. Available from www.washingtonpost.com/wp-dyn/content/article/2010/04/29/AR2010042903669. html (accessed May 25, 2011).

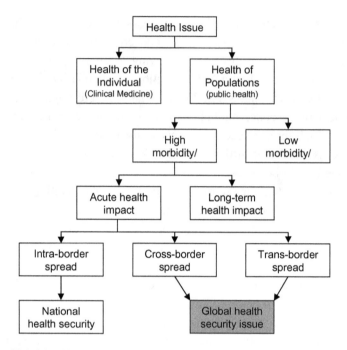

Fig. 1. Global health as a security issue. (Reprinted with permission from Feldbaum and Lee.[5])

a decision tree framework in which a given health issue can be related to a set of criteria and subsequently categorized as a global health security issue as (and if) the criteria are fulfilled (Fig. 1).[5] Feldbaum and Lee used neither the state nor the individual as the main level of analysis; instead, they focused on populations, making a distinction between public health and clinical medicine (i.e. concern with an individual's well-being). Furthermore, they argued that a global health security issue should have a high rather than a low level of morbidity/mortality and acute rather than long-term health impact, and that the problem should cross national borders.[5] In this approach, any health issue that meets these definitions can be considered a global health security issue, but that does not guarantee that it will be viewed as such by the relevant authorities, the wider security community, or the general public. As noted above, the securitization of a certain health issue is often contingent on values other than an objective risk or threat.

David Fidler took another approach to identifying the health issues that may constitute problems for security. Central to his approach is the mobility of the health concern and the possibility for it to cause damage in human populations, which he called the epidemiological elasticity (or "epi-elasticity") of a health issue. Whereas Feldbaum and Lee see mobility as important only if a given health issue poses a national or global security threat, the epi-elasticity approach sees a security threat if (and as) a health problem spreads widely within a given human population. The other factor in this approach is the potential for damage in a human population. Damage in this approach does not limit itself to mortality and morbidity, but also includes material damage such as economic cost. Fidler did not go into detail about the relationship with the two criteria and stated, "[A] public health risk would have a high epi-elasticity if the risk demonstrates mobility within human populations and creates adverse material impact for societies."[12] As an example of a health security issue with low mortality and high material damage, he mentioned a limited bioweapons attack with a noncontagious pathogen. Such an attack would probably inflict a high economic and political cost, but it would still be limited in geographic scope. It would thus satisfy only one of the criteria; nevertheless, Fidler saw this as a health security threat. He recognized that satisfying the two criteria of high mobility and potential for damage does not necessarily turn a health issue into a security threat, because security is contingent on both objective and subjective criteria.

The objective approach to international health emergencies has an institutional home in the WHO's new International Health Regulations of 2005 (IHR). A health concern, detected by a national surveillance system, should meet a set of criteria for it to be defined as a "public health emergency of international concern" and thus be reported to the WHO under the IHR. The criteria include seriousness of the public health impact, risk of international spread, and risk to international travel and commerce.[14] The IHR are an important tool in institutionalizing international cooperation and coordination on emerging health threats and mitigating the effects thereof.

Security and Health in Practice: Some Examples

This section lays out four examples in which security issues and health issues intersect. These examples are by no means exhaustive, but they are intended to illustrate the kinds of policy challenges that draw together security and health concerns and that demand a more comprehensive response informed by a balanced awareness of both security and health issues. They also help illustrate how the normative, subjective, and objective frameworks discussed above can be applied to real-world challenges.

Conflicts and Catastrophes

In her work to conceptualize human security, Mary Kaldor recognized that security is not limited to the absence of physical violence. It is also about "confronting extreme vulnerabilities, not only in wars but in natural and man-made disasters as well."[15] The long-term challenges posed by both natural and man-made disasters extend well beyond the immediate time of crisis. Shortages of essential goods such as food and clean water are major contributors to rapidly deteriorating health conditions, and the destruction of vital infrastructure, including health systems, will inevitably worsen already difficult situations. The 2004 Indian Ocean tsunami, Cyclone Nargis in 2008 in Burma, and the 2010 earthquake in Haiti brought great suffering to the peoples of these regions and resulted in long-term human security challenges, including the deterioration of health and health systems. To build resilience against such disasters, it is important to draw on previous experience and increase global preparedness, not only for the immediate catastrophe but also for the long-term reconstruction of infrastructure and institutions. The international community is fairly well equipped to deal with the immediate demands of search and rescue that are imposed by an unexpected disaster, but it is less effective in delivering humanitarian relief and poorer still at post-disaster reconstruction.

A disaster such as the 2010 Haitian earthquake brings with it all of these challenges (Box 1). For example, when the alert for a humanitarian catastrophe like the one in Haiti is sounded, the International Search and Rescue Advisory Group (INSARG) is activated to coordinate search-and-rescue operations under a UN umbrella. No equivalent to INSARG exists for medical efforts in similar situations. Better coordination between public and private actors on the ground and better preparedness, not only in search and rescue but also for the next step, are badly needed.

Box 1. 2010 Earthquake in Haiti

Even before the catastrophic earthquake struck on January 12, 2010, Haiti was by far the poorest and sickest country in the Americas. The Caribbean country was also plagued by instability, bad governance, and violence. The great challenge for reconstruction work in Haiti was to increase the capacity of the country's institutions to function on their own. In order to increase health care capacity, it is important to have a long-term commitment to strengthen the Haitian health system and thereby improve governance and state legitimacy. Better health is important for economic and political improvement, not only in Haiti, but in the region as a whole. The Dominican Republic, which shares the island of Hispaniola with Haiti, will greatly benefit from both a better health situation and increased political stability in Haiti. The United States and other nations in the Western Hemisphere are greatly concerned about migration from Haiti, and it is within their perceived national security interest to stabilize the situation in the country, which explains in part the massive deployment of resources by the United States to Haiti. Farmer doubts that this kind of venture will have-long term health benefits and has stated that "at best, those of us working in places like Haiti can hope for trickle-down funds if the plagues of the poor are classed as 'US security interests.'"

(Adapted with permission from Feldbaum and Lee, 2004.)

Sanctions

In some circumstances, human security and (inter)national security are in conflict with each other. Political and economic sanctions or embargoes are coercive tools of foreign and security policy that aim to subdue or weaken the targeted state or area. At the same time, sanctions and embargoes can create a state of economic decline and produce a shortage of vital goods such as clean water, food, and medicines; these shortages can have serious impacts on public health and human security. A case in point is the sanctions imposed on Iraq by the UN Security Council after the country's invasion of Kuwait in 1990. The sanctions that effectively were in place until the fall of Saddam Hussein's regime in 2003 are considered among the toughest ever imposed on a country. Certain goods, such as medicines and ("in humanitarian circumstances") foodstuffs, were exempt from the sanctions.[16] Nevertheless, the sanctions took a heavy toll on the health of the Iraqi people and, most notably, on infant and child mortality, which increased significantly.[17] A more recent case is the Israeli blockade of Gaza that has been in effect since June 2007. In response to hostilities originating within the Gaza Strip, Israel imposed controls on all traffic in and out of Gaza, producing shortages of vital supplies within Gaza and also making it difficult for its residents to receive special medical attention in Israel. Fifteen out of 27 hospitals and 43 out of 110 primary health care facilities in Gaza were either damaged or destroyed during the Israeli operation Cast Lead in 2008–2009, and the blockade is seriously obstructing their reconstruction.[18] According to Max Gaylard, the Resident UN Humanitarian Coordinator for the occupied Palestinian Territories, "The continuing closure of the Gaza Strip is undermining the functioning of the health care system and putting at risk the health of 1.4 million people in Gaza. It is causing ongoing deterioration in the social, economic, and environmental determinants of health. It is hampering the provision of medical supplies and the training of health staff, and it is preventing patients with serious medical conditions [from] getting timely specialized treatment outside Gaza."[18]

From a national security perspective, the "collateral damage" caused by sanctions may be accepted as long as the security goals are met. From a human security perspective, however, collateral damage is never acceptable, and sanctions and embargoes that threaten the security of civilians may be as normatively questionable as civilian losses in an armed invasion.

Infectious Diseases

In recent decades, a number of infectious diseases have garnered greater and greater attention for their real and potential impact on political, economic, and social development, not only in the developing world but also in developed countries. The 2003 outbreak of severe acute respiratory syndrome (SARS) in southern China was followed by the spread of avian influenza, and the decade came to a close with worldwide concern over a novel strain of swine flu. The pandemics that seem to befall the world with increasing frequency have sparked serious concern for the security of the worst-affected states. The individual state's ability to deal with the infections has raised both external and internal doubts over state legitimacy, and these doubts have prompted states to engage in negotiations to improve multinational governance structures that can be more responsive to widespread disease outbreaks. Infectious diseases have also put strains on international relations, as, for example, when Indonesia refused to share virus samples from the H5N1 outbreak with the international community or in the case of the worsened bilateral relations between China and Mexico following Beijing's decision to quarantine Mexican citizens in China during the H1N1 outbreak. Concerns have also been raised that emerging infectious diseases can be a contributing cause of state destabilization, as the disease might affect large numbers of otherwise able-bodied citizens and thereby cripple the public and private sectors and their services. A government's response to an emerging infectious disease might also highlight existing inequalities in the affected society, with public disorder a possible result.[19]

The economic impact of emerging infectious diseases has in several cases been enormous, as costs extend well beyond the direct impact on the health system. The economic impact of SARS was heavy not only in China, where the infection originated, but also in countries such as Canada, which suffered loss of travelers and business in heavily affected regions. The H5N1 virus has forced the culling of millions of fowl throughout the world and has been disastrous to the poultry industry, not least in Southeast Asia. The H1N1 scare prompted several countries to stock up on and distribute expensive vaccines in an effort to halt the spread of the disease. The high economic costs associated with an outbreak of an infectious disease may also serve as a disincentive to proper reporting on its occurrence. The failure by the Chinese government to report the emergence of SARS in a responsible manner might have been an example of this (Box 2).

Box 2. SARS in China

When SARS first broke out in the Guangdong province of southern China, the Chinese government initially responded by denying the existence of a novel disease and later tried to downplay its consequences. Following criticism from both the international community and domestic groups, China eventually admitted that there was a problem and proceeded to address it in a more responsible manner. The SARS crisis in China had a great impact on the way that China chooses to cooperate with the international community in the health area, and Beijing has since made a strong commitment to the International Health Regulations. SARS also had important internal political effects: the mayor of Beijing and the Chinese Minister of Health were removed from their posts. With the new Minister of Health, Wu Yi, health became a higher-priority issue in China. After SARS, the Chinese government realized that issues of health that previously were considered "low politics" could potentially have severe political, economic, and social consequences, and this realization was later reflected in their response to both HIV and the H1N1 pandemic.[36]

The single health issue with the most widely discussed security implications is HIV/AIDS. The disease has become a massive humanitarian catastrophe, particularly in sub-Saharan Africa. With infection rates of 15–49-year-olds surpassing 20% in several countries in sub-Saharan Africa at the beginning of the new millennium,[d] HIV/AIDS could not be ignored, even by the countries that were able to bring the epidemic under control. In January 2000, the UN Security Council devoted a whole day to the HIV/AIDS challenge in Africa. Never before had a health issue been given salience as a security threat in such a high-level forum. A report by the US Council on Foreign Relations suggested that bipartisan support for the President's Emergency Plan for AIDS Relief (PEPFAR) would not have been achieved in the United States if HIV/AIDS had not been considered a matter of national security.[20]

---

[d] Countries with a prevalence of more than 20% among 15–49-year-olds in 2008 include Lesotho (23.2%), Swaziland (26.1%), and Botswana (23.9%), according to UNAIDS (www.unaids.org). These figures have been more or less stable since the beginning of the 21st century.

During the past decade, HIV/AIDS was linked not only to human but also to national security in a variety of ways. Claims of links between HIV and security have at times been spectacular and have had little factual support.[21] In an attempt to elucidate the ties between HIV and security, Feldbaum and colleagues constructed a model to show the pathways by which HIV/AIDS affects national security. According to this model, a high HIV prevalence can be detrimental to security if it affects strategically important people, peripheral states and regions, and strategically important states.[22]

High HIV prevalence among strategically important people such as soldiers and international peacekeepers is one of the more debated links between HIV and security. Notwithstanding the difficulty in obtaining reliable information on HIV incidence in national militaries, Laurie Garrett claimed that infection rates are, in fact, slightly higher within militaries than within general populations.[22] Data from which to empirically ascertain the levels of infection within militaries are notoriously difficult to produce, and some reports question both the higher prevalence within African militaries and the suggestion that the infection would seriously undermine the militaries' capacity.[23] As with concerns about national militaries, concerns have arisen about the possibility for international peacekeepers to both acquire and spread HIV. If peacekeepers contribute to the spread of the infection during missions abroad, that could seriously undermine their credibility and put future missions in jeopardy.[24] High HIV prevalence within national militaries could also render recruitment to peacekeeping missions more difficult, because the recruitment base would be diminished.[5,22,25]

The impact of HIV on the security of peripheral states and regions, primarily in sub-Saharan Africa, is often invoked as a major concern by the security community, and yet the link between HIV and state stability is empirically underresearched. High rates of HIV will alter a country's demography, reduce the number of able-bodied men and women who drive the economy, and result in large orphan populations. A shortage of teachers will negatively affect education and training, and the health care system will struggle under added pressure.[5,22] There is no doubt that HIV is imposing a huge humanitarian, economic, and social cost on many countries that are already severely weakened by other factors, such as poverty and conflict. The added burden of a widespread HIV/AIDS epidemic may exacerbate an already unstable situation. The direct implications of HIV/AIDS for state stability, however, largely remain speculative. The case of South Africa suggests that a soaring HIV/AIDS rate among the population does not preclude economic growth. Drawing a comparison between Botswana and Zimbabwe, two of the sub-Saharan countries hardest-hit by HIV/AIDS, suggests that factors such as bad governance are much more detrimental to stability than is HIV.

HIV's impact on strategically important states — most notably, Russia, China, and India — has been a growing concern for the Western security community. These countries all have complex internal dynamics that threaten to take violent expression if power relations shift, and any instability within these countries will have a global security impact. These countries are also part of the "second wave" of HIV, and infection rates are steadily increasing. Since the turn of the millennium, Russia has witnessed a rapid increase in infections, not least within the military, and HIV/AIDS is increasingly perceived as a threat to national security.[26] The fears that China could have had as many as 10 or 20 million people living with HIV by 2010[27] did not materialize, and yet the number of HIV-infected persons in the country continued to rise and was expected to reach around 1.5 million persons in 2010 according to official Chinese estimates.[28] The country has recently gone from downplaying the occurrence of the disease and viewing AIDS activists as threats to national security to a more enlightened and technical approach to the disease. India is also struggling with increasing infection rates, in a complex setting of poverty and cultural heterogeneity. HIV/AIDS has been successfully securitized through both human agency and institutional developments. Powerful securitizing actors such as Richard Holbrooke and Colin Powell have successfully brought HIV/AIDS to the highest priority on the security agenda. The UN and its agencies, such as WHO and UNAIDS (the joint UN Programme on HIV/AIDS), have also been instrumental in elevating HIV and AIDS on the development agenda, and even into the realm of security.

This development reached its pinnacle in the middle of the first decade of this century, and the current trend is to bring the question of

HIV/AIDS back into "normal" politics and approach the issue more from a development perspective rather than from a security perspective. This "desecuritization" of HIV/AIDS has occurred as a result of the poor empirical correlation between the disease and security. There is also an increasing concern that, whereas linking HIV to security may have positive effects such as increased exposure and ensuing funding, it may also contribute to a new type of stigma, as the focus is shifted from humanitarian to security concerns. The perception of HIV as a national security threat could also lead to human rights abuses and nationally exclusive policies that lose track of HIV reduction as a global public good.[29] McInnes and Rushton suggested that the securitizing moves of the first few years of this century were only partly successful, that they had limited beneficial effects, and that the perceived consensus on HIV as a question of security was premature. The lack of solid empirical evidence does not, however, suggest that there are no links whatsoever between HIV and security, but rather that they are more complex than previously anticipated. The fight against HIV/AIDS still needs massive resources. If obtaining these resources can be accomplished by securitization, it must be done in an enlightened way that takes into account the potential pitfalls.[20]

Biological Know-How and Materials

The use of biological agents in warfare is not a novel phenomenon, and yet it is one that has recently received considerable attention. Recent years have seen numerous examples in which a non-state actor acquires and distributes lethal pathogens among civilian populations. In the mid-1990s, there were concerns in the security community that weaponized biological (and chemical) agents, stockpiled in the former Soviet Union and Iraq, would fall into the hands of malicious substate groups or rogue states and be used in terrorist attacks. Whereas these fears have not as yet materialized, non-state actors have in the past successfully produced weaponized biological agents on their own. One of these groups is the Japanese cult Aum Shinrikyo, which in 1995 dispensed sarin gas in the Tokyo subway, killing 12 commuters and seriously debilitating many more. In addition to this sarin gas, the cult was accused of having produced and obtained strains of anthrax, Ebola, and other pathogens.[e] These accusations awakened fears of biological terrorism by suggesting that non-state actors had both the capacity and the will to carry out such attacks with biological agents. Another high-profile incident occurred in 2001, with the mailing of anthrax spores to media outlets and US Senate offices. Coming in the wake of the September 2001 terrorist strikes against the United States, the anthrax attacks were given first priority, and defense against biological weapons was given much attention in the subsequent discussions on increased security and preparedness against future terrorist attacks. In the United States, this approach has taken institutional expressions in the US Public Health Security and Bioterrorism Bill of 2002, which firmly situated public health in the realm of national security. In 2008, the Commission on the Prevention of Weapons of Mass Destruction Proliferation and Terrorism stated that a terrorist attack utilizing weapons of mass destruction was "more likely than not" before 2013, and that the weapons used would likely be biological rather than nuclear.[30]

National health care systems and international health institutions have a double role to play in the defense against biological attacks: ensuring that dangerous biological agents do not fall into the wrong hands (biosecurity) and reducing the negative effects should such an attack occur (biopreparedness). To ensure that public health systems are able to serve their intended purpose and will not be misused for malign intent, a high level of vigilance and close attention to security are necessary within institutions that handle pathogens, toxins, and sensitive materials.[31] Utilizing the national health care system to strengthen biopreparedness may effectively turn this system into an integrated part of a country's national defense, a development that raises several concerns. For example, potentially harmful biological and chemical agents used in research are increasingly being

---

[e]These claims have been widely spread, and they are often credited to one publication: Kaplan DE, Marshall A. (1996) *The Cult and the End of the World.* Arrow, London. The claims have been questioned: see Leitenberg M. (1999) Aum Shinrikyo's efforts to produce biological weapons: A case study in the serial propagation of misinformation. *Terrorism Polit Violence* **11**(4): 149–158.

viewed as a security concern.[32] One critique against programs to increase biopreparedness and defense against biological attacks is that biodefense activities can be used as a cover for an offensive biological weapons program. Another concern is that such defense spending is based on an exaggerated threat and that it diverts much-needed funding from more pressing public health concerns.[33]

Looking Ahead: Building a More Coherent and Useful Field

This chapter has identified three main approaches to security-related health issues that may have implications for our dialogue on health diplomacy. The first approach is the normative approach embodied by the idea of human security, in which security is closely linked with development, and the well-being of the individual is central. This approach is institutionalized in the policies of the UNDP and the MDG, which were negotiated among member states of the UN as an example of health diplomacy. The second approach concerns those issues that have been brought onto the security agenda by human agency and through the exercise of subjective perspectives rather than by dint of their objective threat to national security. The third approach aims to construct frameworks that objectively define the health issues that have significance for security and that may be addressed by negotiations in various health fora. The new IHR take this approach to identifying the events that should be reported to the WHO. This chapter also notes that the securitization framework developed by the Copenhagen School is useful for assessing those health and security issues, of which HIV/AIDS, emerging diseases, and biological terrorism are the most prominent.

Linking health and security is not without complications. The securitization of health issues has a wide variety of institutional implications, because increased attention may lead to more attention and resources. Relating certain health issues to security may raise their status and put them on the agenda; security can in this way work as a "Trojan horse" by which the health community can get the recognition needed so that it can obtain sufficient resources to address the issue as a foreign and security policy priority. Securitizing a health issue is a way to turn it into "high politics" and associate it with the traditionally much more prioritized sphere of security. By tying "the needs of the poor [to] the fears of the rich," in the phrase of Feldbaum and Lee,[5] this approach would in theory motivate the affluent part of the world to contribute to solving the health problems of the poor parts of the world through enlightened self-interest. Stepped-up efforts to address the global HIV/AIDS challenge could be seen, in part, as a successful example of this approach: the intense efforts to relate the disease to security have been followed by massive attention and directed funds and resources from both governments and private initiatives.

In contrast, several good arguments suggest that the health and security linkage be approached with caution and care. The first argument has to do with who is controlling the agenda. Several of the health issues that are currently perceived as security problems are seen this way because they threaten the security of the world's wealthier nations. Potential pandemics of avian or swine flu are perceived as security threats in the developed world, even though they are so far associated with far fewer casualties than are chronic diseases such as cholera and malaria, which overwhelmingly affect poor nations. The attention that HIV has drawn within some institutions in the developed world could be attributed to the perception of the disease's potential to cause state instability, which in the long run could threaten the developed world. The priority given to bioterrorism is especially apparent because the concerns stem from a largely Western security agenda concerned with mass-casualty attacks rather than with promoting better public health. McInnes summarized this argument by stating: "[I]n securitizing health, the national security interests of the West have been prioritized over the human security of the poor elsewhere."[20]

Tying in the security aspect could very well raise the profile of global health issues within institutions that have traditionally given health a somewhat lower priority. In recent years, for example, the European Union (EU) has increasingly identified linkages between global health and the security of the EU.[35] This action may also be true for other organizations that hold security and regional stability in high priority — such as the North Atlantic Treaty Organization (NATO), the African Union (AU), and the Association of Southeast Asian Nations Regional Forum

(ARF) — but that have a less developed view of health in a broader regional and global context and with regard to its relationship to security. Using the security argument is a way to make international institutions and structures for global governance pay attention to the fact that health is indeed global, and that the health situation in one region can have an effect on the political, economic, and security situation not only in that region, but also beyond it.

A risk also exists that securitized health issues are being promoted at the expense of other major killers and a more holistic approach to health. A health systems approach aimed at strengthening health capacity is likely to be more effective in promoting public health than are *ad hoc* measures to resolve isolated issues. When emerging diseases are just a plane ride away from their place of origin, there is no question that health is global today. Recent disease outbreaks show that the closing of borders is not a very effective way of dealing with disease, and that international openness and cooperation through diplomatic efforts are essential. Global public goods, such as immunization, will benefit all mankind, as opposed to global public "bads," such as excessive use of antibiotics which leads to the emergence of resistant strains. It is important that perceived national security concerns do not stand in the way of promoting better public health. The securitization of disease should not occur at the expense of the consideration of health as a global public good. Securitization of health and health as a global public good are not two mutually exclusive approaches, however. Caballero-Anthony, for example, has advocated an integrated approach by which the attention gained by securitization is complemented by the inclusiveness of the global public goods.[35]

One important step ahead would see current, emergent, and future governance structures that are concerned with health and security beginning to more actively examine the linkage between the two. For example, organizations such as the UN, the EU, NATO, AU, ARF, and the Organization for Economic Cooperation and Development, as well as the Group of 20 process and others should devote greater resources to understanding and assessing the interrelatedness of health and security. This kind of work can be carried out in cooperation with the private sector and civil society organizations that are also grappling with this issue.

On the whole, the linkage between health and security should bring benefits to both sides of the equation. In the end, an enlightened, informed, and balanced approach to the relationship between health and security is necessary in order to avoid an overemphasis on one at the expense of the other. But more work is needed in the research and policy community to understand this balance of pluses and minuses and to translate it to policies that help achieve maximum benefit for both. At present, the field continues to struggle in developing a coherent approach to what "health and security" is and what the primary areas of policy and research interest should be. The review of three approaches to the field — the normative, the subjective, and the objective — suggests that a certain incoherency and even controversy around issues of security and health will continue for the foreseeable future. In the meantime, it will be important to continue bringing together scholars and policymakers from such diverse fields as public health, bioscience, development, and security so they can interact, exchange views, and come to better understand the interests, expertise, and experience their counterparts can contribute to enhance both health and security.

References

1. US Government, Executive Branch. (2002) *The National Security Strategy of the United States of America.* September. Available from www.information-clearinghouse.info/article2320.htm (accessed May 14, 2011).
2. Aldis W. (2008) Health security as a public health concept: A critical analysis. *Health Policy Plann* **23:** 369–375.
3. Youde J. (2005) Enter the fourth horseman: Health security and international relations theory. *Whitehead J Diplom Int Relat,* winter/spring, pp. 193–220.
4. McInnes C, Lee K. (2006) Health security and foreign policy. *Rev Int Stud* **32:** 5–23.
5. Feldbaum H, Lee K. (2004) Public health and security. In: Ingram A (ed.), *Health, Foreign Policy, and Security: Towards a Conceptual Framework for Research and Policy.* Nuffield Trust, London, pp. 19–28.
6. Roosevelt FD. (1941) State of the Union Address to the Congress of the United States of America. January 6. Available from http://docs.fdrlibrary.marist.edu/od4Frees.html (accessed May 15, 2011).

7. United Nations Development Programme. (1994) *Human Development Report 1994*: *New Dimensions of Human Security*. Oxford University Press, New York City. Available from http://hdr.undp.org/en/reports/global/ hdr/1994 (accessed May 14, 2011).

8. Chen LC. (2004) Health as a human security priority for the 21st century. Paper presented to Human Security Track III, Helsinki Process. December 7. Available from www.helsinkiprocess.fi/netcomm/2mg/Lib/24/89/LCHelsinkiPaper12% 5BI%5D.6.04.pdf (accessed May 15, 2011).

9. Commission on Human Security. (2003) *Human Security Now*. United Nations.

10. Paris R. (2001) Human security: Paradigm shift or hot air? *Int Security* **26(2):** 87–102.

11. Buzan B, Waever O, de Wilde J. (1998) *Security: A New Framework for Analysis*. Lynne Rienner, London.

12. Fidler DP. (2007) A pathology of public health securitism: Approaching pandemics as security threats. In: Cooper AF, Kirton JJ, Schricker T (eds.), *Governing Global Health* [Global Environmental Governance Series, Kirton JJ (series ed.)]. Ashgate, Aldershot, UK, pp. 41–64.

13. National Intelligence Council. (2000) The global infectious disease threat and its implications for the United States. *National Intelligence Estimate,* NIE 99-17D. Available from www.fas.org/irp/threat/nie99-17d. htm (accessed May 15, 2011).

14. World Health Organization. (2008) *International Health Regulations 2005*, 2nd edn. WHO Press.

15. Kaldor M. (2007) *Human Security*. Polity, Cambridge, UK.

16. United Nations Security Council. (1990) *Resolution 661*. August 6. United Nations.

17. Ronsmansa C, Campbella O, Fawzib MCS, *et al.* (1996) Sanctions against Iraq. *Lancet* (Letter to the Editor) **347(8995):** 198–200.

18. UN Humanitarian Coordinator and Association of International Development Agencies (AIDA). (2010) The closure of the Gaza Strip puts at risk the health of people in Gaza and undermines the functioning of the health care system. January 20. Available from http://reliefweb.int/node/341788 (accessed May 15, 2011).

19. McInnes C. (2008) Health. In: Williams P (ed.), *Security Studies: An Introduction.* Routledge, Abingdon, UK, pp. 274–286.

20. McInnes C, Rushton S. (2010) HIV, AIDS and security: Where are we now? *Int Aff* **86(1):** 225–245.
21. Garrett L. (2005) *HIV and National Security: Where are the Links?* Council on Foreign Relations, New York City.
22. Feldbaum H, Lee K, Patel P. The national security implications of HIV. *PLos Med* **36(6):** e171. doi:10.1371/journal.pmed.0030171.
23. Whiteside A, de Waal A, Gebre-Tensae T. (2006) AIDS, security and the military in Africa: A sober appraisal. *Afr Affairs* **105(419):** 201–218.
24. Wiharta S. (2009) The legitimacy of peace operations. In: *SIPRI Yearbook 2009.* SIPRI, Stockholm, pp. 95–116.
25. International Crisis Group. (2001) HIV/AIDS as a security issue. Available from www.crisisgroup.org/en/regions/africa/001-hiv-aids-as-a-security-issue.aspx (accessed May 14, 2011).
26. Sjöstedt R. (2008) Exploring the construction of threats: The securitization of HIV/AIDS in Russia. *Secur Dialogue* **39(1):** 7–29.
27. Schneider M, Michael M. (2002) *The Destabilizing Impacts of HIV/AIDS: First Wave Hits Eastern and Southern Africa; Second Wave Threatens India, China, Russia, Ethiopia, Nigeria.* CSIS, Washington, DC.
28. Gill B, Okie S. (2007) China and HIV — A window of opportunity. *N Engl J Med* **356:** 1801–1805.
29. Elbe S. (2006) Should HIV be securitized? The ethical dilemmas of linking HIV/AIDS and security. *Int Stud Q* **50(1):** 119–144.
30. Commission on the Prevention of Weapons of Mass Destruction Proliferation and Terrorism. (2008) *World at Risk: The Report of the Commission on the Prevention of Weapons of Mass Destruction Proliferation and Terrorism.* Vintage, New York City.
31. Clevestig P. (2008) *Handbook for Applied Biosecurity for Life Science Laboratories.* SIPRI, Stockholm.
32. Hart J, Clevestig P. (2009) Chemical and biological materials. In: *SIPRI Yearbook 2009.* SIPRI, Stockholm, pp. 413–433.
33. Sidel VW. (2002) Defences against biological weapons. In: Wright S (ed.), *Biological Weapons and Disarmament: New Problems/New Perspectives.* Rowman & Littlefield, Lanham, MD., pp. 77–101.
34. European Commission. (2009) *The EU Role in Global Health.* European Commission.

35. Caballero-Anthony M. (2006) Combating infectious diseases in Asia: Securitization and global public goods for health and human security. *J Int Aff* **59(2):** 195–127.
36. Chan L-H, Chen L, Xu J. (2010) China's engagement with global health diplomacy: Was SARS a watershed? *PLoS Med* **7(4):** e1000266. doi: 10.1371/journal.pmed.1000266.

8

Military Health Diplomacy

Eugene V. Bonventre, MD,* and
Lt Col Valérie Denux, MD, PhD†

Introduction

War is a mere continuation of policy by other means.

— General Carl von Clausewitz, *On War*

It is generally recognized that war negatively affects the health of civilians in conflict zones.[1,2] This effect is largely indirect: more civilians die of infectious disease, poor sanitation, and lack of access to safe water and medical care, than die of traumatic injuries.[3] Less well appreciated, seldom studied, and sometimes denied are the ways in which militaries can positively affect both global health and international relations. When Egypt and the United States broke diplomatic relations during the Arab–Israeli Six-Day War in 1967, the US military research laboratory in Cairo was the only American facility that Egypt allowed to continue operating;[4] today, that laboratory is a highly respected institution that contributes to health in Africa and to bilateral and regional relations. The challenge for policy-makers and diplomats is to understand military strategy enough to recognize the strengths and weaknesses of military health diplomacy,

*Global Health Consulting, Washington, DC.
†Allied Command Transformation Medical Staff Officer, NATO.

191

which will enable them to maximize the positive impact on global health and on foreign policy and to reduce unintended consequences.

In this chapter, we demystify the techniques that militaries use to influence global health and international relations. We examine military strategies in contexts ranging from peacetime to open warfare. We consider ethical issues of military involvement in health diplomacy and scrutinize the role of coordination with the global health community.

Military Diplomacy

To seduce the enemy's soldiers from their allegiance and encourage them to surrender is of especial service, for an adversary is more hurt by desertion than by slaughter.

— Flavius Vegetius Renatus, *The Military Institutions of the Romans*

Military diplomacy is not a new idea; nations have used military might throughout recorded history to directly support political objectives or to accomplish security objectives in indirect support of political objectives. Militaries build relationships with other militaries and civilian governments to develop mutual confidence and to increase the effectiveness of working together in an alliance or coalition.[a] They do so during wartime (i.e. through prisoner-of-war exchanges, peacekeeping activities, and psychological warfare) and peacetime (i.e. through training exercises with allies, visits of senior officers, and exchanges of military academy students). The Berlin Airlift, for example, successfully reassured not only the population of Germany, but also the populations of other nations, in ways that are still felt today.[b]

---

[a] An alliance is a formal relationship between two or more nations, based on an agreement or treaty, to accomplish broad, long-term objectives; a coalition is an *ad hoc* arrangement between nations to accomplish specific short-term objectives. Most wars are waged by alliances or coalitions.

[b] The United Kingdom, the United States, France, Canada, New Zealand, Australia, and South Africa contributed to an airlift of supplies to the citizens of Berlin in 1948–1949, after the Soviet Union blockaded the Western-controlled sectors of that city. In "Operation Vittles," allies flew almost 300,000 flights and delivered more than 2 million tons of

The United Kingdom's Ministry of Defence noted that "influence is achieved when we change the behavior of the target audience through the coordination of all military actions, words, and images;" a combination of word and deed is most effective, and audiences interpret messages "through a lens of their own culture, history, and tradition."[5] After the 2005 earthquake in Kashmir, the US military and the North Atlantic Treaty Organization (NATO) supported the civilian response; "Chinook diplomacy" — military helicopters ferrying relief supplies to isolated villages — complemented military field hospitals in providing care to quake victims. The primary audience was the affected people, but the military also intended to influence relations with the government of Pakistan and to reassure allies and Muslim populations around the world. Former US Secretary of Defense Robert Gates has noted: "[S]uccess will be less a matter of imposing one's will and more a function of shaping the behavior of friends, adversaries, and, most importantly, the people in between."[6]

Military Health Diplomacy

Military health diplomacy refers to health activities implemented by militaries (or their contractors or civilian employees) that are intended to influence bilateral, regional, or global relationships and to improve the health of foreign military or civilian populations. Few militaries have specific policies on military health diplomacy, but many militaries deliver health care to civilians simply because of the altruistic nature of medical personnel. The target audience of military health diplomacy may be civilian government agencies, military forces, the general population, or a combination. For instance, the Colombian Navy used "gunboat diplomacy" in the 1960s: military patrol vessels provided medical and dental care to civilians in territories where guerilla warfare was common.[7] The Indian Army provides health care to civilians in occupied Kashmir.[8] Just

---

supplies. Then-First Lieutenant Gail (Hal) Halvorsen began dropping candy during the approach to Tempelhof Airport in Berlin; ultimately, 3 tons of candy were delivered during "Operation Little Vittles." Germans today still speak of the "candy bomber" when discussing that period in history.

as European nations of the 19th century used military health activities to "win the hearts and minds of the people" and to reduce violent extremism, the US military of today delivers health care to counter the rise of transnational terrorist groups. US military medical personnel provide health care in Ethiopia, near the Somali border, to gain information about the activities of extremists and undermine their popular support. In Muslim majority areas of Mindanao in the Philippines, the US military trains and equips the Filipino military to fight insurgents. Such missions include medical and veterinary activities, such as the vaccination of cattle, and have reported anecdotal success.[9] Neither the impact of such activities on health nor their effectiveness in achieving political objectives has been rigorously studied.

Historical Perspectives

If the doctor understands his role, he is the first and most efficient agent to provide peace among the population.

— Marshal Louis Hubert Lyautey

To facilitate the withdrawal of foreign troops after a conflict and avoid the recurrence of violence, donors implement reconstruction and development activities. In 2005, the United States' national strategy in Iraq asserted "the value of building and rehabilitating health care facilities." This is not a new concept: during the colonial wars of the 19th century, military commanders noticed the potential value of such an approach. Joseph Gallieni, military commander and administrator in French colonies in Africa, Indochina, and the Caribbean, emphasized the necessity of state building and modernizing the colonized countries.[10] For him, "[D]estroying is easy but rebuilding is more difficult, however more politically useful." This novel vision made the colonial wars a real change in the military's approach toward the population. The commanders came to understand that "the inhabitants are at the heart of the conflict." Marshal Lyautey recommended three aspects of war:[11] continuity of military action, the link between military and policy, and the well-being of the population. In line with this vision, he declared: "A doctor is worth a battalion." In Morocco, for instance, French military doctors had an important position in diplomacy: they managed clinics to treat the indigenous population and opened services to combat trypanosomiasis, leprosy, and tuberculosis. In Algeria, the efficiency of the French Military Health Service strongly contributed to the success of Algerian colonization. In 1924, colonial politicians recognized that the French Military Health Service played a prominent role in building the French Empire.[10]

Militaries provided medical assistance to local populations as a counterinsurgency strategy during the wars of independence that followed World War II. For example, during the Algerian War (1954–1962), the French Military Health Service was the only organization to provide medical and social assistance in the southern desert of Algeria. The relationship with the population was so good that the Military Health Service stayed after independence (until 1976) to ensure reconstruction and development of the country. Even if medical diplomacy alone was not able to offer France the possibility of keeping Algeria as a French colony, it influenced and maintained bilateral relations for years after independence.

Militaries were involved in the origins of public health. The US Marine Hospital system that was established in 1798 evolved into the US Public Health Service,[12] and the Army's Malaria Control in War Areas program became the US Centers for Disease Control and Prevention.[13] The US military used public health to achieve political objectives of "nation building" and "pacification" in the Philippines insurgency of 1898.[14] The government of the military occupation established a Board of Health to provide safe water and sanitation, vaccinate civilians, build medical infrastructure, and supply essential drugs in a program referred to as "medical charity." National mortality rates were reduced by 50% during the first year of the program; senior leadership deemed it, paired with coercion of hardcore insurgents, successful in pacifying the population and improving civilian health.

The US military used military health diplomacy in South Vietnam, and the principles developed 50 years ago are used today in Iraq, Afghanistan, and elsewhere. The Medical Civic Action Program (MEDCAP) I began in 1963 to build the capacity of the South

Vietnamese government to deliver health services, to increase civilian confidence in their government and its army, and to promote the government's legitimacy.[15] American soldiers advised local providers and Ministry of Health officials, delivered health care in rural areas, and drilled wells, usually sharing credit with local leaders and government officials. As the United States' troop commitment grew, the US Marines began MEDCAP II in 1965. It differed substantially from MEDCAP I by attempting to establish trust in the American military presence, rather than in the South Vietnamese government. At that point, significantly larger numbers of American troops provided health care in villages and provincial hospitals; local government officials and health care providers were rarely involved. The more involved that US personnel became, the more that local hospitals depended on their services.[16] MEDCAP II missions to villages lacked followup, however, so chronic health conditions were not treated; the Vietnamese population's expectations were raised but not met. Lack of security impeded continuity, as medical teams withdrew to the safety of their bases at night, leaving the population exposed to insurgent attack. The US Agency for International Development (USAID) also launched medical projects under MEDCAP II, but that program duplicated effort, lacked coordination, and caused interagency rivalries.[16] The Civil Operations Revolutionary Development Support program was established in 1966 to resolve these difficulties.[c] Its activities focused on improving public health services, including the establishment (credited to the Saigon government) of the National Institute of Public Health. Overall effectiveness was limited, because the program was underresourced and because public health activities had no immediately visible impact at the local level.[17] The program succumbed to corruption, local bureaucracy, increasing dependency on US staff, and lack of continuity.

Although no formal evaluations of Vietnam era military health diplomacy programs took place, personnel involved claimed that civilian health

---

[c] Experts from the Department of State, Department of Defense (DoD), Central Intelligence Agency, and Department of Agriculture were included to synchronize interagency activities. DoD oversaw the program, because its primary objective was security, and because DoD had greater capacity than did the civilian agencies.

improved (as measured by the number of patients treated: 40 million[d] by the end of the war in 1973[17]) and that activities were "enthusiastically received by all," thus "winning hearts and minds." [15] In reality, health outcomes were not measured, the population did not associate American health activities with the South Vietnamese government, and the outcome of the conflict was not affected.[16]

Military Health Diplomacy: Strategy and Techniques

Military health diplomacy has simultaneous goals of achieving military objectives, influencing international relations, and improving health, and it often is difficult to determine which goal is primary. In this section, a handful of examples illustrate this balance.

Conventional Warfare

Militaries are obliged under International Humanitarian Law to minimize the effect of combat on civilian populations and on the medical and public health systems. European militaries use Civil–Military Co-operation (CIMIC) to minimize the negative effects of health emergencies on the force and to address the urgent health needs of a population in a conflict zone. CIMIC may involve coordination with international organizations, nongovernmental organizations, or local authorities.[18] Danish CIMIC teams in Iraq reported the success of employing civilians from the Danish Ministry of Foreign Affairs, an example of diplomatic personnel supporting military objectives.[19] Similarly, US military medical personnel may work with the Office of Civil Affairs to conduct "medical civil–military operations" to accomplish military objectives, influence relationships with allies and the civilian population, and improve civilian health.[20] CIMIC can shape public perceptions to encourage the population to support the mission of military troops, and so it helps to protect those troops.[21]

---

[d] The total cost of the military health diplomacy programs in Vietnam was estimated (by Wilensky[17]) at US$350 million, or (as Malsby calculated[14]) about US$1.9 billion in 2008 dollars.

The United Kingdom used military health diplomacy effectively in Sierra Leone as that country's civil war ended in 2002. After rescuing 11 UN troops who had been kidnapped by rebels, Britain launched a training and assistance mission[e] that effectively took control of the army of Sierra Leone.[22,23] The political objectives were to restore order and security; the military objectives were to train and mentor the Sierra Leonean Army to be a competent and accountable fighting force.[f] British military medics mentored their Sierra Leonean Army counterparts and restored health infrastructure, gradually raising the quality of military health care. The United Kingdom paid the salaries of local military physicians and nurses to discourage a brain drain and to recruit quality personnel to replace a military health workforce that had been decimated by war.[g] Britain recruited the United States, Canada, and Bermuda into the coalition to enhance the legitimacy of their mission. Nearly a decade on, the peace in Sierra Leone has survived two peaceful transitions of power. The military medical mission, while it certainly cannot be credited with stabilizing the country, certainly can boast of making a contribution to the health of soldiers and family members, as well as to boosting the image of the United Kingdom as a world power that is interested in the health and well-being of its former colonies.

Indirect Strategies to Counter Violent Extremism

Although counterterrorism and counterinsurgency are quite different,[h] the United States-led coalitions in Iraq and Afghanistan are evolving similar

---

[e] This team was called the International Military Assistance & Training Team (see www.operations.mod.uk/africa/imattsl.htm). The UK-led military health assistance team has only seven members and an annual budget of about £200,000 — an extremely low cost to mentor a Sierra Leonean army of about 15,000 that protects a country of 3.5 million.

[f] This was no small task in a country whose military had launched two successful coups in the previous decade.

[g] Of the 70 British military physicians before the war, only seven remained at the end, four of whom were in administrative positions.

[h] Organizations such as Al-Qaeda use terrorism as a tactic to achieve global aims, whereas insurgents compete with national governments for control of a population.

strategies that have global implications. Military health diplomacy plays a supporting role in this political strategy.

As the security situation in Iraq deteriorated in 2003, US military medical personnel used the Vietnam era MEDCAP model of providing health care to Iraqi civilians, in an effort to win their hearts and minds. The population had witnessed the destruction — first by sanctions and then by looting — of a health care system that was one of the best in the region. Under Muqtada al-Sadr, the health system was used to support the Mahdi Army and to identify and kill Sunni leaders, including one provincial health director.[24] US commanders began to see that the MEDCAPs model was wholly inadequate to the task of gaining popular support; not only did such "band-aid medicine" or "drive-by health care" not contribute significantly to health, it also presented targets of opportunity for suicide bombers and undermined the legitimacy of the Iraqi government.[25] One military medical officer developed an alternative to MEDCAPs in Tal Afar, Iraq, in 2005. The local hospital was a frequent site of sectarian violence; in one instance, a Shi'ite boy's corpse was booby-trapped, and his father was killed when he came to collect the body. US troops guarded the hospital and created safe lanes for patients and staff to access the facility, and they then transitioned the security mission to the Iraqi army and police. US military personnel delivered medical supplies and textbooks, repaired infrastructure and ambulances, and helped Iraqi physicians to establish a professional medical society. The health impact was quantifiable: outpatient visits to the Tal Afar hospital increased from 10 per day in 2005 to more than 800 per day in 2006, as civilians regained trust in Iraqi medical professionals and Iraqi security forces. The hospital director observed: "I see peace in the faces of the people for the first time in two years."[25] Local ownership, sustainability, and capacity-building contributed to the success of this approach.

In Afghanistan, international military troops help the Afghan army and police to develop capable medical systems. A quality military health care system is a recruiting and retention tool, and healthier soldiers are better able to provide the security that is necessary for development to proceed.[26] In remote areas, Afghan army clinics and hospitals provide health care to civilians; international assistance to the military health system complements civilian health assistance.[i] Although the United States tried the MEDCAP model in Afghanistan, it had limited impact on the military mission and no measurable impact on civilian health.[27] NATO troops emphasized medical activities that contributed to a civilian-led effort to build capacity of the Afghan health system in areas which civilian organizations cannot reach because of insecurity or lack of resources; this approach avoids duplication of effort, follows development principles,[j] and pays careful attention to local standards of care and cultural norms.[28]

Egypt's military hospital at Bagram Air Base treats up to 500 Afghan civilians per day. Although the Egyptian physicians use the MEDCAP model, they likely provide more culturally appropriate care than do Americans.[29] Egypt's intentions are to convince Afghans to support coalition military operations and to improve civilian health; officials note a degree of success in both.

Complex Humanitarian Emergencies

Bernard Kouchner (former French Foreign Minister) and Professor Mario Bettati, among others, have defended the idea of humanitarian interventions in fragile or failed countries.[30] From the 1990s, more and more states have intervened in humanitarian crises by using their military capabilities to provide humanitarian corridors. Two operations illustrate this approach: "Operation Restore Hope" in Somalia (1992–1993) and the French "Operation Turquoise" in Rwanda (July–August 1994). Restore Hope, operated by a task force led by the United States, was charged with carrying out UN Security Council Resolution 794: to create

---

[i] The Afghan Army Surgeon-General and the Police Surgeon-General reported that their health systems serve 900,000 Afghan civilians; while this number is probably an exaggeration, it indicates a situation found in a variety of developing countries (and some developed ones), in which the military provides health services to civilians.

[j] As described by Andrew Natsios, former USAID administrator, the development principles are ownership, capacity building, sustainability, selectivity, assessment, results, partnership, flexibility, and accountability (http://www.carlisle.army.mil/usawc/parameters/articles/05autumn/natsios.pdf).

a protected environment for conducting humanitarian operations in the southern half of Somalia. The aim of Operation Turquoise was "… protection of displaced persons, refugees and civilians in danger in Rwanda, by [all possible] means, including the establishment and maintenance, where possible, of safe humanitarian areas."[31] The French Military Health Service was widely involved in the humanitarian mission. These types of operation are sometimes questionable with regard to international law, but public opinion is in favor of them because of their humanist character. The military health services are fundamental tools in such operations because they treat populations. Without the medical component, justification of these operations would be difficult. In this case, military medical participation is really a part of the global diplomacy effort.

Medical civil–military operations also play important roles in other UN Security Council operations. For instance, France deployed military medical facilities to support the population during "Operation Libage" in Kurdistan in 1992. The objective was to protect, feed, and treat Kurdish refugees that were being threatened by Iraqi forces. In 2008, the European Union (EU) launched the bridging military operation, led by France in Chad and the Central African Republic, that was mandated by UN Security Council Resolution 1778. In conducting this operation, the EU is stepping up its long-standing action in support of efforts to tackle the crisis in Darfur. One objective was to facilitate the delivery of humanitarian aid and the free movement of humanitarian personnel by improving regional security. In this case, the overlap between military and humanitarian objectives is important. The French concept is "to place the military contribution in support of both civil and military and in a complementary approach," and that objective is the reason that the French Military Health Service is systematically involved in assisting civilians during such an operation. The lack of civilian medical facilities is profound; 80% of the activity in the French Military Medical Facilities in Chad is provided to the local population, and only 20% is devoted to supporting the military force. This type of humanitarian assistance represents a long tradition in Africa for the French Military Health Service,[10] which has played a strong role in the close relationships between France and Africa.

Natural Disaster Response

At the end of the 1960s, France created a rapid-intervention medical military element to provide medical assistance after disasters. This element was used in Biafra (1968–1970), after earthquakes (Peru in 1972, Mexico in 1975, and Armenia in 1988), and in Colombia (1985).

The 2005 earthquake in Kashmir destroyed the military hospital in Muzaffarabad, the sole source of secondary health care for the region. The US Mobile Army Surgical Hospital (MASH) arrived three weeks after the earthquake, so only 2% of the patients the hospital treated had earthquake-related injuries. But the presence of MASH enabled the United States to reassure a new ally in its global counterterrorism campaign and to demonstrate its willingness to take humanitarian action in Muslim countries. Opinion polls showed a doubling of favorability toward the United States among Pakistanis, from 23% in May 2005 to 46% in November 2005, and a drop in support for Osama bin Laden, from 51% to 33%.[32] However, the relief effort did not affect Pakistanis' opinions of the United States' fight against terrorism: opposition actually rose to 66% in 2006, compared with 52% before the quake,[33] The criticisms expressed by the Pakistani public were relatively minor: free medical care and pharmaceuticals undermined local physicians and pharmacies, and created dependence on American assistance.[34]

After the deployment of the US Navy hospital ship *Mercy* in response to the 2004 Indian Ocean tsunami, favorable opinions among Indonesians toward the United States increased from 15% to 44%, and support for Osama bin Laden fell from 58% to 23%.[35] During the deployment of the hospital ship *Comfort* to Haiti after the January 2010 earthquake, the US military used electronic media to promote its mission. The task force had RSS feeds, podcasts, fan pages on Facebook and Twitter videos on YouTube, and photographs on Flickr, and the task force commander had a personal blog.[k] Such media saturation implies a desire to reach an audience far beyond Haiti.

---

[k] Two weeks after the quake, the military's Haiti diary on Twitter had 3000 followers, the Pentagon channel on YouTube had had 50,000, and the DoD Facebook site had 17,000 fans.

Preventive Diplomacy in Peacetime

Tommy Thompson, US Secretary of Health and Human Services during the George W. Bush administration, stated, "America has the best chance to win the war on terror and defeat the terrorists by enhancing our medical and humanitarian assistance to vulnerable countries."[l] Although the Obama administration dropped the term "war on terror," military health diplomacy outside conflict zones has grown to "encourage the development of relationships that can build trust and help prevent the spread of terrorism.[36–39] Critics highlight the scant evidence that a lack of health care causes violence, extremism, or terrorism;[m] even fewer examples exist in which health diplomacy has reduced the risk of violence.[40] Whether health diplomacy undermines extremism or not, Stewart Patrick laments a leading role for the military: "[W]hat the military calls phase 0 is what we used to call foreign policy."[n] The militarization of foreign policy may increase the resources available for health assistance. One often-mentioned disadvantage of such militarization is a potential risk to humanitarian aid workers, as a result of the perception that they are closely aligned with the military; this risk has not been well-studied, and it may be limited to highly politicized environments.[41]

The US Africa Command uses military health diplomacy to prevent violence. The Office of Civil Affairs provides veterinary, dental, and health care in the Horn of Africa, using the MEDCAP model to gather information regarding extremists.[42] The effectiveness of such operations is difficult to document, and no attempt is made to assess their impact on health.

---

[l] Thompson defined medical diplomacy as "the winning of hearts and minds of people in the Middle East, Asia, Africa, and elsewhere by exporting medical care, expertise, and personnel to help those who need it most." See www.boston.com/news/globe/editorial_opinion/oped/articles/2005/10/24/the_cure_for_tyranny

[m] See "Winning 'hearts and minds' in Afghanistan: Assessing the effectiveness of development aid in COIN operations" (https://wikis.uit.tufts.edu/confluence/pages/viewpage.action?pageId=34085650).

[n] Statement at the Humanitarian Action Summit in Boston, 2009. See http://hhi.harvard.edu/programs-and-research/program-on-humanitarian-effectiveness/humanitarian-action-summit

Effective military health diplomacy features coordination with civilian-led health diplomacy. The US military spends $100 million per year from the President's Emergency Plan for AIDS Relief, and it can show an increase in knowledge regarding HIV prevention in African militaries, a reduction in HIV prevalence, and an improvement in bilateral military relationships.[43] Military research laboratories in Thailand, Kenya, Egypt, and Peru contribute to global disease detection and response, and they build the local capacity to respond to malaria, tuberculosis, and other diseases of importance to both military and civilians;[o] this action helps developing nations to meet their obligations under the International Health Regulations, an activity that has inadequate donor funding.[44]

Ethical Issues in Military Health Diplomacy

When signatories to the Geneva Conventions are involved in conflict, they are obliged to protect the local public health and medical systems.[45] Countries that are not signatories are still responsible for following humanitarian principles that are outlined in national law, international human rights law, treaties, and customary law.[46,47] However, medical standards that are taken for granted in developed countries are not uniformly applied during many MEDCAP-style military health activities, even in peacetime, and the principle of "do no harm" is often ignored.[48] Treatment compliance rates and complication rates are seldom measured, because followup and continuity of care are lacking. The physician–patient relationship that represents the core of ethical modern medical care is frequently absent.[48]

NATO is the first military organization to include a "do no harm" clause in its civil–military medical doctrine, recognizing that, even with the best of intentions, military health assistance risks undermining the work of aid agencies and the host government. NATO has stated: "[T]he provision of direct patient care in exchange for information that is to be utilized for purely military purposes is ethically unacceptable and contravenes international humanitarian principles."[49] European militaries separate health activities from intelligence activities in order to avoid placing

---

[o] See the Armed Forces Health Surveillance Center website (http://afhsc.army.mil/home).

physicians in the position of violating the Hippocratic oath; the collection of information is limited to disease surveillance for the determination of health and environmental risks to the military force. If the military delivers health care according to needs and if beneficiaries share information as a result, such passive collection of information may be acceptable as a secondary benefit under the ethical principle of "double effect,"[50] but it should not be the primary reason that the military delivers care.

Military medical personnel face the challenge of dual loyalty — they must address the medical needs of their patients, while also meeting the requirements of the military mission. For instance, a military physician who treats a pilot for chest pain may need to violate patient confidentiality by informing the pilot's commander of the patient's condition, to avoid endangering that pilot's crew and aircraft. Military physicians face similar challenges when they treat civilians during military heath diplomacy activities, although ethical dilemmas of treating patients on the basis of their perceived vulnerability to extremist influence, rather than on the basis of medical need, are seldom discussed. Tensions can exist when commanders order military medical personnel to treat patients to gather information or because the patients belong to a specific ethnic group, even though surrounding areas may have a greater medical need.

Such dilemmas raise the following question: Is the goal of military health diplomacy to improve health, to improve security, or both? Ideally, militaries should strive to achieve the two goals simultaneously. NATO's health principles are timely but, ultimately, commanders and military medical personnel should discuss specific situations as they arise. NATO advises that military health activities should be clinically appropriate, culturally sensitive, coherent with other aspects of development, sustainable, coordinated with the host nation's medical authorities and other appropriate agencies, and — above all — undertaken only when there is no civilian alternative. Because the US military has no such explicit policy, its health activities are *ad hoc*, which makes it more difficult to analyze ethical issues. Failure to publish and follow ethical guidelines can have negative effects on military objectives and international relations, as was the case when US military medical personnel were accused of being complicit in abuse at Abu Ghraib prison in Iraq.[51]

Coordination Among Stakeholders

Western governments are improving interagency cooperation to address complex political problems. After the Iraq War, the White House gave the State Department additional resources and authority to coordinate interagency approaches to stability operations.[p] This "comprehensive approach" is gaining momentum in NATO, and civil–military coordination is improving in Sudan, Somalia, Afghanistan, Iraq, and elsewhere. However, health is often seen as a low-priority technical issue, separate from the main debate on the advantages, disadvantages, and risks of a closer civil–military relationship. In the absence of civil–military coordination, military health professionals often see gaps in health coverage in insecure or underserved environments, and they act in accordance with the principle of humanity that their profession demands. Better interagency coordination can increase the likelihood that military health diplomacy will improve civilian health and international relations, and it also may reduce the negative impact that conflict has on global health. Greater oversight of military health diplomacy by professional diplomats may help ensure that military health activities support political objectives and that the right message reaches the right audience.

Greater transparency and coordination of military health diplomacy would make it easier to determine the impact of military health activities on health and security. Military health professionals are part of the global health community, even in politically sensitive regions. In Afghanistan, the military is understandably not part of the Health Cluster led by the World Health Organization to reduce conflict-related morbidity and mortality and fill gaps in health services.[52] However, despite the cluster's principles of partnership and inclusiveness and its mandate to improve effective coordination, a lack of communication between the cluster and military health professionals is common. The risk to NGO staff is usually given as an excuse, even though some experts suggest. "[A]id organizations are being attacked not just because they are perceived to be cooperating with Western political actors, but because they are perceived

---

[p] See National Security Presidential Directive 44 (www.fas.org/irp/offdocs/nspd/nspd-44.html).

as wholly a part of the Western agenda. It would seem that the undeniably Western nature and orientation of much of the international aid community is at the root of the insecurity [that] aid workers face in countries such as Somalia and Afghanistan."[41] Curtailing dialogue with the military will not make aid workers more secure. The UN Office for the Coordination of Humanitarian Affairs (OCHA) describes civil–military coordination as essential and necessary;[q] appointing a trusted agent as a liaison between the Health Cluster and military health professionals would facilitate this dialogue. In Haiti, a less politicized and more secure environment, military health professionals were members of the Health Cluster; this structure allowed aid agencies to better understand the capabilities and limitations of military health assets, and to directly address challenges with medical logistics and the rehabilitation of patients from the hospital ship *Comfort*.

Donor agencies and their NGO implementing partners are the primary experts on the development principles. Whether by intent or by default, they often must deal with the long-term effects of military health diplomacy activities. Improving relationships between development agencies and the military has been challenging because of very different organizational structures and values. Increased coordination must find a balance between the intimate relationship that USAID had with the military during the Vietnam conflict and the attitude of avoidance that some agencies and organizations have today. It should be extremely easy for health professionals from different agencies to communicate, because health is a universal language. Donor agencies must take into account the impact of coordination on implementing partners; policy-makers should seek a practical, evidence-based approach that preserves the independence and impartiality of NGOs, while permitting the military

---

[q] UN OCHA defines civil–military coordination as "the essential dialogue and interaction between civilian and military actors in humanitarian emergencies that is necessary to protect and promote humanitarian principles, avoid competition, minimize inconsistency, and, when appropriate, pursue common goals. Basic strategies range from coexistence to cooperation. Coordination is a shared responsibility facilitated by liaison and common training." See the report "Civil–Military Relationship on Complex Emergencies," Inter-Agency Standing Committee, Geneva, January 2006 (www.unocha.org/what-we-do/coordination-tools/UN-CMCoord/overview).

to achieve its mission.[53] The ultimate goal of civil–military coordination is not the "unity of effort" that militaries often seek, but a "unity of understanding."

Academia can play a unique role in military health diplomacy. Although measuring civilian mortality in conflict zones is controversial, challenging, and imperfect, such research sheds light on the significance of excess civilian mortal.[54,55] The next step is to work with militaries to refine techniques to minimize the impact of war on civilian health, both during and after conflict, and to describe methods that the military can use to protect civilians and preserve the capacity of the civilian health sector.

Civil society plays an important role as well. Human rights groups should continue to insist on transparency of military health diplomacy and should expand existing ethical guidelines to include such activity.[56] Military health activities are well funded and popular with military leaders and politicians alike; calls for the military to stop conducting these activities will likely fall on deaf ears. Militaries seem more open to constructive criticism now than they have ever been, so civil society should use this opportunity to positively influence military health diplomacy activities.

Summary

The nation that will insist on drawing a broad line of demarcation between the fighting man and the thinking man is liable to have its fighting done by fools and its thinking done by cowards.

— Sir William Francis Butler

Nations have used military health diplomacy for centuries to accomplish military and political objectives by improving relationships with the armed forces of allied and coalition nations. Relationships improve mutual understanding and familiarity with tactics and strategies (what militaries call interoperability), and they can benefit the health of soldiers in partner militaries. Military health diplomacy may also influence the attitudes and the health of civilian populations. Such activities can support civilian health diplomacy; when properly planned and coordinated, these activities complement and improve the effectiveness of donor programs and bring additional resources to bear in support of political objectives and global health. Military health diplomacy intended to influence the attitudes of governments or civilian populations has had mixed results; little evidence exists to suggest that these efforts have reduced the drivers of extremism, prevented or mitigated violence, or improved stability and security. The effectiveness of military health diplomacy is improved when all target audiences are considered, when personal contacts and relationships are emphasized, and when the development principles of local ownership, cultural and medical appropriateness, and sustainability are kept in mind.

Poorly coordinated, *ad hoc* military health diplomacy has unintended consequences, ranging from undermining local health capacity to risking the lives of aid workers. Activities that seek to achieve short-term military objectives but ignore global health principles risk undermining long-term development. Military health activities that meet needs but ignore political objectives are usually more expensive, less culturally appropriate, and less sustainable than are activities conducted by development experts. Militaries should measure, qualitatively and quantitatively, the impact of military health diplomacy on political and military objectives and on global health by using well-established monitoring and evaluation techniques and by developing new techniques.

Military health diplomacy is one tool in the toolbox of many militaries. Greater transparency and improved coordination may mitigate the risks and improve the effectiveness of military health diplomacy and facilitate further study of ethical issues.

References

1. Coghlan B, Brennan RJ, Ngoy P, *et al.* (2006) Mortality in the Democratic Republic of Congo: A nationwide survey. *Lancet* **367(9504):** 44–51.
2. Roberts L, Lafta R, Garfield R. (2004) Mortality before and after the 2003 invasion of Iraq: Cluster sample survey. *Lancet* **364:** 1857–1864.
3. Burkel FM, Greenough PG. (2008) Impact of public health emergencies on modern disaster taxonomy, planning, and response. *Disaster Med Public Health Prep* **2:** 192–199.
4. Badeau JS. (1970) Diplomacy and medicine. *Bull New York Acad Med* **46(5):** 303–312.

5. United Kingdom Ministry of Defence. (2009) *A Guide to the Military Contribution to Security and Stabilization.* UK Ministry of Defence, London.
6. Robert Gates, as quoted in Atwood BJ, McPherson MP, Natsios A. (2008) Arrested development. *Foreign Aff* **87(6):** 123–132.
7. Carey HL. (1970) A war we can win: Health as a vector of foreign policy. *Bull New York Acad Sci* **46(5):** 334–350.
8. Cariappa MP, Bonventre EV, Mohanti BK. (2008) Operation Sadbhavana: Winning hearts and minds in the Ladakh Himalayan region. *Mil Med* **173(8):** 749–753.
9. No author. (2010) Front-line vets: American forces in the Philippines. *The Economist.* Available from www.economist.com/world/asia/displaystory.cfm?story_id=15393857 (accessed May 12, 2011).
10. Roberts SH. (1929) *The History of French Colonial Policy (1870–1925)* (London: P.S. King).
11. Hoisington, William A Jr. (1995) *Lyautey and the French Conquest of Morocco.* Palgrave Macmillan.
12. United States Public Health Service. (No date.) About the commissioned corps: History. Available from www.usphs.gov/aboutus/history.aspx (accessed May 12, 2011).
13. Centers for Disease Control and Prevention. (No date.) Our history — our story. Available from www.cdc.gov/about/history/ourstory.htm (accessed May 12, 2011).
14. Malsby RF. (2008) "Into which end does the thermometer go?" Application of military medicine in counterinsurgency: Does direct patient care by American service members work? Master's thesis, US Army Command and General Staff College, Fort Leaventworth, KS.
15. Wilensky RJ. (2004) *Military Medicine to Win Hearts and Minds: Aid to Civilians in the Vietnam War.* Texas Tech University.
16. McMaster HR. (1997) *Dereliction of Duty: Lyndon Johnson, Robert McNamara, The Joint Chiefs of Staff, and the Lies That Led to Vietnam.* HarperCollins, New York City.
17. Wilensky RJ. (2001) Medical Civic Action Program in Vietnam: Success or failure? *Mil Med* **166(9):** 815–819.
18. North Atlantic Treaty Organization. (2003) *Allied Joint Publication 9: NATO Civil–Military Co-operation (CIMIC) doctrine.* NATO. Available from www.nato.int/ims/docu/ajp-9.pdf (accessed May 11, 2011).

19. Buchholz B. (2009) *Battalion-Level Civil–Military Operations — Danish Style.* US Army Infantry School, Fort Benning, GA.
20. Joint Chiefs of Staff. (2006) *Joint Publication 4-02: Health service support.* Joint Chiefs of Staff, Washington, DC.
21. United Kingdom Chiefs of Staff. (2006) *Joint Doctrine Publication 3–90: Civil–Military Co-operation (CIMIC).* UK Chiefs of Staff, London.
22. Bentham M, Sherwell P. (2000) Jungle search after kidnap of British soldiers. *The Telegraph.* Available from www.telegraph.co.uk/news/worldnews/africaandindianocean/sierraleone/1367871/Jungle-search-after-kidnap-of-British-soldiers.htm (accessed May 11, 2011).
23. Smith M. (2000) Britain sends extra troops to "advise" Sierra Leone army. *The Telegraph.* October 11, 2000. Available from http://www.telegraph.co.uk/news/uknews/1369831/Britain-sends-extra-troops-to-advise-Sierra-Leone-army.html
24. Paley AR. (2006) Iraqi hospitals are war's new "killing fields." *The Washington Post.* Available from www.washingtonpost.com/wp-dyn/content/article/2006/08/29/AR2006082901680.html (accessed May 14, 2011).
25. Baker JB. (2007) Medical diplomacy in full-spectrum operations. *Mil Rev*, Sep.–Oct., pp. 67–73.
26. Bricknell MC, Thompson D. (2007) Roles for international military medical services in stability operations (security sector reform). *J R Army Med Corps* **153(2):** 95–98.
27. Beitler AL. (2006) Humanitarian assistance in Afghanistan: A prospective evaluation of clinical effectiveness. *Mil Med* **171(9):** 889–893.
28. Bricknell MC, Gadd RD. (2007) Roles for international military medical services in stability operations (reconstruction and development). *J R Army Med Corps* **153(3):** 160–164.
29. Cloutier G. (2008) Egyptian hospital in Afghanistan provides care, changes attitudes. American Forces Press Services. Available from http://fhp.osd.mil/intlhealth/article.jsp?articleID=6 (accessed May 14, 2011).
30. Bettati M, Kouchner B. (1987) *Le devoir d'ingérence: peut-on les laisser mourir?* Denoël, Paris. (Influential statement arguing for the right to provide assistance to alleviate suffering caused by human-made disasters, without the consent of the state.)
31. United Nations. (1992) United Nations Security Council Resolution 794 (Granting the Secretary-General Discretion in the Further Employment of

Personnel of the United Nations Operation in Somalis), S.C. res 794, 47 U.N. SCOR at 63, U.N. Doc. S/RES/794.

32. Terror Free Tomorrow. (2005) A dramatic change of public opinion in the Muslim world: Results from a new poll in Pakistan. Available from www.terrorfreetomorrow.org (accessed May 15, 2011).

33. Terror Free Tomorrow. (2006) Humanitarian assistance key to favorable public opinion in world's three most populous Muslim countries: Results from new polls of Indonesia, Bangladesh, and Pakistan. Available from www.terrorfreetomorrow.org (accessed May 15, 2011).

34. Mosier W. Orthner W. (2007) *Military Medical Support for Humanitarian Assistance and Disaster Relief: Lessons Learned from the Pakistan Earthquake Relief Effort*. Joint Center for Operational Analysis, Suffolk, VA.

35. Terror Free Tomorrow. (2006) Unprecedented Terror Free Tomorrow polls: World's largest Muslim countries welcome US Navy. Available from www.terrorfreetomorrow.org (accessed May 15, 2011).

36. Amundson D, Lane D, Ferrara E. (2008) Operation Aftershock: The US military disaster response to the Yogyakarta earthquake May through June 2006. *Mil Med* **173(3):** 236–240.

37. Mancuso JD, Price EO, West DF. (2008) The emerging role of preventive medicine in health diplomacy after the 2005 earthquake in Pakistan. *Mil Med* **173(2):** 113–118.

38. Timboe HL, Holt GR. (2006) Project HOPE volunteers and the Navy hospital ship *Mercy*. *Mil Med* **171(10):** 34–36.

39. Vanderwagen W. (2006) Health diplomacy: Winning hearts and minds through the use of health interventions. *Mil Med* **171(10):** 3–4.

40. Bradbury M, Kleinman M. (2010) *Winning Hearts and Minds? Examining the Relationship Between Aid and Security in Kenya*. Feinstein International Center, Medford, MA.

41. Stoddard A, Harmer A, DiDomenico V. (2009) *Providing Aid in Insecure Environments: 2009 Update*. Humanitarian Policy Group, London.

42. Buxbaum P. (2009) Soft power with guns. *INS Security Watch*. Available from www.isn.ethz.ch/isn/Current-Affairs/Podcasts (accessed May 15, 2011).

43. Serafino NM. (2008) *Department of Defense Role in Foreign Assistance: Background, Major Issues, and Options for Congress*. Congressional Research Service, Washington, DC.

44. Bonventre EV, Peake JB. (2010) The role of the US Department of Defense in preparing for global pandemics and natural disasters. In: *From Conflict to*

Pandemics: Three Papers from the CSIS Global Health and Security Working Group. Center for Strategic and International Studies, Washington, DC. Available from http://csis.org/publication/conflict-pandemics

45. International Committee of the Red Cross. (1949) *The Geneva Conventions of August 12, 1949*. ICRC.

46. Rubenstein LS, Bittle MD. (2010) Responsibility for protection of medical workers and facilities in armed conflict. *Lancet* **375:** 329–339.

47. Thieren M. (2007) Health and foreign policy in question: The case of humanitarian action. *Bull World Health Organ* **85(3):** 218–224.

48. Ritchie EC, Mott RL. (2003) Military humanitarian assistance: The pitfalls and promise of good intentions. In: Beam TE, Sparacino LR, Pellegrino ED, *et al.* (eds.), *Military Medical Ethics*. Uniformed Services University of the Health Sciences, Bethesda, MD, pp. 805–830.

49. Allied Command Operations. (2009) *Strategy for NATO Military Medical Services Involvement with Humanitarian Assistance, and Support to Governance, Reconstruction and Development*. North Atlantic Treaty Organization. Available from http://www.aco.nato.int/page1420733.aspx

50. Jonsen AR, Siegler M, Winslade WJ. (2006) *Clinical Ethics*. Macmillan, New York City.

51. London L, Rubenstein L, Baldwin-Ragaven L, Van Es A. (2006) Dual loyalty among military health professionals: human rights and ethics in times of armed conflict. *Cambridge Q Healthcare Ethics* **15(4):** 381–391.

52. The United Nations and the Humanitarian Coordination Mechanisms in Afghanistan. (2008) Health Cluster Afghanistan Terms of Reference. Available from http://ochaonline.un.org/OCHALinkclick.aspx?link=ocha& docid=1112403

53. US Agency for International Development. (2009) *Civilian–Military Relations: An LTL Strategies Study Group, 2009*. USAID, Washington, DC.

54. Brownstein CA, Brownstein JS. (2008) Estimating excess mortality in post-invasion Iraq. *N Engl J Med* **358(5):** 445–447.

55. Mills EJ, Burkle FM. (2009) Interference, intimidation, and measuring mortality in war. *Lancet* **373:** 1320–1322.

56. International Dual Loyalty Working Group, Cape Town, South Africa. (2002) *Dual Loyalty and Human Rights in Health Professional Practice: Proposed Guidelines and Institutional Mechanisms*. Physicians for Human Rights and School of Public Health and Primary Health Care, University of Cape Town, Health Sciences Faculty, Cape Town, South Africa.

9

Health Diplomacy in Humanitarian Action

Valerie Percival, MA, DrPH

Introduction

During humanitarian emergencies, access to health care means the difference between life and death for thousands of civilians. Yet the delivery of that health care requires humanitarian actors to quickly and effectively navigate complex — and sometimes dangerous — local, national, regional, and international processes and negotiations. Diplomacy is therefore a critical, yet often overlooked process, which must be used by humanitarian workers in order to accomplish their mission.

As dialogue has always been integral to humanitarian action, the concept of *humanitarian diplomacy* evolved, advocated by humanitarian actors such as the International Committee of the Red Cross (ICRC). Its objective is to encourage humanitarian actors to develop and utilize diplomatic skills to promote respect for international humanitarian law and facilitate access to civilian populations in need of humanitarian assistance.[1,2] From this perspective, humanitarian diplomacy "… encompass[es] the activities carried out by *humanitarian organizations* to obtain the

*Assistant Professor of International Affairs, Norman Paterson School of International Affairs, Carleton University, Tel.: 613-520-2600 x. 6658, Office: 5319 River Building, 1125 Colonel By Drive, K1S 5B6, Ottawa, Canada
E-mail: valerie_percival@carleton.ca

space from political and military authorities within which to function with integrity. These activities comprise such efforts as arranging for the presence of international humanitarian organizations and personnel in a given country, negotiating access to civilian populations in need of assistance and protection, monitoring assistance programmes, promoting respect for international law and norms, supporting indigenous individuals and institutions, and engaging in advocacy at a variety of levels in support of humanitarian objectives".[3] (*Emphasis added by the author.*)

While a useful tool for humanitarian workers, we argue that this conceptualization of humanitarian diplomacy, with its restricted focus on those organizations that deliver humanitarian assistance, is too limited. It does not sufficiently capture the range of diplomatic activities present during humanitarian crises and the involvement of actors that facilitate the humanitarian response. As we demonstrate below, diplomacy in humanitarian action involves dialogue among a multitude of state and non-state actors within a variety of forums, at the international and local levels.

In this chapter, we apply the less restrictive concept of health diplomacy to international engagement in humanitarian crises. We examine the processes through which state and non-state actors use health diplomacy to achieve their objective — the delivery of medical assistance to civilians in need. While precise definitions vary,[a] global health diplomacy broadly encompasses international cooperation on issues related to global health. Health diplomacy is the "policy-shaping processes through which states, intergovernmental organizations, and non-state actors negotiate responses to health challenges or utilize health concepts or mechanisms in policy-shaping and negotiation strategies to achieve other political, economic or social objectives."[6]

This chapter explores health diplomacy in humanitarian settings, examining the characteristics it shares with traditional forms of global health diplomacy as well as its distinguishing features. We frame our inquiry by examining the following six issues:

- Why — the objectives of that diplomacy.
- When — its timeframe.

---

[a]Several papers review the various definitions of global health diplomacy.[4–6]

- Where — the forums where that diplomacy takes place.
- Who — the actors that undertake that diplomacy.
- What — its tools.
- How — the key processes of health diplomacy in humanitarian crises.

While this overview presents the "ideal": how health diplomacy would work in a perfect world, the reality is far messier, particularly during humanitarian crises. We conclude with illustrations from recent cases that demonstrate the challenges as well as the potential of health diplomacy in humanitarian settings.

Objectives of Health Diplomacy in Humanitarian Action

A humanitarian emergency occurs when the survival of a significant portion of the population is threatened by a natural disaster, by violence and armed conflict, or by a combination of the two.[7–9] The state may lack the ability or willingness to provide basic services and emergency assistance to such endangered populations. As a result, a variety of actors step in to fill this void.

Humanitarian assistance is the provision of life-saving interventions — medical care, food, shelter, and sanitation. Its objective is to reduce the suffering of civilians and to limit the loss of life, and as a result, medical interventions are a significant and highly visible component of humanitarian engagement. The objective of health diplomacy in humanitarian action is to ensure that effective medical and other health assistance reaches civilians in need during complex emergencies and other humanitarian crises.

Achieving this objective is not easy. Humanitarian assistance can be impeded by logistical challenges such as poor roads and terrain, inclement weather, and the challenges of identifying recipients within urban environments. In addition, regulatory barriers imposed by visa requirements and customs laws; challenges of in-country corruption and lack of professionalism among some humanitarian workers; limited financial resources; and security challenges may impact the success of humanitarian assistance.

The ability to access civilian populations also varies dramatically among different types of crises or conflicts. Within intrastate conflicts, characterized by one-sided violence and the intentional killing of civilians, the ability of humanitarian actors to access those populations may be very limited. Insurgencies also pose a challenge to humanitarian action, as insurgent groups often engage in highly politicized, violent tactics designed to change the perception of and support for the government.[10] This violence has included the targeting of humanitarian assistance providers. Internationalized conflict, where conflict protagonists receive support from one or more states or international military alliances,[11] can also be problematic, as the perception of the independence, impartiality and neutrality of international humanitarian organizations can be undermined.

While the response to natural disasters may not be as politically charged as in conflict situations, the scope, scale, and implementing environments for these disasters are also extremely challenging. Many events, such as earthquakes or hurricanes, occur quickly with little warning and incur widespread, indiscriminate damage that necessitates a very rapid response. Moreover, natural disasters that require significant international assistance often occur in fragile states, and there is evidence that disasters can also contribute to future state instability.[12]

Although the contexts of humanitarian emergencies vary, there are several common characteristics. First, the objective of assistance is to rapidly intervene to protect the civilian population through the direct delivery of health care assistance. Improvements in the quality and effectiveness of medical assistance during humanitarian emergencies have benefited from a growing evidence base on best practices, the development of technical standards, and better coordination of such assistance.[13] Second, actors other than the recipient state provide much of this assistance, although they rely on states and conflict protagonists to facilitate its delivery. Third, in all of these environments, diplomacy is an essential process through which humanitarian actors may achieve their objective of protecting the health of civilians while navigating a complex implementing environment.

Timeframes: When Diplomacy Takes Place

Diplomacy traditionally involves long, iterative bilateral and multilateral dialogues, and global health negotiations are no exception. Countless diplomatic sessions within multinational organizations, such as the World Health Organization (WHO), often make only incremental progress over time on global health priorities. It can take years to reach agreements, and several more years for those agreements to be implemented. Even with pressing issues such as influenza virus sample sharing, WHO Member States took almost two years to reach an agreement.[12]

However, in humanitarian settings, the timeframes for diplomacy are compressed, particularly for rapid-onset emergencies linked to natural disasters such as earthquakes and hurricanes. The failure to initiate dialogue and discussions, to quickly reach agreement on humanitarian priorities, and to efficiently and effectively fund and deliver humanitarian assistance can immediately translate into excess civilian mortality and morbidity.

For acute, rapid-onset natural disasters, humanitarian health diplomacy must take place immediately after the disaster strikes, and should continue throughout the crisis. During conflict, the timeframes for health diplomacy are less predictable. The toll on civilians is not constant; it takes time to assess the impact of conflict on civilians, to determine if a humanitarian emergency exists and the severity of that crisis, and to galvanize international actors to respond.

Forums for Humanitarian Diplomacy — Where Health Diplomacy Takes Place

International diplomacy, including diplomacy related to global health, takes place in multiple forums — the same issue can be debated at the United Nations General Assembly, the World Health Assembly of the WHO, the World Trade Organization, or at the board meetings of multilateral organizations such as the Global Fund for AIDS, TB, and Malaria. Negotiations take place at the international level, within regional organizations, at the national level, and at the subnational level.

This multiplicity of forums is also reflected in humanitarian action. Forums at the international, regional, national, and local levels are all critical for achieving the objective of humanitarian action — delivering assistance to populations in need. Due to the rapid-onset timeframes for humanitarian crises, dialogue at these various levels must be simultaneous, or must occur within days or weeks of each other. As a result, diplomacy at these various levels and forums is often mutually reinforcing, and in some cases catalytic. These key forums are outlined in Fig. 1 and described below.

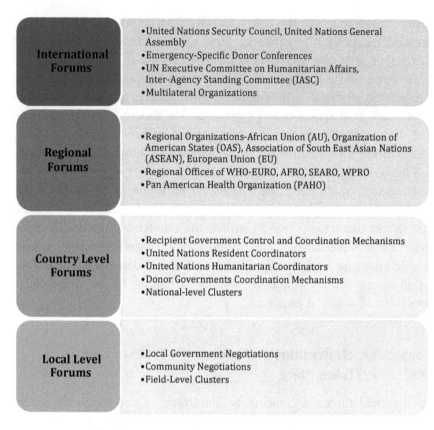

Fig. 1.   Forums for diplomacy in humanitarian action.

International forums

At the international level, the United Nations Security Council (UNSC) and the General Assembly (UNGA) call the attention of member states to the humanitarian emergency, reiterate the importance of international humanitarian norms, and galvanize action by calling for member states to respond. In cases where international funds are quickly needed to avert a large loss of life, donor conferences specific to that emergency can be convened, held most typically for high profile emergencies. Other key forums at the United Nations include the Executive Committee on Humanitarian Affairs, chaired by the Emergency Relief Coordinator

(ERC), who also holds the position of Under Secretary for Humanitarian Coordination and heads the UN Office for the Coordination of Humanitarian Affairs (OCHA). The Executive Committee on Humanitarian Affairs brings together representatives of UN humanitarian agencies with UN political, security, and peacekeeping departments.

The Inter-Agency Standing Committee (IASC), composed of multilateral organizations with representation from some transnational NGOs, helps determine the priorities for humanitarian action and sets relevant technical standards. Multilateral organizations that act as the lead agencies of the Country Cluster System (see below) also undertake dialogue and negotiation within their specific area of responsibility: with health at the WHO, water and sanitation and education at the United Nations Children's Fund (UNICEF), and food security and agriculture at the World Food Programme (WFP) and the Food and Agriculture Organization (FAO).[b]

Regional forums

The African Union (AU), the Association of East Asian Nations (ASEAN), and the European Union (EU) can also provide a forum for diplomacy in humanitarian settings, particularly if agreement is blocked at the international level or if specific action is needed from countries in the "neighborhood" of the specific humanitarian crises. These organizations can raise awareness of the impact of the humanitarian emergency, compel their members to commit resources to humanitarian action, pressure recipient governments to facilitate the delivery of that assistance, and uphold their obligations under international humanitarian agreements.

---

[b] For more information on the cluster system, see the One Response website: *http://oneresponse.info/Coordination/ClusterApproach/Pages/Cluster%20Approach.aspx*. For a useful diagram on how the various elements of the Cluster System work together, see p. 3 of the IASC "Handbook for RCs and HCs on Emergency Preparedness."[14] IASC. Handbook for RCs and HCs on Emergency Preparedness and Response. Geneva: IASC; 2010. This handbook is also available on the IASC website: http://www.humanitarianinfo.org/iasc/pageloader.aspx?page=content-news-newsdetails&newsid=146

Country-level forums

Within the recipient state, the UN Humanitarian Coordinator (in his/her absence, the UN Resident Coordinator), together with lead humanitarian organizations, implements the Cluster System at the country level, with meetings most often held in the capital city of the recipient state, where the country-level headquarters of various international organizations are located. This system establishes national-level forums for each cluster that include relevant multilateral and nongovernmental organizations, representatives from the donor state, and representatives from the recipient country to facilitate coordination and information-sharing. While the government of the recipient state may also establish separate processes at the country level, they are encouraged to participate in the Cluster System.

Local level forums

The Cluster System is also implemented at the subnational level, close to the location of the humanitarian crisis, with processes established to share information and facilitate coordination for organizations actively working in the field and for local government officials and leaders of civil society. In addition, local-level government and community leaders may establish formal forums for dialogue to provide input into humanitarian assistance and ensure access to affected populations.

Actors — Who Undertakes This Diplomacy?

While global health diplomacy has traditionally focused on the role of states, multiple actors at the international and national levels are critical participants in health diplomacy during humanitarian action. Many of these actors straddle international, regional, national, and local forums, while the reach of others (particularly local actors and local governments) is more limited. Figure 2 outlines the main humanitarian actors, and the lines indicate the forums that they are able to influence. The solid line indicates a strong influence, while the dashed line refers to more limited influence. We divide these actors into those who deliver humanitarian assistance and those who facilitate if and how humanitarian assistance reaches those in need.

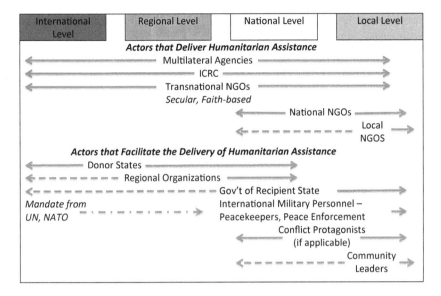

Fig. 2. Main actors in humanitarian diplomacy.

Actors delivering humanitarian assistance

There are four key sets of actors that engage in the delivery of humanitarian assistance: multilateral agencies, the ICRC, transnational NGOs, and local and community NGOs.

Multilateral agencies

At the international level, health diplomacy is often led by multilateral organizations, such as OCHA and the WHO. These organizations convene and coordinate donors and NGOs, provide a forum for the mobilization of assistance at the international level, and provide technical guidance on best practices to meet those needs. Multilateral agencies are also independent actors with offices and staff within the country affected by the crises, actively taking part in diplomatic processes at the national and local levels to secure access for humanitarian agencies and facilitate the delivery of assistance.

OCHA is part of the UN Secretariat, and as such reports to the UN Secretary General. It leads the negotiation of a Consolidated Appeal

Process with relevant multilateral agencies and nongovernmental organizations that collectively identify needs and priorities.[c] Multilateral organizations that lead a Cluster, such as the WHO, are also critical to the Appeal, facilitating the flow of information between the field and headquarters; they help set priorities and ensure that proposed interventions are based on the best available evidence. As a result of these roles, multilateral agencies can effectively straddle the international- and national-level forums. While their influence extends from the global to the local level, multilateral organizations are large and complex bureaucracies, with reporting relationships to their governing boards, which ultimately extends to UN member states.

International Committee of the Red Cross

While the ICRC is a non-state organization, and its involvement in the International Red Cross and Red Crescent Movement provides it with a reach that resembles that of transnational NGOs, it is a separate and special entity. As the custodian of the Geneva Conventions, the ICRC works to promote and strengthen respect for international humanitarian law and principles in situations of conflict and violence.

In relation to health, the ICRC strives to provide those affected by conflict and violence with access to health care, and to remind parties to the conflict of their legal obligations to protect health care facilities and personnel during armed hostilities. Its influence as a diplomatic actor has arguably been both facilitated and hindered by its policy of confidentiality. While acting as an advocate for international humanitarian law and human rights, the ICRC does not speak publicly regarding specific cases of abuse. This facilitates the ICRC's access to monitor violations of international law and to present those violations to the countries concerned as a reminder of their responsibilities under the Geneva Conventions. However, they will not share specific violations of the Geneva Conventions

---

[c]The Consolidated Appeal Process (CAP) brings together humanitarian organizations to identify needs and priorities in the humanitarian crisis, plan and coordinate the response of multiple humanitarian actors, and issue a collective appeal for funds. For information on the CAP, see the OCHA website: http://ochaonline.un.org/humanitarianappeal/webpage.asp?Page=1243

publicly, which enhances their ability to perform "silent diplomacy," but also undermines their ability to mobilize other states and non-state actors in public advocacy campaigns.

Transnational NGOs

Transnational NGOs include secular organizations such as MSF and CARE, and also faith-based transnational NGOs, such as World Vision, Catholic Relief Services, and Islamic Relief, which provide assistance in a diversity of settings.

Lacking rigid bureaucracies, NGOs tend to be more flexible and adaptable than either states or international institutions, and this flexibility gives them the ability to navigate and influence domestic, regional, and international humanitarian actions. They mobilize international campaigns to heighten awareness of emergencies, and they raise funds for the humanitarian response. They are key participants in coordination forums at both the international level and the local level. Some NGOs focus on improving the accountability of various institutions through monitoring humanitarian action and reporting on results. Many NGOs are able to link to national-level organizations and thus facilitate their involvement in national and international campaigns.[15]

National and local NGOs

National organizations are also critical actors in the delivery of humanitarian assistance. They often have better access to populations at risk during hostilities, greater ability to navigate the complexities of local culture and politics, and working with these organizations can build local capacity. National and local NGOs can be important implementing partners for international organizations and also independent providers of health-related assistance in humanitarian settings.

Actors facilitating the delivery of humanitarian assistance

While much of the focus on health diplomacy has been on those groups actively engaged in the delivery of medical assistance, other actors enable the delivery of health assistance during humanitarian crises.

Donor states

Donor states play a crucial role. Not only do they fund humanitarian action, they also assist in mobilizing international action by championing humanitarian responses at the UNSC and UNGA, hosting donor conferences, undertaking *démarches* with like-minded states to request financial support for the humanitarian effort, reminding parties of their obligations under international law, and monitoring humanitarian assistance in the recipient state. Donor states also sit on the governing boards of multilateral organizations, provide bilateral assistance to recipient states, and fund the activities of many transnational organizations. As a result, donors are able to influence international priorities during the humanitarian response, and encourage adherence to international norms, coordination mechanisms, and accountability structures. While they can have a significant influence on humanitarian response at the international and national levels, their ability to shape actors and processes at the local level is less clear.

Regional organizations

The role of the African Union (AU), European Union (EU), Organization of American States (OAS), and Association of South East Asian Nations (ASEAN) in shaping diplomacy within the humanitarian response has not been studied in depth. Yet, as we will see in the case study section below, regional organizations can play an important role in raising awareness of crises in international forums, promoting adherence to international humanitarian law, negotiating access for humanitarian personnel, and encouraging their member states to provide financial re-sources to support the humanitarian effort. Their influence ranges from international forums to country-level mechanisms.

Recipient states

The state in which the humanitarian crisis unfolds is also a crucial diplomatic actor. While its influence is most strongly felt at the national and local levels, it can also have limited influence on regional and international processes. The recipient country hopefully facilitates the entry of humanitarian goods and personnel, facilitates access to affected populations and participates in country-level coordination meetings. Internationally, the recipient state represents its interests at meetings of the United Nations, outlining its needs, defending its own response to the emergency, and in some cases advocating a more robust international response.

International military personnel

International military personnel mandated by international and regional organizations, including representatives of the North Atlantic Treaty Organization (NATO), and peacekeeping troops from the UN, the AU, and the EU are also important actors in humanitarian diplomacy. They facilitate the entry of humanitarian goods/personnel; help maintain the neutrality, independence, and impartiality of humanitarian health workers; and ensure that health workers and infrastructure are protected. As noted in the chapter by McInnes and Rushton, in an increasing number of contexts their involvement extends beyond the provision of a safe and secure environment to the provision of medical assistance and other forms of humanitarian aid.

Conflict protagonists

The protagonists of war are often not perceived as actors engaged in health diplomacy. However, their role is critical. They can either facilitate or impede the delivery of humanitarian assistance, and they may provide protection of health workers and the civilians seeking assistance.

What are the Tools of Health Diplomacy? The Instruments of Humanitarian Action

We have established that the objective of health diplomacy in humanitarian action is to provide emergency, life-saving medical assistance to civilians; outlined the urgency of the timeframe for this diplomatic action; identified the key forums in which that diplomacy takes place; and reviewed the actors that deliver assistance as well as those that facilitate its delivery. But how do humanitarian actors in these various forums navigate this complex universe? How do they persuade donors, the recipient state, and conflict protagonists that health assistance will be effective and in their best interests? The key tools of diplomacy within humanitarian action include international norms and agreements, coordination mechanisms, and technical standards. These tools facilitate collaboration among actors engaged in humanitarian assistance and are critical for reaching the objectives of humanitarian assistance to civilian populations.

International norms

International norms (and related agreements) are "shared expectations about appropriate behavior held by a community of actors."[16] They range from treaties with sanctions that punish defection, to norms that are agreed upon by states but have no enforcement mechanisms. Norms influence international cooperation by providing models for expected behavior and practice; they identify appropriate and inappropriate actions of states.[17] They are developed either through explicit negotiation and agreements among states or through years of international practice. International norms related to humanitarian assistance include rules governing the behavior of parties to the conflict, the responsibilities of states, and guidelines for humanitarian organizations engaged in delivering the humanitarian assistance. A separate set of norms has been developed for humanitarian engagement in conflict situations.

Four norms in particular emerged as central defining characteristics of humanitarian organizations, developed over decades of humanitarian action and affirmed in Resolutions of the United Nations General Assembly:[d]

- Humanity: Humanitarian action must protect the health and life of, and promote respect for, civilian populations.
- Neutrality: During hostilities, humanitarian actors must not take sides, or "engage in controversies of a political, racial, religious or ideological nature."

---

[d]See UN General Assembly (UNGA) Resolution 46/182, which was passed in 1991; and UNGA Resolution 58/114, in 2004.

- Impartiality: Humanitarian assistance must be provided on the basis of need, with aid prioritizing situations of distress, with no distinctions related to race, nationality, religion, or ideology.
- Operational independence: Humanitarian assistance must be autonomous from political, economic, and military objectives.[18]

The Geneva Conventions (agreed to in 1949) and its Additional Protocols, as well as human rights law, include the following measures to enable civilians to access health services and protect health facilities:[19]

- The wounded, the sick, and civilians must be protected from the effects of war, no one should be willfully left without medical assistance and care, and the wounded, the sick, the infirm, and expectant mothers should receive particular protection.
- Health care personnel cannot be attacked, harmed, or hindered in the performance of medical tasks.
- Health care personnel cannot be harassed or punished for "performing activities compatible with medical ethics," compelled to "perform activities contrary to medical ethics," or to refrain from "performing acts required by medical ethics."
- Medical personnel decide, in accordance with medical ethics, which patients receive priority treatment.
- Health care facilities must be protected against attack, provided that they are not used to commit acts harmful to the enemy, such as storing arms and ammunition or sheltering able-bodied combatants.[19]

These norms are important tools for both sets of actors — those that deliver health assistance, and those that facilitate delivery of assistance. They provide guidelines for the behavior of those actors that deliver humanitarian assistance, as well as those actors that can facilitate or impede that delivery, including conflict protagonists, donor states, and recipient governments. While they are not always respected, they are an important benchmark regarding the access to civilians in need and the delivery of humanitarian assistance. International norms facilitate diplomacy during humanitarian crises. They are shared expectations regarding the behavior of parties to the conflict toward civilians; how humanitarian organizations should provide emergency assistance; and the behavior of all actors toward those humanitarian organizations.

Humanitarian coordination

Given the number of actors engaged in humanitarian assistance in different forums, the compressed timeframe for humanitarian action, and the urgency of the response, ensuring that aid is delivered in an effective and efficient manner is paramount. Coordination mechanisms have been established as nonbinding guidelines to facilitate aid delivery. These guidelines clarify the roles and responsibilities of various actors, outline how these actors should work together, and provide a forum and mechanism for discussion and dialogue. Such guidelines also provide a useful reference point for humanitarian actors monitoring that assistance.

The Cluster System is one key coordination mechanism. Clusters are groups of humanitarian organizations operating in the main sectors of humanitarian action, such as health, water and sanitation, and protection. Organizations that are part of a cluster agree to share information and coordinate their response during a humanitarian emergency. A cluster is headed by one or two organizations, which usually remain the consistent leads at both the global and the national level. This consistency helps build capacity and facilitates the transfer of lessons and experiences from crisis to crisis. Globally, cluster leads work to strengthen preparedness and coordinate technical capacity in their area of responsibility. At the country and field levels, cluster lead agencies coordinate the activities of their members and are the main point of contact for the recipient state.[14] Their objective is to maximize the collective work of their organizations and facilitate the effective delivery of humanitarian assistance.

The CAP is another important diplomatic tool for coordinating the activities of multiple actors in complex emergencies and for achieving the objective of efficiently delivering humanitarian assistance. Through it, the humanitarian community and the host governments assess the humanitarian needs, including health, of the civilian population; they develop a strategy for how these needs will be met in a coordinated manner; and they identify and cost out complementary projects that respond to these needs. As outlined above, the head of OCHA — the Emergency Relief

Coordinator — manages the CAP at the global level; while, within the recipient country, the process is managed by the Humanitarian Coordinator. Within the health sector, WHO leads the discussions on health priorities and projects within the CAP.

Technical standards

Another essential diplomatic element in humanitarian action is the application of technical standards on the quantity, quality, and methods of delivering humanitarian assistance. Technical guidelines include "The Humanitarian Charter and Minimum Standards for Disaster Response," better known as the *Sphere Handbook*, developed by a group of NGOs and the Red Cross and Red Crescent Movement in 1997 and frequently updated,[20] or the guidelines developed and endorsed by the IASC on various aspects of the health response in humanitarian action, including guidelines on mental health and psychosocial support, gender-based violence interventions, and HIV interventions in emergency settings.[21-23] The objective of these tools is to increase the quality and effectiveness of medical interventions in humanitarian engagement. They also form an important standard for those monitoring humanitarian assistance.

How Does Diplomacy Unfold? The Key Processes of Health Diplomacy in Humanitarian Action

Utilizing the language of health diplomacy, there are five key "processes through which States, intergovernmental organizations, and non-state actors negotiate responses" to reach the objective of providing humanitarian assistance to civilian populations.

Declaration of a humanitarian emergency

Multilateral organizations, donor states, and NGOs must first determine if a humanitarian crisis exists. While this determination is often *ad hoc*, the official definition of an emergency is if the crude mortality rate is over 1 death per 10,000 per day, and the under 5 mortality rate is over 2 deaths per 10,000 per day.[20] With such basic information, multilateral organizations and NGOs can document the scale and scope of the crises and determine if external intervention is required. With this declaration, multilateral organizations may remind donor states, recipient states, humanitarian actors, and other relevant actors of their obligations under international law, the importance of coordination mechanisms, and the role of technical standards in the response.

Establish health priorities

Ideally, multilateral organizations, NGOs, and the recipient state work to determine humanitarian needs and set priorities for humanitarian action, including the specific health response. Together they determine the most vulnerable groups, the best approaches to reaching those vulnerable groups, and the appropriate evidence-based interventions. The CAP is one mechanism that the humanitarian community utilizes to establish priorities and plan the humanitarian response. Through it, OCHA works to reinforce coordination and the application of technical standards in the humanitarian response. However, the process is often complicated by a lack of data. It is also iterative, as ongoing needs assessments are conducted in the field.

Raise funds

The response to humanitarian emergencies is expensive: mobilizing multilateral agencies and transnational NGOs requires paying for salaries, travel costs, humanitarian supplies, and operational expenses. Therefore an important component of humanitarian diplomacy is the multi-party negotiations for funding from the donor community and the public to support the humanitarian response.[e] Multilateral agencies and transnational donors also engage in their own efforts to mobilize funds.

---

[e] As the mobilization of funds can take time, and as time is of the essence, an important component of the humanitarian reform effort was the establishment of a prepositioned fund within the United Nations. The Central Emergency Response Fund enables early response to humanitarian emergencies and facilitates humanitarian action in underfundedv crises.

Deliver medical assistance

Diplomacy is also a critical process in mobilizing civilian populations to deliver humanitarian assistance to those in need. To deliver that assistance, multilateral agencies and transnational NGOS must navigate customs and visa requirements, arrange for transportation of assistance, and negotiate access with community leaders, the military, and conflict protagonists to serve the affected populations.

Monitor the effectiveness of medical assistance

To ensure that humanitarian assistance is of the appropriate quality and reaches those in need, it is critical to monitor that assistance, report any irregularities, and negotiate with implementing agencies, donors, or those impeding the effective delivery of assistance. Figure 3 summarizes the "ideal" progression of health diplomacy in humanitarian action. However, as outlined below, the process is never so smooth.

The Key Debates in Humanitarian Action

Despite its altruistic nature, humanitarian assistance is not without its acrimonious debates. While these debates take multiple forms, they are

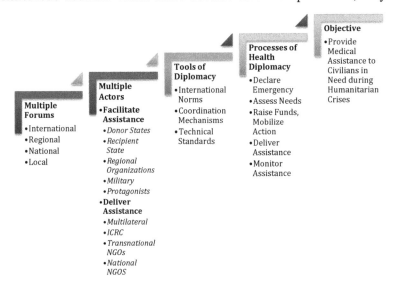

Fig. 3. Health diplomacy in humanitarian action.

reflections on the same theme: the ability and the desirability of humanitarian actors to maintain their adherence to the humanitarian norms of operational independence, impartiality, and neutrality in the face of changing conflict dynamics. There are three main elements in this larger debate: the instrumentalization of health for political purposes; the concept of humanitarian space, its perceived erosion, and the causes of that erosion; and the role of the military in providing or facilitating the delivery of humanitarian aid. As shown in the case studies, these debates are frequently played out in humanitarian diplomacy.

Health for diplomacy or diplomacy for health?

The health and foreign policy literature generally assumes that putting health on the foreign policy agenda is positive, contributing to greater international cooperation to achieve health objectives. From this perspective, not only does instrumentalization elevate health to the level of "high politics," it also helps mobilize political, financial, and institutional resources to address a broad range of global health priorities.[24] Yet there is discomfort within the humanitarian community regarding the framing of health as a foreign policy objective. International diplomacy to achieve health objectives is quite different than using health assistance during humanitarian emergencies to achieve diplomatic objectives. While humanitarian norms, coordination, and technical standards are the necessary "tools" of health diplomacy in humanitarian actions, with the explicit politicization of health, there is no guarantee that states will adhere to these norms, particularly when the provision of humanitarian assistance is associated with political goals and objectives.

The role of the military

The role of the military in providing humanitarian assistance has received increased scrutiny. The military's involvement with humanitarian assistance can take one of three forms. First, the military can work to provide as secure an environment as possible for humanitarian actors to work (securing humanitarian space), while maintaining their distance from the sites of humanitarian activity so as to respect the neutrality of such intervention. Second, the military can provide more active security for humanitarian action, such as security escorts and armed guards for humanitarian actors that deliver assistance. Third, as noted in the chapter by McInnes and Rushton, the military actively provides humanitarian services through the use of military medics and army hospitals — described by some as "tailgate medicine" — or through hospital ships such as the United States Navy Ships (USNS) *Comfort and Mercy*. As noted above, in conflict contexts tailgate medicine may violate the humanitarian norms of impartiality and neutrality, and may not be independent of related political objectives.

The military has many incentives to move beyond securing humanitarian space to the direct provision of medical services. It has significant prepositioned resources at its disposal, an effective command-and-control structure, soldiers organized to work together and take orders, access to heavy equipment and transportation infrastructure, and extensive logistical support resources. These resources ensure that the military can efficiently and effectively provide emergency assistance at short notice. Particularly in the context of a rapid onset natural disaster, these attributes can save many lives. However, the military's association with humanitarian assistance can have both positive and negative externalities in conflictaffected states. As noted by McInnis and Rushton, in the context of a counterinsurgency strategy, the military might use an association with humanitarian assistance to help win the hearts and minds of the local population, and thus make them less prone to support insurgents. Yet, humanitarian actors warn that the provision of humanitarian assistance by the military can erode the neutrality of all humanitarian actors. This erosion of neutrality can make those delivering assistance, as well as those receiving it, the target of attack by other combatants.

Integrated missions and humanitarian space

Humanitarian space is a concept used by the humanitarian community to describe the need for a physical space where humanitarian workers are able to evaluate the needs of civilians, to distribute and monitor assistance, and to maintain dialogue with the civilian population through respect for the neutrality, impartiality, and independence of humanitarian workers. Many scholars debate if and whether humanitarian space is constricted as a result of the changing nature of conflict. More specifically, what is the impact of integrated missions where the international community implements a strategy to increase security, protect civilians, deliver humanitarian assistance, and build political and social institutions to achieve the objective of stabilizing a recipient society?[25] The United Nations is a key political actor in such contexts. Security Council Resolutions frequently direct UN representatives and agencies to coordinate their activities and work together toward the goal of the cessation of violence and the stabilization of society.[26] Bosnia, Kosovo, the Democratic Republic of Congo, and Darfur are all examples of integrated UN missions with stabilization goals.

While promoting efficient use of UN resources, and collaboration toward common UN objectives, how do integrated missions impact on humanitarian agencies affiliated with the UN, as well as the broader humanitarian community? In these missions, the UN builds and supports state institutions, extending that support to whatever government has been elected or selected to occupy those institutions. Protagonists frequently view this support as the UN picking a side, and from their perspective the international community is not neutral. Such erosion of neutrality impacts humanitarian actors as protagonists are unable to distinguish the political arm of the UN [the Special Representative of the Secretary General (SRSG)], the Department of Peacekeeping Operations, and the Office of Political Affairs] from the humanitarian arms of the UN, namely OCHA, WHO, UNHCR, and WFP. The tendency of all international actors to drive white, four-wheel-drive cars does not help distinguish those actors with a humanitarian role from those with a political mandate.

The Application: Health Diplomacy in Action

To analyze health diplomacy in humanitarian action, we examined the humanitarian response to the 2011 hostilities in Libya, the 2010 floods in Pakistan, the 2010 earthquake in Haiti, and the 2008 cyclone in Burma/Myanmar.[f] These cases included the humanitarian response to natural

---

[f] An in-depth analysis of these findings can be found in: Percival V, Bollettino V, Sondorp E, (2011). Speak softly and carry a stethoscope? Health Diplomacy in Humanitarian action. Working Paper, October 2011.

disasters in fragile states (the 2010 earthquake in Haiti), the response to disasters in states with ongoing instability (the 2008 response to Cyclone Nargis in Burma/Myanmar and the 2010 flooding in Pakistan), and the response to civilians impacted by an internationalized civil war (the 2011 rebellion in Libya).

These cases reveal the complexity of health diplomacy in humanitarian action. Assistance was delivered in countries with a devastated capital city and disabled state (Haiti), within a country whose government deeply distrusted any form of international engagement (Burma), in the context of an insurgency (Pakistan), and when NATO was actively engaged in an aerial campaign (Libya). As a result of this complexity, the cases show the critical role that diplomacy, often undertaken simultaneously in multiple forums, plays in securing the delivery of assistance to civilians in need. They also demonstrate the multitude of actors engaged in diplomacy, both in delivering assistance and in facilitating its delivery, and how all these actors are critically important in varying ways to medical assistance in humanitarian action. Yet much of this diplomacy is undocumented, and is also not necessarily recognized as diplomacy.

Below, we summarize the cases, and outline the key humanitarian and health issues. We conclude with an analysis of how health diplomacy facilitates the understanding of these cases, and the contribution of this study of humanitarian action to health diplomacy research. These cases demonstrate that health diplomacy in humanitarian action is complex. It is characterized by multiple forums, where actors who deliver and facilitate the delivery of assistance use the tools and processes of diplomacy to work toward the objective of providing medical assistance to those in need. This is not *ad hoc* diplomacy: these forums, actors, processes, and tools are well established, as they are utilized in most humanitarian responses. Yet the success of these efforts is not guaranteed. Table 1 summarizes the findings of the case studies.

Libya

Protests broke out in Libya on February 17, 2011, as part of the Arab Spring uprisings that spread across the North Africa/Eastern Mediterranean region. The response by the Gaddafi regime was swift and violent,

Table 1. Health Diplomacy in Action

	Libya	Haiti	Pakistan	Burma
Objective: Access to Populations	Extremely limited access to civilian populations — access mainly in rebel areas	Access achieved — impediments were scale of devastation and number of NGOs	Partial access achieved — impediments were scale of disaster, role of military	Access achieved after 25 May Yangon meeting
Timeframe	Hostilities began February 11, 2010 Flash appeal March 7	Earthquake struck January 12, 2010 Flash appeal January 15	Monsoon rains began July 22, 2010 Flash appeal August 11	Cyclone Nargis May 2, 2008 Flash appeal May 9
Forums				
• *Int'l*	UNSC — several resolutions IASC — Principals' meetings	UNSC — resolution UNGA — resolution IASC — principals' meeting Haiti Donor Conference	UNGA — meeting and resolution IASC — Principals' meeting	Joint UN–ASEAN Donor Meeting
• *Regional*	Libya Crisis Network (OCHA) African Union — not helpful	OAS PAHO	N/A	ASEAN
• *National*	Cluster approach	Cluster approach	Cluster approach National disaster Management authority	Tripartite Core Group — TCG (UN, ASEAN, Burmese government) Humanitarian Coordinator

(Continued)

Table 1. (*Continued*).

	Libya	Haiti	Pakistan	Burma
• **Local**	Cluster approach	Cluster approach	Cluster approach Provincial disaster Management authority	TCG recovery hubs
Actors				
• ***Delivering Assistance***	Multilateral agencies (WHO) ICRC MSF Islamic Relief Libyan Red Cross	Multilateral agencies (PAHO supported by WHO) ICRC Transnational NGOs	Multilateral agencies ICRC Transnational NGOs Local NGOs	Multilaterals (WHO) MSF
• ***Facilitating Assistance***	OCHA (Head of OCHA & Libyan Humanitarian Coordinator) Donors NATO Libyan rebel forces	OCHA — Haiti's Humanitarian Coordinator Haitian Government Donors MINUSTAH	OCHA — Pakistan's Humanitarian Coordinator Pakistan National Disaster Management Authority	UN Secretary General (meeting with Burmese authorities May 23) Humanitarian Coordinator
• **Tools**	Norms Coordination — Cluster System	Norms Coordination — Cluster System Attempts to implement technical standards	Norms Coordination — Cluster System	Norms of impartiality and nonpoliticization of aid important to Myanmar Coordination (TCG)

triggering an armed rebellion and the intervention of the United Nations Security Council. On March 17, UNSCR 1973 authorized member states "acting nationally or through regional organizations" to take all necessary measures to protect civilians. On March 24, NATO began an extensive air campaign to enforce a no-fly zone and to protect civilians. As a result of NATO's involvement, the conflict became internationalized.

Over 860,000 civilians, the majority of them non-Libyans, fled Libya during the fighting, while tens of thousands were displaced within the country. The Ministry of Health reported that an estimated 50,000 were injured as a result of the fighting (there is lack of clarity as to whether the injured were civilians or combatants), with 20,000 of those injuries assessed as severe.[27] Hospitals and clinics were short of essential medical supplies and medicines,[28] and struggled to function with shortages of fuel and water.[27]

The humanitarian response was relatively swift. The IASC held an *ad hoc* meeting of their Principals — the heads of IASC member organizations — on February 28. A consolidated appeal document was launched on March 5, 2011; which identified and prioritized humanitarian needs,[g] appealed for funds, outlined the establishment of coordination mechanisms and the launch of the cluster system, and identified how the humanitarian response would meet technical standards.[29] The appeal received significant support from donors.[30,h] OCHA also set up an informal network of humanitarian agencies working in Libya, Egypt, and Tunisia — known as The Libya Crisis Network.[31]

Yet one key actor, the Libyan state, refused to cooperate, and obstructed health and other forms of humanitarian assistance. As part of its effort to negotiate access, OCHA sent its humanitarian coordinator for Libya, Rashid Khalikov, to Tripoli from[13-16] March to request humanitarian access in government controlled areas. He reported: "The government was of the view that there are no humanitarian needs, that the situation is under control, and that the humanitarian requirements are limited to food and

---

[g]This assessment of humanitarian needs was not based on a widespread assessment mission; the assessment team could access only the eastern part of Libya.
[h]The total amount funded was 60%, yet the health sector received only 30% of the requested funds.

medical supplies. And they have plenty of those, according to them. Yet despite the consensus regarding the existence of a humanitarian emergency, the ability to assess needs and raise funds, humanitarian actors had tremendous difficulty negotiating access to deliver assistance to civilians, particularly in conflict affected areas."[32]

While the Security Council repeatedly reminded parties to the conflict of their obligations under international humanitarian law, including "ensuring safe passage of humanitarian and medical supplies, and humanitarian agencies and workers, into the country,"[33] hospitals, medical workers, and patients were too frequently the target of violence.[34] Snipers attacked hospitals, patients attempting to access hospitals, and ambulances.[35] Five members of the Libyan Red Cross were killed while providing medical assistance.[34]

After the April 17 visit of Valerie Amos, UN Under Secretary General for Humanitarian Affairs and head of OCHA, the Gaddafi government reached an agreement to allow humanitarian organizations to access civilians in need.[36] However, this agreement was repeatedly violated. Even NATO was reluctant to suspend the bombing campaign to allow the delivery of humanitarian assistance.[37] Humanitarian access was facilitated in rebel-controlled areas, but many cities and towns under the control of the Gaddafi regime remained too dangerous for humanitarian action. The various actors, forums, tools, and processes outlined above were evident in Libya. Critical international forums included the UNSC and the IASC, and local forums included the initiation of the cluster system. Regional forums, such as the African Union, were less helpful in terms of health diplomacy because of the close relationship of African leaders with Gaddafi.[38] Multiple actors engaged in health diplomacy at the international, national, and local levels, attempting to use the tools of international norms and coordination to deliver medical assistance to civilians in need. Internationally, multilateral organizations and states reminded parties to the conflict of their obligations under international humanitarian law, most visibly through resolutions at the United Nations Security Council and through *démarches* by OCHA envoys. At the national level, OCHA, the ICRC, and NGOs such as MSF continuously pressed parties to the conflict to assure humanitarian access to victims.

This case demonstrates the clear limits of health diplomacy within internationalized conflicts. The Gaddafi regime restricted humanitarian access, placing the lives of thousands of civilians at risk, while NATO was reluctant to grant a ceasefire to assure access to affected populations. The internationalized nature of the conflict, where the UNSC and NATO intervened on behalf of civilians, made this an integrated mission, where the political role of the UN was hard to distinguish from its humanitarian role. Even the evocation of the tools of health diplomacy — first and foremost, humanitarian norms — did not always work, and humanitarian organizations were not always able to achieve its objective of providing medical assistance to civilians in need.

Haiti

On January 12, 2010, a magnitude 7 earthquake struck Haiti, with the epicenter in Leogane, just west of the capital city of Port au Prince. The devastation was immediate and severe. The earthquake killed an estimated 220,000 people, injured over 300,000,[39] and left 1.3 million displaced in 1354 spontaneous settlements.[39] Of a total Haitian population of 10 million, 3 million were affected. Needs assessments estimated that 105,000 homes were completely destroyed and over 208,000 damaged.[40] The total damage and economic losses from the earthquake are estimated at US$7.8 billion, which was slightly more than the entire Haitian GDP in 2009.[40]

The earthquake also devastated the capacities of the Haitian government, civil society groups, and international organizations already active on-site. To complicate these challenges, Haiti was also emerging from decades of political violence and instability. Prior to the earthquake, 86% of the Haitian population lived in slums, with 40% lacking access to health care. Only 25% of Haitian women gave birth in a health facility.[41] The health system in Haiti was largely supported by NGOs and outside donors.

Although the capacity of many international organizations was undermined by the impact of the earthquake, in general the humanitarian response was swift. The timeframe for action was critical: the nature (trauma) of the injuries and the scope of the devastation required immediate action.

The humanitarian community quickly moved to mobilize teams to rescue the injured and assess the humanitarian needs. A flash appeal was issued on January 15, and OCHA moved to implement the cluster system within the Haitian response at the national and local levels, although coordination was a challenge in the days following the earthquake given the destruction of communication networks, blockage of roads, and displacement of large populations.

Multiple forums were utilized almost simultaneously to mobilize international assistance. The IASC Principals held a consultation on Haiti on January 15. Both the UNSC and the UNGA released resolutions on the situation in Haiti, with the UNSC increasing the size of the peace-keeping force (MINUSTAH) on January 19,[42] while on January 22 the UNGA asked member states to support the flash appeal and to "to ensure that the humanitarian assistance provided is timely, adequate, effective and coherent and coordinated among all humanitarian actors, in particular the Government of Haiti, and in accordance with the principles of humanity, neutrality, impartiality and independence."[43] Regional forums were also utilized to mobilize support, with the Organization of American States (OAS) providing aid and requesting member states to contribute. Donor conferences were held in Montreal (January 25) and New York (March 31).

By the end of January, 396 international health agencies were engaged in a broad range of health activities in Haiti.[39] The Pan-American Health Organization (PAHO), the regional office of the WHO in the Americas, reported that by May 2010, 900,000 vaccine doses had been administered, 17 field hospitals (11 run by the military) had been established, and the PROMESS (Programme des Médicaments Essentiels) warehouse had distributed 345,000 boxes of medical supplies.[39] Twenty-one international organizations provided emergency health services to 266 IDP sites,[39] and in Port au Prince 90% of internally displaced persons (IDPs) had access to health clinics.[40]

Unlike in Libya, the blending together of political and security objectives and the reinforcement of the MINUSTAH mission did not undermine health diplomacy. Transnational NGOs and multilateral agencies were able to ensure that the majority of Haitians were able to access medical assistance. Yet questions were raised about the efficiency of this response.

While the humanitarian community quickly established coordination mechanisms and identified relevant technical standards, the over 400 NGOs registered with the health cluster made coordination and monitoring of assistance almost impossible, particularly at the local level. The feasibility of coordination, as well as the technical quality, and the effectiveness and efficiency of assistance given this large number of health actors in Haiti were also questioned, with one humanitarian querying: "Should we always aim to coordinate all health actors in a major disaster or should we coordinate the major actors?"[44]

While the response to the earthquake is an example of global health diplomacy, meeting its immediate objectives, the cholera epidemic that struck Haiti in late 2010 underscored concerns regarding the effectiveness of the humanitarian response. In little over a month, the outbreak killed more than 2000 people.[45] Despite the presence of hundreds of nongovernmental organizations, the functioning of a PAHO-led health cluster, the inflow of donor resources, and the ease and availability of treatment for cholera, the case fatality rate for hospitalized patients in the early days of the outbreak was 9%, falling to 3.5% several weeks later.[45] This fatality rate raised serious concerns regarding the implementation of technical standards and the quality of the health response.

Pakistan

In 2010, Pakistan was hit by the worst flooding in memory. The flooding began on July 22 in the north, affecting some of the same areas where 2.1 million had previously been displaced by a military offensive against insurgents (2008–2009), and where the military remained actively engaged in counterinsurgency activities.[46] Many individuals living in this region were already vulnerable, with many previously affected by poverty and food insecurity.[47]

The scope and scale of the disaster posed difficulties for humanitarian action. Early estimates placed the number of affected people at 14 million, with 1200 killed in the first weeks of the floods.[48] Beyond the hardship of displacement, the floods had a devastating impact on livelihoods throughout the region. Access to health care was undermined, with 236 health facilities damaged and 200 facilities destroyed across the flooded region.[46] By the time the water receded, the floods had killed 1980 people, impacted one-third of Pakistan's geographic area, affected 18 million people (one-tenth of the Pakistani population), destroyed 2.2 million hectares of crops, killed half-a-million livestock, and damaged or destroyed 1.7 million homes and schools.[47]

The slow response of the Pakistani government, as well as the international community, was criticized.[49] A flash appeal was launched on August 11, and the cluster system was operationalized. Yet the donor response to the floods remained sluggish, prompting a Special Session of the UN General Assembly, held on August 18,[50] and a UNGA Resolution, which called on the international community to provide financial support to humanitarian efforts.[51] The IASC did not hold consultations on Pakistan until August 19, when they held a teleconference of Emergency Directors, while the IASC Principals did not meet to discuss the crisis until August 20.

Within Pakistan, the Humanitarian Coordinator worked with the National Disaster Management Authority, which was responsible for the coordination of the national disaster response by both the international community and the Pakistani government.[47] Over 20,000 Pakistani troops and 2,500 international troops also participated in the relief efforts.[47] At the local level, the Provincial Disaster Management Authorities coordinated the response.[47] Yet the capacity of these local actors was very limited: the National Disaster Management Authority reportedly received insufficient financial support from the government, with an annual budget of only US$740,000 and a full-time staff of 21 officers.[52]

The ability of humanitarian actors to access those affected by the floods was undermined by several factors. Within many of these areas, international NGOs had a limited presence due to ongoing security concerns, and the humanitarian response faced a critical shortfall of human resources.[47] Coordination between local authorities and UN agencies was reportedly hampered by language difficulties.[52] In addition, the Pakistani military attempted to control relief efforts. Particularly in the areas previously affected by conflict, the military restricted the access of humanitarian actors to affected civilians.[49] Moreover, there were concerns regarding the military's adherence to humanitarian principles, with allegations that during the IDP crises in the north the military forcefully returned IDPs to areas that lacked sufficient services.[49]

By January 31, 2011, medical assistance had been provided to 10 million people, with 9.3 million people receiving essential medicines.[47] A year later, 70% of the funding requirements set out in the CAP had been met, with the health cluster funded at 56%.[46] Yet there remains deep dissatisfaction among the population and humanitarian workers with the response, as approximately 800,000 remained displaced a year after the flooding, and high food prices and few job opportunities characterize much of the region.[53] At the international level, health diplomacy was successful in ramping up the initially slow international response. However, at the local level, many humanitarian actors were constrained by the military's control over affected areas, the challenges of coordinating with national authorities, and the scale and scope of the disaster. These factors impeded their ability to effectively reach populations in need.

Burma

Burma, like Pakistan, experienced a natural disaster while dealing with internal strife. Cyclone Nargis struck Burma on May 2–3, 2008, bringing a 12-foot storm surge that devastated the delta region southwest of Yangon. The cyclone killed over 84,000 people with 53,000 missing, injured 19,000, and severely affected 2.4 million people.[54] The Burmese government was simultaneously fighting a rebellion against several ethnic groups, including the Karen, in the border area with Thailand. In addition, they faced a democratization movement at home, led by Aung San Suu Kyi, and the cyclone struck one week prior to a national vote on a new constitution.[55] The military regime that controlled Burma was fearful of any international engagement. As a result of the UN's condemnation of the actions of the Burmese military government, that distrust extended to the UN itself.

While the existence of a humanitarian emergency was not in doubt, the Burmese government initially refused to issue visas for additional humanitarian personnel, relax the procedures to allow internationals to travel outside of Yangon, or allow international assistance into Burma unless that assistance was provided through bilateral channels "with no strings attached."[55] When an ICRC plane filled with relief supplies landed in Yangon on May 8, the supplies were distributed by the Myanmar

Red Cross.[56] Yet the international community was wary of channeling assistance through the Burmese government, for fear that the government would not adhere to humanitarian norms to provide assistance on the basis of neutrality and impartiality.

Despite the protestations of the government that it could handle the crisis, it lacked the logistical capacity to respond. As a result, three weeks after the cyclone, only a quarter of the affected population had received assistance.[57] The condemnation from some members of the international community was swift, and included a call from French Foreign Minister Bernard Kouchner to evoke the Responsibility to Protect Doctrine and hold a special meeting of the United Nations Security Council (which was thwarted by China).

As an example of why regional forums can be so critical to health diplomacy, the Association of South East Asian Nations (ASEAN) stepped in to mediate in this dispute. On May 8, the Burmese government and the ASEAN Secretariat agreed to the deployment of an ASEAN Rapid Assessment Team.[58] The Team undertook its field assessment from May 9–18, and submitted its report to a special meeting of the ASEAN Foreign Ministers.[59] The ASEAN Humanitarian Task Force was established, chaired by the Secretary-General of ASEAN, and comprised officials from ASEAN member states, with an advisory group consisting of neighboring countries, the Red Cross, the World Bank, and NGOs.[59] To facilitate the distribution of humanitarian assistance within an environment of distrust, ASEAN proposed to the Burmese government the creation of the Tripartite Core Group (TCG), consisting of the government of Burma, ASEAN, and the United Nations.[59] This group would oversee the humanitarian operation, including coordination, resources, operations, monitoring, and reporting.[58]

On May 25, an ASEAN–UN pledging conference was held in Yangon, where the TCG was announced, and the Burmese government agreed to important international norms regarding humanitarian assistance.[59] The Chairmen's Summary included the following statement: "There was unanimous agreement on the need to scale up urgently and very significantly the current relief efforts, to ensure that *all those in desperate need* are reached quickly and with adequate life-saving relief supplies, and that an *effective flow of these supplies is maintained* for as long as is necessary, through the establishment of the necessary logistical arrangements and an acceleration of the arrival and distribution of vital relief goods. The agreement of the Government of Myanmar to *facilitate international relief workers* to enter and operate in the country, will undoubtedly contribute to the necessary immediate stepping up of the relief operation."[60] (Emphasis added.)

The Burmese case provides us with an example of how humanitarian actors utilized diplomacy in multiple forums to ensure that medical and other forms of humanitarian assistance reached civilians in need. This accomplishment is noteworthy given the strained political relationship between the UN and the Burmese government.

Conclusion: Health Diplomacy as a Framework for Analyzing Humanitarian Action

These cases demonstrate the enormity, and complexity, and messiness of the health response to humanitarian crises. Forums at the international, regional, national, and local levels are utilized to raise awareness of the need for health engagement, raise resources, identify needs, determine the appropriate technical response, and deliver and monitor that assistance. A multitude of actors are engaged in these processes, including those actors that facilitate health assistance and those that deliver it. Instruments of health diplomacy, including humanitarian norms, technical standards, and coordination mechanisms, are utilized to persuade actors that the delivery of assistance will be efficient, effective, and in their best interest. Given the complexity of international engagement in humanitarian crises, it is a diplomatic achievement that medical and other forms of humanitarian assistance reach civilians in need in such challenging conditions.

What is exceedingly clear from the cases is that despite efforts by multilateral organizations and NGOs to underscore their adherence to humanitarian norms and principles, political relations between donor states and recipient countries are critically important in determining the ability of humanitarian actors to reach civilian populations. Where political relations are strained, it is more challenging to deliver medical assistance to civilians in need, as the cases of Libya and Burma clearly demonstrate. Moreover, in situations where donor states were engaged in supporting a government fighting an insurgency (Pakistan), efforts to ensure that humanitarian assistance remained neutral, impartial, and independent were under pressure, as underscored by the efforts by the Pakistan military and government to control access to populations in need.

These case studies also demonstrate that health diplomacy is a useful lens through which to examine humanitarian action, as it facilitates a broad focus on diplomatic activities within international, regional, national, and local forums and among those actors that deliver assistance as well as those that facilitate its delivery. In addition, the health diplomacy lens highlights the specific tools and processes of health diplomacy within the humanitarian response. Moreover, the comparative studies of health diplomacy, as summarized in Table 1, highlight the consistency in the forums, actors, tools, and processes of health diplomacy across case studies.

What is striking about all the case studies is how quickly diplomacy unfolded. Within days and weeks of the recognition of a humanitarian crisis, the international community had identified needs and established coordination mechanisms through the CAP, pressed international donors for support, and reminded all parties of their obligations under humanitarian norms and principles. This compressed diplomatic timeframe, while a challenge, also opened doors for those organizations with the capacity to navigate a multitude of forums — from the international to the local — to influence the process through their ability to identify those humanitarian needs, articulate those needs to donors, and initiate the humanitarian response. As a result, health diplomacy often occurred simultaneously across various forums. While international-level forums were utilized to raise awareness of the crises and remind actors of their normative obligations, at the local level organizations were engaged in the exercise of identifying needs and the appropriate technical responses. Forums were also used as catalysts for action. In some cases, such as Burma, new forums such as ASEAN were needed to enable access to populations in need. In others, such as Pakistan, high-level forums such as the UNGA were needed to raise awareness of the scope of the crises and the importance of international response.

While the diplomatic processes were the same in all cases, some cases were more complex than others. In Burma, the government initially refused to acknowledge that the damage brought by Cyclone Nargis exceeded its capacity to respond. The identification of needs and priorities can be extremely challenging when there is little access to that population (Libya) or when the military attempts to control that access (Pakistan). Raising funds is easier in sudden-onset emergencies (Haiti) but more challenging in slower-onset natural disasters (Pakistan). The delivery of assistance, and convincing parties to the conflict of the neutrality, impartiality, and independence of medical assistance, is more challenging in situations of internationalized conflict (Libya) or when the United Nations has taken a politically active role in critiquing the government (Burma). Monitoring and accountability is very challenging when coordination mechanisms are overwhelmed by the sheer scale of the disaster and the number of NGOs engaged in the response (Haiti).

More research is needed to examine the specifics of the medical response to humanitarian crises. This desk study of Libya, Haiti, Pakistan, and Burma did not illuminate if and how the health dimension of humanitarian response differs from other humanitarian sectors. Is it easier to negotiate access to civilians to deliver medical assistance, than other forms of assistance? Field research is needed to determine if and how health assistance differs from other forms of humanitarian action. Such studies could contribute to a broader understanding of health diplomacy, to determine if and how it is distinct from other forms of diplomacy, and the conditions for its success.

Acknowledgments

The author would like to thank Michael Brisson and Shannon Rosset for their invaluable research assistance during the preparation of this chapter.

References

1. Minear L, Smith H. (2007) *Humanitarian Diplomacy: Practitioners and Their Craft.* United Nations University Press, Tokyo.
2. Mancini-Griffoli D, Picot A. (2004) *Humanitarian Negotiation.* Centre for Humanitarian Dialogue, Geneva.
3. Minear L, Smith H. (eds.) (2007) *Humanitarian Diplomacy: Practitioners and Their Craft.* United Nations University Press, Tokyo.
4. Feldbaum H, Michaud J. (2010) Health diplomacy and the enduring relevance of foreign policy interests. *PLOS Med* **7(4)**.

5. Kickbusch I, Silberschmidt G, Buss P. (2007) Global health diplomacy: The need for new perspectives, strategic approaches and skills in global health. *Bull World Health Organ* **85(3):** 230–232.

6. Smith R, Fidler D, Lee K. (2009) *Global Health Diplomacy Research*. WHO Network on Global Health Diplomacy, Geneva.

7. Noji EK. (1997) *The Public Health Consequences of Disasters*. Oxford University Press, Oxford.

8. Levy BS, Sidel VW. (1997) *War and Public Health*. Oxford University Press, New York.

9. Burkle F. (2006) Complex humanitarian emergencies: A review of epidemiological and response models. *J Postgrad Med* **52:** 110–115.

10. Fearon J. (2008) Economic develoepnt, insurgency and civil war. In: Helpman E (ed.), *Institutions and Economic Performance*. Harvard University Press, pp. 292–328.

11. HSRP. (2008) *Miniatlas of Human Security*. Myriad, Brighton.

12. Nel P, Righarts M. (2008) Natural disasters and the risk of violent civil conflict. *Int Stud Quart* **52:** 159–185.

13. Spiegel P, Checchi F, Columbo S, Paik E. (2010) Health-care needs of people affected by conflict: Future trends and changing frameworks. *Lancet* **375:** 341–345.

14. IASC. (2010) *Handbook for RCs and HCs on Emergency Preparedness and Response*. IASC, Geneva.

15. McCoy D, Hilson M. (2009) Civil society, its organizations, and global health governance. In: Buse K, Hein W, Drager N (eds.) (2009) *Making Sense of Global Health Governance*. Palgrave Macmillan, Houndsmills.

16. Finnemore M, Sikkink K. (1998) International norm dynamics and political change. *Int Organ* **52(4):** 887–917.

17. O'Neill K, Balsiger J, Van Deveer S. (2004) Actors, norms and impact: Recent international cooperation theory and the influence of the agent-structure debate. *Annu Rev Polit Sci* **7:** 149–175.

18. IASC. (2000) *International Humanitarian Norms & Principles: Guidance Materials*. IASC, Geneva.

19. ICRC. (2011) Health Care in Danger: Making the Case. ICRC, Geneva.

20. The Sphere Project. (2011) *The Sphere Project: Humanitarian Charter and Minimum Standards in Humanitarian Response*. Practical Action Publishing, Rugby.

21. IASC. (2009) *IASC Guidelines on Mental Health and Psychosocial Support in Emergency Settings*. IASC, Geneva.
22. IASC. (2005) *Guidelines for Addressing HIV in Humanitarian Settings*. IASC, Geneva.
23. IASC. (2005) *Guidelines for Gender-based Violence in Humanitarian Settings*. IASC, Geneva.
24. Horton R. (2007) Health as an instrument of foreign policy. *Lancet* **369:** 806–807.
25. Collinson S, Elhawary S, Muggah R. (2010) States of fragility: Stabilisation and its implications for humanitarian action. *Disasters.* **34(s3):** s275–s296.
26. Egeland J, Harmer A, Stoddard A. (2011) *To Stay and Deliver: Good Practice for Humanitarians in Complex Security Environments*. United Nations, New York.
27. WHO. (2011) *Health and Nutrition Cluster Bulletin: Crisis in Libyan Arab Jamahiriya*. WHO, Geneva.
28. OCHA. (2011) Libya: Mirsata is difficult to access. Humanitarian assessment finds people in need of medical supplies. OCHA, Geneva (cited October 5). Available from http://www.unocha.org/top-stories/all-stories/libya-misrata-difficult-access-humanitarian-assessment-finds-people-need-med
29. OCHA. (2011) *Regional Flash Appeal for the Libyan Crisis*. OCHA, New York.
30. Walmsley L. (2011) *Libya Crisis #1*. Global Humanitarian Assistance, Wells.
31. OCHA. (2011) *Libyan Arab Jamahiriyah: Situation Report No. 2*. OCHA, Geneva, New York.
32. Schlein L. (2011) Libya: No need for international aid. *Voice of America*, March 23.
33. UNSC. (2011) Resolution 1970. United Nations.
34. Michel B. (2011) Libya: Humanitarian challenges six months on. ICRC, Geneva (cited October 5). Available from: http://www.icrc.org/eng/resources/documents/interview/2011/libya-interview-2011-08-12.htm
35. CNN wire staff. (2011) Doctors operating without anesthesia in Misrata hospital. *CNNWorld*, March 24.
36. UNSG. (2011) Secretary-General's press conference after meeting President Pal Schmitt of Hungary. United Nations (cited October 5). Available from http://www.un.org/apps/sg/offthecuff.asp?nid=1787

37. Clark C. (2011) Crack's showing in NATO's Libya strategy. *Globe and Mail*, June 22.

38. Has the African Union got Libya wrong? *Reuters Africa News Blog*, August 31.

39. PAHO. (2010) *Situation Update: Nine Months After the Earthquake in Haiti*. Washington, PAHO2010, October 4.

40. IASC. (2010) *Response to the Humanitarian Crisis in Haiti Following the 12 January 2010 Earthquake: Achievement, Challenges and Lessons to Be Learned*. IASC, Geneva.

41. Lewis C. (2010) Learning from experience: Haiti. Presentation to Wellcome Trust, June 2010, London.

42. UNSC. (2010) Resolution 1908. UNSC, New York.

43. UNGA. (2010) Resolution 64/250: Humanitarian assistance, emergency relief and rehabilitation in response to the devastating effects of the earthquake in Haiti. United Nations.

44. IASC. (2010) Global Health Cluster Meeting. International Federation of Red Cross and Red Crescent Societies, Geneva.

45. PAHO. (2010) *Health Cluster Bulletin: Cholera Outbreak in Haiti #5*. PAHO, Port au Prince.

46. United Nations Office in Pakistan. (2011) *Pakistan Floods: One Year On*. United Nations Office in Pakistan, Islamabad.

47. Report of the Secretary General. (2011) Strengthening emergency relief, rehabilitation, reconstruction and prevention in the wake of devastating floods in Pakistan. United Nations General Assembly.

48. OCHA. (2010) *Pakistan: Initial Floods Emergency Response Plan*. OCHA, New York.

49. Crisis Group. (2010) *Pakistan: The Worsening IDP Crisis*. International Crisis Group, Islamabad/Brussels.

50. UNGA. (2010) *General Assembly Calls for Strengthened Emergency Relief to Meet Pakistan's Urgent Needs after Massive Destruction Caused by Unprecedented, Devastating Floods*. United Nations, New York.

51. UNGA. (2010) Resolution adopted by the General Assembly: Strengthening emergency relief, rehabilitation, reconstruction and prevention in the wake of devastating floods in Pakistan. UNGA, New York.

52. Ahmed I. (2011) One year after its worst flooding, is Pakistan ready for monsoon season? *The Christian Science Monitor*, June.

53. Oxfam. (2011) *Ready or Not: Pakistan's Resilience to Disasters One Year on from the Floods*. Oxfam, Oxford.

54. Tripartite Core Group. (2008) *Post-Nargis Joint Assessment*. ASEAN Secretariat, Jakarta.

55. Belanger J, Horsey R. (2008) Negotiating humanitarian access to cyclone-affected areas of Myanmar: A review. *Humanitarian Exchange Magazine* **41** (December).

56. Red Cross. (2008) *First Red Cross Relief Flight Lands in Myanmar*. Red Cross, Ottawa.

57. Stover E, Vinck P. (2008) Cyclone Nargis and the politics of relief and reconstruction aid in Burma. *JAMA* **300**(6).

58. Creac'h Y-K, Fan L. (2008) ASEAN's role in the Cyclone Nargis response: Implications, lessons and opportunities. *Humanitarian Exchange Magazine* **41** (December).

59. ASEAN. (2010) *A Humanitarian Call: The ASEAN Response to Cyclone Nargis*. ASEAN Secretariat, Jakarta.

60. ASEAN–UN International Pledging Conference on Cyclone Nargis. (2008) ASEAN, Yangon.

10

Key Factors in Negotiations for Health

Kelley Lee, DPhil, MPA, MA*

Introduction

Negotiation is the process of bargaining between two or more interested parties for the purpose of reaching agreement on a matter of mutual concern. Within public health, negotiation may take place on a daily basis and on many different levels, from the interpersonal to the global. For example, negotiation might be used to secure participation by a local community in a new health initiative; to agree on the distribution of limited public resources to address multiple health needs; to agree on the specific intervention to be used to tackle a health issue such as childhood obesity or illicit drug use; or to resolve a conflict over the sharing of authority and responsibility among countries affected by a cross-border disease outbreak. In such situations, analysis usually focuses on the substantive issues that give rise to negotiations. This process of negotiating agreement on health issues has so far received limited attention in the

*Director of Global Health, Associate Dean, Research, Faculty of Health Sciences, Simon Fraser University, Room 11322, Blusson Hall, 8888 University Drive, Burnaby, BC V5A 1S6, Canada.
Tel.: 1 778 782 9039; Fax: 1 778 782 5927.
E-mail: kelley_lee@sfu.ca
URL: http://www.fhs.sfu.ca/portal_memberdata/klee

scholarly literature. Better understanding of the way that health negotiations are conducted is needed, especially when health issues have come to be addressed as a part of foreign policy at the bilateral or multilateral level.

This chapter discusses the key factors for consideration in negotiating agreement on health issues. Whereas many of the considerations described are generic to negotiations in any setting, health issues are often highly technical, involve diverse and multiple stakeholders, are subject to particular accountability demands, may take place under time constraints, and can be characterised by significant uncertainties. Moreover, because health issues increasingly are influenced by globalization, by which many health determinants and outcomes do not conform to the territorial boundaries of states, negotiations to address health issues in this global context have grown in importance. This chapter examines the particular challenges faced in negotiating at the global level and provides examples throughout from a variety of health-related negotiations.

Preparing for Negotiation

The start of any effective negotiation process occurs long before formal discussions by the interested parties. The image of the senior official sitting down with his or her counterpart to sign an agreed document is usually the culmination of substantial preparations that began much earlier. Indeed, whether negotiations do or do not lead to a formal agreement can critically depend on the quality of those preparations.[1]

One of the first tasks in preparing for negotiations is to ensure that there is a clear and shared understanding of the issue to be resolved. With luck, it may be discovered that disagreement is due to a lack of information or perhaps a misunderstanding and prenegotiation discussions may lead to early consensus. In stark contrast, preparations may reveal a political environment that precludes opportunities to negotiate agreement given a sufficient lack of common ground on which to proceed. Determining the situation beforehand can save substantial effort in preparing for, and then conducting, negotiations. If disagreement is indeed confirmed, clarifying the specific points of disagreement helps to focus efforts. An agenda of subissues that break the problem into manageable pieces might be drawn up, especially when the larger problem may seem a considerable task to resolve. It may even be possible to resolve one or more points of disagreement ahead of time and thus to focus subsequent negotiations on the "sticking points." For example, the dispute over the sharing of influenza virus samples initially focused on the broader controversy over the World Trade Organization (WTO) Agreement on Trade-Related Intellectual Property Rights and its protection of pharmaceutical patents. Negotiations over Indonesia's withholding of virus samples have since, however, reached agreement on the principle of equitable access and have moved to establishing a new system of influenza virus and benefits sharing (e.g. stockpiling) that would ensure equitable access in the event of an influenza pandemic.[2]

Once the interested parties have agreed on an agenda of points for negotiation, preparations for discussion of substantive matters can be undertaken. Negotiators must think about the information that is needed to facilitate an understanding of the problem and its resolution. Such analysis might be undertaken by the diplomatic corps, whose role is to gather and analyse background information for policymakers. Such information is used to analyse the contextual environment: what are the factors likely to influence negotiations, who are the key interests involved, and how might the prevailing political or economic environment be relevant? Background analyses should focus on the issue at hand and yet cast their inquiry sufficiently broadly to identify the reasons behind a disagreement and, equally important, the likelihood that specific options will resolve the disagreement, given a particular context. For example, as described in the chapter in this volume by Feldbaum, an understanding of the domestic political aspirations of Indonesian politicians has been important in furthering virus-sharing negotiations.

In addition to the assistance of diplomats, that of technical experts is usually required for the conduct of negotiations on health issues. Health issues often require some knowledge of clinical matters (e.g. impact on human health) or options for intervention (e.g. clinical effectiveness or cost-effectiveness). Or health issues may require knowledge of legal matters and processes such as human rights law or existing international obligations. When a health issue involves other policy sectors, such as trade, agriculture, or the environment, cross-sectoral knowledge is also needed. A good example is the 2007 dispute between the Ministry of Health in Thailand and the pharmaceutical company Abbott Laboratories over the compulsory licensing of the HIV/AIDS drug Kaletra (a combination of ritonavir and lopinavir). Negotiations between the ministry and the private company required specialist knowledge of the drugs themselves and of their effectiveness, as well as a detailed understanding of the legal flexibilities available under the Trade-Related Aspects of Intellectual Property Rights (TRIPS) Agreement and their interpretation under the subsequent Doha Declaration on the TRIPS Agreement and Public Health[3] and the Implementation of paragraph 6 of the Doha Declaration on the TRIPS Agreement and Public Health.[4]

Once an appropriate level of understanding of the substantive content of a health issue under negotiation is achieved, it is essential for negotiators to identify a clear sense of the desired outcome. What form of agreement are negotiators seeking that would signal successful completion? In other words, how would the negotiating parties know when they have reached agreement? This question relates both to a procedural matter and to a matter of due process. Careful planning is required beforehand with regard to those who will be involved in making the decision and how decision-making will take place during negotiations. For example, during the final stages of the Framework Convention on Tobacco Control (FCTC) process, heads of member state delegations were requested to sign the final document indicating agreement with its painstakingly negotiated content. This requirement was an important first step signalling the closure of negotiations on the main text. This document was followed by an agreement that 40 countries would have to ratify the FCTC (formal approval by domestic legislatures) before the treaty could officially come into force as international law. The decision to adopt the framework convention model, instead of a single, detailed treaty for tobacco control, derived from anticipation of strong opposition from the tobacco industry. This approach allowed for additional protocols to be subsequently negotiated on issues that were expected to yield a lower level of consensus.[5] In contrast, the International Code on the Marketing of Breastmilk Substitutes was adopted by a vote of member states at the World Health Assembly in 1981. Whereas the code received the support of an overwhelming majority of member states (with only the United

States abstaining) and had an immediate effect, its status as a nonbinding recommendation meant that it has no legal force to ensure implementation by member states or food companies.[6] The form of agreement reached, in other words, can vary considerably, depending on the issue to be resolved, the stakeholders and interests involved, and the prevailing political context.

Knowing what you want from the negotiations is also essential. The question of what you ideally want may seem relatively straightforward, but effective negotiation is about "give and take," and it is likely that some "giving" will be needed for an agreement to be reached. What is more helpful in preparing beforehand is identifying a range of options — including best- and worst-case scenarios — that would be acceptable outcomes. Negotiators should identify the goals they seek to achieve and then rank them by relative value. For example, in negotiations for new trading arrangements under the Cotonou Agreement, the 15 small states of the Caribbean Forum (CARIFORUM) have sought to decelerate the erosion of the trading advantage for their goods in the European Union (EU) market and to enhance their trading access to the services sector. At the same time, CARIFORUM countries have indicated a need to ensure an appropriate balance between the level of protection granted to intellectual property rights and the level of development of their economies, particularly in the area of innovation.[7] These negotiations illustrate the ways in which different policy goals can compete for attention and showed the need to decide beforehand which goals are to be given higher priority or where there may be opportunities for tradeoffs between different policy goals.

A ranking of what you must have (sometimes known as non-negotiables or "deal breakers"), what you would be willing to give up in order to gain those must-haves, and under what conditions you could compromise is also helpful to have clarified before entering negotiations. At what cost is agreement or disagreement acceptable? In international relations, the territorial integrity of a sovereign state is generally viewed as non-negotiable, and any position that may be perceived as threatening sovereignty is unacceptable. In the realm of public health, a publicly funded health system might be seen as a "sacred cow" that is not to be negotiated. As in a chess game, when even one's opening position can influence how the contest will eventually play out, one's starting place in a negotiation must leave some "wiggle room." An experienced negotiator does not generally start with his or her optimal outcome and then refuse to move from that position throughout negotiations. Rather, the negotiator may begin with a more extreme position, knowing that it is likely to be unobtainable, and then negotiate with knowledge of an acceptable outcome in mind. Establishing in advance the concessions you are and are not willing to make and how these options are likely to play out within a given political context is a key task of pre-negotiation preparations. The likely outcome will not be the best-case scenario for all interested parties, but rather one that is acceptable to them.

Equally important is arriving at an understanding of what other interested parties or your counterparts are likely to want from the negotiations. Anticipating what other parties are likely to want, what they are likely to give up to achieve those goals, and what they will hold firm on will inform your own negotiation strategy. Ahead of the negotiations, you should consider these questions: What positions are negotiating counterparts likely to take? What is important to them? What flexibility in position might the different parties have? Where might there be possible compromises? The more you can anticipate negotiation positions and how they might unfold, the less likelihood that you will be pressured to make snap decisions and risk giving too much or gaining too little in the process. Indeed, negotiators can sometimes be under pressure to make a decision within a certain timeframe or to conform to certain normative pressures, or they may simply get caught up in the process. In the cold light of day, the resultant agreement may not be optimal and, in fact, negotiators might even have difficulty gaining subsequent support for it from stakeholders. Making poor decisions can create new problems when it comes to implementing them. Better decisions during negotiations are more likely to be made, in short, by well-informed, well-prepared interested parties. For a good example, consider the Millennium Development Goals (MDGs) adopted in 2000. They were hailed as "the most broadly supported, comprehensive and specific development goals the world has ever agreed upon,"[8] but reviews of progress toward the MDGs suggest that subsequent efforts to reach the eight time-bound goals agreed upon by world leaders have met with limited success.

As Hulme wrote: "[T]he MDGs were the outcome of a fragmented conversation between critics of neo-liberalism, loosely grouped around the idea of 'human development,' and non-fundamentalist neo-liberals, moving toward a post-Washington consensus.[a] The MDGs emerged at a time when (i) the previously dominant model for world development, neo-liberal capitalism, was being heavily questioned, but there was no clearly articulated alternative; and (ii) world leaders and multilateral institutions were coming under pressure to generate a vision of 'how' the world would be different and better in the new millennium."[9]

An important dynamic — as is usually the case in health diplomacy — is that the interested parties negotiate on behalf of a collective rather than an individual interest. For the negotiator, it is imperative therefore to clearly understand whose interests you represent and where that party or parties are likely to stand on a particular issue. There is no use in reaching agreement on an issue only to find that the stakeholders involved, who may be critical to successful implementation, oppose the terms of the agreement. In this respect, good negotiation is about good governance. What means exist for ensuring that negotiators understand and represent relevant stakeholders? Should there be a consultation process, and, if so, who should be consulted, and how? Depending on the available time and resources for pre-negotiation preparations, this structure might range from a policy analysis of the health issue to provide background to negotiators, to a formal referendum canvassing the opinions of the relevant constituencies. Ensuring the consideration of stakeholders that may not be immediately apparent, or of those less able to voice their interests, can be particularly challenging but is no less important. When key constituencies are excluded from negotiations, as in the absence of public health representatives during the negotiation of the TRIPS agreement, problems of implementation can ensue (see Box 1). Consultation can also help build alliances, especially when vested interests may raise opposition to negotiations. Brazil's effective contribution to the FCTC negotiations was built on

---

[a]The Washington Consensus describes a set of ten relatively specific economic policy prescriptions that constitute the "standard" reform package promoted for developing countries by Washington, DC-based institutions, such as the International Monetary Fund (IMF), the World Bank, and the US Treasury Department.

a process of widespread consultation across and beyond the public health sector.[14] Public hearings held by the World Health Organization (WHO) before the FCTC negotiation, inviting the submission of evidence and views by interested parties not directly involved in formal negotiations, served a similar purpose. In contrast, the fragility of the alliance of non-governmental organisations (NGOs), international organisations, and governments, and the formation of that alliance after intellectual property (IP) protections under the TRIPS agreement were negotiated, led to prolonged debate.[15] Overall, the effectiveness of outcomes from negotiations is dependent on negotiators having the authority of relevant stakeholders to act on their behalf.

Box 1. Public Health Representation in the Negotiation of the Agreement on Trade-Related Aspects of Intellectual Property Rights

The Agreement on Trade-Related Aspects of Intellectual Property Rights (TRIPS) is an international agreement administered by the World Trade Organization (WTO) that sets down minimum standards for many forms of intellectual property (IP) regulation as applied to nationals of other WTO member states. It was negotiated at the end of the Uruguay Round of the General Agreement on Tariffs and Trade (GATT) in 1994. The agreement introduced IP law into the international trading system for the first time, and it remains the most comprehensive international agreement on IP to date.

   While the TRIPS Agreement is ostensibly not about pharmaceutical patents, from the mid-1990s, concerns among developing countries, scholars, and nongovernmental organisations began to arise over the implications of the TRIPS for agreement for access to medicines. Some of the criticisms were aimed at the WTO as a whole, but many regarded the agreement itself as bad policy.[10] The effect of TRIPS on wealth redistribution, from developing countries to copyright and patent owners in developed countries, and its imposition of artificial scarcity on countries that would otherwise have weaker IP laws are common bases for such criticisms.

   During the ensuing debates, it became apparent that the process of negotiating the TRIPS agreement allowed limited input by developing countries and no input by the public health community. Indeed, Drahos went as far as to argue that this was a deliberate strategy by which "the [United States] embarked on a strategy of forum shifting" away from the World Intellectual Property Organization (WIPO), where developing countries could assert greater influence by virtue of their numbers.[11] In contrast, as described by Enyart, the corporate sector exerted significant influence over the negotiations in the GATT and the form it eventually took: "We went to Geneva, where we presented [our] document to the staff of the GATT Secretariat. What I have described to you is absolutely unprecedented in GATT. Industry has identified a major problem in international trade. It [industry] crafted a solution, reduced it to a concrete proposal, and sold it to our own and other governments.... The industries and traders of world commerce have played simultaneously the role of [the] patient, the diagnostician, and the prescribing physician."[12]

Concerned that advocates of TRIPS were insisting on an overly narrow reading of its provisions, critics initiated negotiations at the 2001 WTO Ministerial Conference on the interpretation of the agreement in relation to public health and access to medicines. The resultant special Ministerial Declaration, known as the Doha Declaration on the TRIPS Agreement and Public Health, which was adopted by WTO member states, affirmed that "the TRIPS Agreement does not and should not prevent Members from taking measures to protect public health." In this respect, as stated by WHO, "[T]he Doha Declaration enshrines the principles [that] WHO has publicly advocated and advanced over the years — namely, [it reaffirms] the right of WTO Members to make full use of the safeguard provisions of the TRIPS Agreement in order to protect public health and enhance access to medicines for poor countries."[13]

Overall, while it may be argued that the exclusion of critical voices, including public health representatives, from the TRIPS negotiations facilitated [the reaching of that] agreement, the ensuing and prolonged debates, legal cases, and trade disputes over access to medicines have raised fundamental questions about due process.

Thus, preparing well for negotiations is a key factor in their longer-term effectiveness. Given the usually complex nature of global health negotiations, this preparation requires giving sufficient resources for this purpose in terms of time, money, and technical capacity. Being better prepared than one's counterpart can be an initial advantage. But negotiating with others who are less prepared can also lead to agreements that must eventually be re-negotiated. Due process is thus integral to effective pre-negotiation preparations in the form of stakeholder analysis, consultation, and information gathering. This effort will require greater commitment from the interested parties, but how well this phase is undertaken is likely to influence the outcome of negotiations and their longer-term effectiveness.

Let the Negotiations Begin: The Importance of Process

Health negotiations seek to achieve many different goals; whether these goals are actually achieved is strongly influenced by procedural decisions defining how the negotiations are to be conducted. "Process" sets out the terms of engagement of the parties concerned.

Who Should Participate?

The first of these considerations is: Who should participate in negotiations? Negotiations can be undertaken by a single individual (such as a minister of health) or by large delegations representing a diverse range of backgrounds and experience (as during the FCTC negotiations). The number of people involved may reflect the importance of the issue to be discussed, the need for specialist expertise, the diversity of the interests that need to be represented, or simply the available resources. When multiperson delegations are involved, a nominated head of delegation usually acts as the chief negotiator, who is responsible for communicating with his or her counterparts in other delegations, as well as with government officials back home. The rank of the chief negotiator for each party involved, in terms of authority and experience, should be roughly equivalent to the ranks of all other chief negotiators. It is important that the person who has the authority to make a decision on behalf of each of the parties involved be considered. If a negotiator does not have the authority to make decisions, but has to defer to a higher authority each time a position is tabled, negotiations will be considerably slowed.

In relation to global health negotiations, whether that lead role should be fulfilled by a public health expert or diplomat will depend on the context. Ideally, the individual should bring both types of experience to the table, although this is rarely possible. When an issue to be discussed is likely to involve political wrangling, perhaps even spilling beyond the issue at hand, an experienced diplomat may be more suitable. When negotiations involve detailed and specialized subject matter, as in the negotiation of the revised International Health Regulations (IHR), someone holding relevant technical knowledge may be more appropriate. A good example of the need for both types of participants is the Biological Weapons Convention (BWC) Conference, which takes place every five years. With intersessional expert and annual meetings taking place during the interim that deal with more-detailed matters, such as the oversight of pathogens, capabilities for responding to and investigating alleged uses of biological weapons, mechanisms for disease surveillance and response, and codes of conduct for scientists, the five-yearly BWC Conference has become a high-level meeting led by senior diplomats for taking stock and building common political ground on sensitive issues concerning foreign policy and national security.

In some negotiations, a chair may be nominated to preside over proceedings overall, especially when there is likely to be substantial disagreement or when many interested parties are involved. While the chair's position is perceived as relatively neutral, Tallberg wrote that the position of a chair in international negotiations is still politically influential: "[C]hairmanship [is]… a source of independent influence in international cooperation. Formal leaders perform functions of agenda management, brokerage, and representation that make it more likely for negotiations to succeed, and [they] possess privileged resources that may enable them to steer negotiations toward the agreements they most prefer."[16]

The chair should be someone who is perceived as knowledgeable about the technical matters involved, but also having the necessary experience and skills in diplomacy. Such a combination is especially important in health-related negotiations. Indeed, the growing importance of health agreements has given new prominence to processes of global health diplomacy that require a special combination of technical knowledge and negotiating skills that often is difficult to find in a single individual. Prominent individuals who have played this dual role in recent times include Gro Harlem Brundtland, who, as well as being medically qualified, has been a high-level politician and diplomat. Besides serving as Prime Minister of Norway and Director-General of WHO, Brundtland chaired the World Commission on Environment and Development and was a UN Special Envoy for Climate Change.

Where Should Negotiations Take Place?

The second important procedural consideration is the location where the negotiations will take place. If the negotiation process will extend over more than one session, as is usually the case for an international agreement, alternating venues might be agreed to avoid giving one side "home advantage." Or, if political tensions run high, finding neutral ground might help to ease the situation. Holding negotiations in locations other than Geneva or New York has become increasingly favoured as a way to enhance the capacity of low- and middle-income countries to participate. For this reason, the four sessions so far of the Conference of the Parties (COP) of the FCTC, comprising all Parties to the Convention, have been held in Geneva; Bangkok; Durban, South Africa; and Punta del Este, Uruguay. The specific surroundings might also be given careful consideration. A relaxed and informal setting can help build rapport among negotiators. A venue away from public attention, such as a geographically isolated location, can help negotiators feel more relaxed and protected from potential interruptions. For more than 50 years, the Rockefeller Foundation's Bellagio Centre in Italy, for example, has served as a key venue for negotiating agreements on a wide range of global health issues,[17] such as the Global Alliance for Vaccines Initiative (GAVI).[18] Alternatively, a particular type of venue might be needed to ensure that the required resources, such as communication facilities, information, and expertise, are close at hand. The four sessions so far of the Intergovernmental Negotiating Body (INB) on a Protocol on the Illicit Trade in Tobacco Products have been held in Geneva because of the proximity of relevant international organizations, such as the FCTC Secretariat and World Customs Organization (Belgium).

How Should Negotiations be Timed?

The third of the important procedural considerations is timeframe — that is, when should negotiations take place, and how much time should they be permitted to take? Timeframe is dictated by the nature of the issue at hand and the time available to resolve it. In an emergency situation, the time available for negotiations will be more limited. For example, if the WHO needed to negotiate access to the site of a suspected disease outbreak, relatively rapid agreement would be required to enable timely intervention. In contrast, the negotiation of the FCTC took place over six INB sessions from 1999 to 2003, as each word was carefully considered and agreed on by 192 member states. Another consideration is the availability of the required participants. The diaries (calendars) of senior officials are invariably very full. If agreement requires their participation, scheduling can be challenging. Oftentimes, negotiations might commence with less senior officials, who hammer out the details over an agreed period of time leading up to the arrival of senior officials. As well as making optimal use of the limited time of senior officials, their impending arrival can put pressure on negotiators to reach agreement by a given time. A good example is the two-week UN Climate Change Conference that was held in December 2009, which was intended to reach agreement on the Copenhagen Accord, a framework for climate change mitigation beyond 2012. The Copenhagen conference was, in fact, the 15th session of the COPs, following a series of meetings to draft the negotiating text. The impending arrival of key world leaders, such as US President Barack Obama, on the final day of the conference was intended to push deadlocked negotiators to reach a compromise. In the end, after eight draft texts and all-day talks between 115 world leaders, the differences proved too much, and the weak nonbinding document signed was widely seen as a failure.[19]

A consideration related to timeframe is that negotiators understand the other issues that may be vying for policymakers' attention. Negotiations can raise public awareness of a given issue but, to do so, that issue must compete successfully for the attention of policy-makers. According to the Organization for Economic Co-operation and Development, the health sector has become a major recipient of development assistance, going from just over US$6 billion in 1999 to US$13.4 billion in 2005.[20] The financial, energy, climate change, and food crises at the end of the 21st century's first decade, however, pushed global health downward on the policy agenda.[21] When health-related negotiations form part of a broader agenda, such as the environment or development, effort must be made to ensure that health concerns are represented appropriately. For example, von Schirnding wrote about the 2002 World Summit on Sustainable Development (WSSD):

"The major outcomes of WSSD included a negotiated Plan of Implementation, a Political Declaration and a number of implementation partnerships and initiatives.... New targets and agreements were negotiated in a number of important areas, for example in sanitation. Previous agreements, such as those relating to the achievement of the Millennium Development Goals... were also reaffirmed, making the Johannesburg Plan of Implementation a somewhat eclectic mix of new and past agreements and affirmations, albeit with many important implications for health."

"While relatively modest in its achievements, and with difficulties in achieving consensus in key areas such as energy, trade, finance, and globalization, WSSD nevertheless succeeded in placing sustainable development back on the political agenda.... Health was singled out as one of five priority areas, along with water, energy, agriculture, and biodiversity, and...a separate chapter [was devoted to it] in the resulting Plan of Implementation, which highlighted a range of environmental health issues as well as issues relating to health services [and] communicable and noncommunicable diseases.... From the perspective of health, WSSD must be seen as a reaffirmation of the central place of health on the sustainable development agenda, and in the broader context of a process which began in Rio and was given added impetus with the Monterrey Financing for Development conference and the World Trade Organisation meeting held in Doha."[22]

Conversely, events can fortuitously elevate certain global health issues and thus facilitate negotiations. For example, negotiations to revise the International Health Regulations were initiated by a resolution of the World Health Assembly in 1995 amid concerns about emerging and re-emerging diseases. A revision process commenced, but progress proved glacial, given a lack of interest and support by key member states. It was not until the outbreak of severe acute respiratory syndrome (SARS) in 2003 and 2004 that sufficient political priority was forthcoming. That crisis led to concerted efforts under the auspices of an Intergovernmental Working Group on the Revision of the International Health Regulations, which reached agreement on the revised International Health Regulations (2005), which countries have adopted.

To what extent proceedings will be reported publicly is an important consideration. Intergovernmental negotiations that take place under the auspices of UN organizations are generally recorded, either verbatim or in summary form, in several working languages, to enable a historical record. Such records vary in their level of detail and attribution, and they can be sound-recorded or documented in a written record. Oftentimes, however, while public interest might be high, negotiators may welcome an environment in which they can be open and frank in their discussions with their counterparts; that cannot occur if negotiations take place in a public forum. Thus, negotiations may adopt so-called "Chatham House rules," whereby statements are not attributed to individuals and proceedings are not reported in detail.

It is good practice to formally document in writing the proceedings and the terms of the agreement and then to have all relevant parties sign the agreement. This document serves as a record to enable transparency and accountability, as well as a way of resolving disagreements or obtaining clarification in the future. For this reason, the document should set out the agreement in some detail, notably the obligations of each party, they way in which the implementation of the agreement would be undertaken, the resources that will be needed and the sources of those resources, and the timeframe for compliance. The word-smithing of such agreements can be time-consuming and can require specialised, legal, expertise.

Overall, negotiations can take many forms, and the process agreed on can strongly influence the outcome of a negotiation. Indeed, the negotiation process can itself become subject to negotiation among the parties concerned, given its strategic importance.

The Challenges of Negotiation Within a Global Health Context

Whereas any negotiations can be challenging at the best of times, conducting such negotiations within a global health context poses its own specific challenges. Perhaps the most obvious challenge in global-level negotiations is the ways in which culture is likely to influence negotiation styles. Negotiations are often prompted by differences in perspective and interests on a particular issue. This dynamic can be intensified when cultural differences such as language, values, normative frameworks, and beliefs are added to the mix. There is a substantial literature on different styles of negotiation, varying by culture, personality, and the issue being addressed.

In their well-known book, *Getting to Yes* (and its followup, *Getting to No*), Fisher and colleagues described styles of negotiation with the aim of improving the quality of negotiation, from the interpersonal to the international level.[23] Such differences can lead to misunderstanding and can even give offense. One of the most famous examples of this is the 1960 incident of shoe-banging by then Soviet Premier Nikita Khrushchev. Forty years later, his granddaughter recalled the episode[24]:

> "Dismissing him as a worthy opponent, capitalists thought of Khrushchev as a vaudeville character. Very well then, he would become one. He needed the UN stage to make an important statement: it is better to take the socialist world seriously. He wanted to be heard. But, next to the noble Macmillan, smart Eisenhower, refined De Gaulle, and wise Nehru, the short Nikita Khrushchev couldn't help looking a wag."
>
> "Instead of trying to act and speak according to traditional diplomacy, he broke the ritual and created his own manner. The manner, which suited his goal, was to be different from the hypocrites of the west, with their appropriate words but calculated deeds. He would do it the other way — say more than he meant. A tragi-comic act of shoe-banging was intended to separate two superpowers not only in terms of their politics, but also in their diplomatic methods."

"As a good performer, Khrushchev needed a strong, convincing exit, true to the role he chose, and that is what happened: in the excitement of fist-banging, his watch fell off. Meanwhile, his shoes, made of durable Soviet leather in a special shoe atelier for the Soviet *nomenklatura*, were too new and too tight, and he removed them. He bent down to pick up the watch and saw his empty shoes. How lucky!"

Appreciating cultural differences in negotiation style is also important for understanding the pressures faced by counterparts from their own constituencies. Whereas a negotiator might approach the process as mortal combat, seeking maximum gain at the expense of maximum loss by the opponent, effective global-level negotiations cannot resemble a medieval battlefield. Treating your counterpart as a defeated adversary might play well back home, but crowing about how you destroyed your fellow negotiator risks their capacity to achieve support from their own stakeholders.

Admittedly, there can be a degree of posturing by negotiators for the benefit of home audiences. As Belford wrote, then Indonesian Minister of Health Siti Fadilah Supari "turned the fight against avian influenza into a broader struggle over the soul of globalisation,"[25] framing the withholding of influenza virus samples as a wider battle between rich and poor countries: "Then the virus is turned into vaccines [that are sent to] Indonesia, and Indonesia has to buy them, and, if they don't buy them, they have to go into debt, and it turns and turns again, and, in the end, developed countries make new viruses, which are then sent to developing countries. The conspiracy between superpower nations and global organisations is a reality. It isn't a theory, isn't rhetoric, but it's something I've experienced myself.... What Indonesia has been doing so far is to save humankind, and Indonesia is of the view that [under] the current system, which is unfair, untransparent, and not equitable, the danger is much more than the pandemic itself."

Tapping into existing resentment in the country and region toward economic globalization, Supari's resultant status as a hero to many Indonesians made it necessary for any negotiating process on virus sharing to appropriately address those local sensitivities. Regardless of negotiating style, negotiators are more likely to reach agreement if there is recognition that terms must be acceptable to the home audiences of both sides. At the global level, where a greater number and diversity of interested parties may be involved, sensitivity to cultural differences is needed. An effective negotiator is one who recognizes that all parties share an interest in reaching agreement. Recognising that both sides must "save face" increases the likelihood that an agreement will be accepted and implemented by stakeholders.

A related challenge of negotiating within a global health context is language. French was the language of diplomacy in Europe from the 17th century. Today, six official languages and two working languages are used within the UN system. As Kappeler has written: "Documents exchanged between countries in the past were written in the single... language then in use [throughout] Europe: Latin. In the 18th century, French had become the generally accepted diplomatic language, so much so that even diplomatic notes addressed to the British Foreign Office by the Legation of the United States were written in that language. The 20th century saw a gradual emergence of English as a second and, later, even dominant diplomatic language. At the same time, a growing number of countries insisted on the use of their own language in diplomatic correspondence and joint diplomatic documents. As a result, the United Nations [agreed to use] five languages at its inception (Chinese, English, French, Russian, and Spanish), to which Arabic has later been added by informal agreement. In the European Union, all twelve languages of the members are currently in use, and their number is bound to grow as new members [are] admitted. Translation and interpretation have therefore become a major element in present-day diplomatic life."[26]

In global health diplomacy, the use of any of the world's languages in negotiations is complicated further by the often complex and technical subject matter. Reaching terms of agreement is dependent on a shared understanding of the issue, agreed definitions of key terms, the articulation of relative positions, and the exchange of detailed technical information. All of these processes are influenced by the precise, and often subtle, use of language. When more than one working language is involved in global health negotiations, additional resources in terms of technical staff, translators, and time should be allowed. Of particular importance is ensuring that any agreement reached is translated accurately, and that the subsequent interpretation is to the mutual satisfaction of interested parties.

A further challenge of global health negotiations is ensuring appropriate involvement by relevant stakeholders. Interest groups, and their representation around negotiating tables, do not necessarily conform to national borders in an increasingly globalised world. Regional coalitions, for example, have become increasingly prominent. A good example is the new European External Action Service, created by the Lisbon Treaty, which will play an increasingly important role in diplomacy. Eventually, the European Union (EU) will be represented in many international organisations, and even in national capitals, by a European diplomatic corps. When participation in international negotiations is required, EU delegations would need to reflect the interests of member states, while coordinating their positions beforehand to enable the EU to "speak with one voice."[27] Within the context of global health, intersessional meetings for the FCTC process played a critical role in developing regional positions that were then taken forward at subsequent meetings of the INB.[28]

Moreover, the term *global negotiations*, as opposed to *international* (or *intergovernmental*) *negotiations*, suggests the participation of both state and non-state actors. For example, the Global Forum on MSM & HIV was launched at the 16th International AIDS Conference in 2006 "to advocate for equitable access to effective HIV prevention, care, and treatment services tailored to the needs of gay men and other men who have sex with men (MSM), while promoting their health and human rights worldwide."[29] Similarly, the Women's Global Network for Reproductive Rights is an autonomous, independent, grassroots-led network of more than 1000 members worldwide that advocates sexual and reproductive health rights.[30] Although not necessarily taking part in formal negotiations, non-state global actors serve a range of functions (e.g. advocacy, information dissemination, and norm generation) that influence wider processes of negotiation. The process of negotiating, within a global context, must thus adapt to this greater political complexity. The formal negotiation of international treaties within the UN, involving 192 member states, has already raised concerns about logistics. Negotiations can become prolonged, lasting many years, and unwieldy, requiring reams of documentation, long and detailed drafting sessions, and hence substantial capacity (and stamina) on the part of the participating delegations. The incorporation of non-state actors into such processes, without adding further to this unwieldiness, remains a major governance challenge.

As well as the question of who should negotiate, variation in the capacity of interested parties to participate remains problematic. Alongside greater complexity of negotiations has been the continued inequity of resources available to many stakeholders to engage in preparatory work, negotiations, and the implementation of resultant agreements. Whereas this situation might be seen as a welcome advantage by some parties who are seeking an edge in negotiations, the lack of capacity of interested parties to participate meaningfully is likely to reduce the quality and, ultimately, the sustainability of any agreement reached. Such an eventuality, in turn, may lead to disagreements arising again and the need for further negotiation. The need for meaningful representation in global health diplomacy, and more generally in the building of good governance of global health, is beginning to be recognized. During the FCTC process, the WHO's support for regional consultations and the involvement of civil society organisations (often supporting developing country delegations) have been critical to strengthening the voices of Asia, Africa, and Latin America. Patel wrote that, in the WTO, coalition building within and across states has become increasingly important for leveraging influence: "Historically, trade negotiations in the WTO and prior to that [in] the GATT have proceeded through the creation of 'consensus' within restricted inner-circle group meetings, traditionally dominated by the Quad — the [United States], Japan, the EU, and Canada. The lack of transparency and exclusivity of these meetings, combined with the limited resources of weak states, meant that developing countries found themselves isolated from many decision-making processes. In the face of these disparities and institutional pressures, developing countries have now increasingly sought to build coalitions as the primary means of improving their representation in the WTO."[31]

The use of new information and communication technologies in diplomacy has been another means of coping with ever-greater complexity. The progressive advent of the telegraph, telephone, facsimile machine, satellite, and Internet have enabled each generation of diplomats to receive, analyse, and disseminate information more effectively. Today, terms such as "cyber diplomacy," "digital diplomacy," "Internet diplomacy," "online diplomacy," and "electronic diplomacy" ("e-diplomacy") denote new capabilities that may bring significant changes to the ways in which diplomats carry out their daily work. For example, Roberts has argued that "digital age diplomacy" is facilitating the "need for embassies to carry out the necessary spadework for a successful ministerial visit or to keep their capitals informed about other countries' negotiating positions."[32] Using technologies such as videoconferencing could also overcome limited capacity, and thus enhance diplomatic processes, by reducing the need to maintain a substantial presence in Geneva or New York.

Conclusion

Negotiation, the process of bargaining between two or more interested parties for the purpose of reaching agreement on a matter of mutual concern, is more likely to be successfully undertaken if careful attention is given to preparation and the negotiation process itself. With due consideration given to practical matters, such as clearly defining the problem, the possible and desired solutions, and the procedures for reaching a negotiated agreement, the likelihood of success is enhanced.

Particular challenges are raised when negotiations are required to resolve a health-related issue. Appropriate technical expertise becomes critical for informing the substantive discussions, which, in many cases, can be highly complex. Health expertise is diverse, embracing the biological sciences, clinical practice, and the social sciences. Additional knowledge may be required from those skilled in law, management, systems analysis, and economics. For example, to negotiate an agreement concerning the control of disease outbreaks worldwide, all of these types of expertise may be needed simultaneously.

Negotiation within a global context poses further challenges because of the diversity of stakeholders involved and the resultant complexity of the political environment. Undertaking negotiations involving all 195 countries of the world has meant that venues, such as the UN, have to perform an increasingly difficult logistical feat. The increased participation of non-state actors, either directly or indirectly in global negotiations, has added to this complexity. Moreover, inequities remain in the capacity of many state and non-state actors to participate meaningfully in such proceedings. Addressing these problems, as a key pillar of "good" global governance, remains fundamental for achieving effective collective action on matters of shared global concern.

References

1. Drager N, McClintock E, Moffitt M. (2000) *Negotiating Health Development: A Guide for Practitioners*. WHO/Conflict Management Group, Geneva.
2. Fidler D. (2010) Negotiating equitable access to influenza vaccines: Global health diplomacy and the controversies surrounding avian influenza H5N1 and pandemic influenza H1N1. *PLoS Med* **7(5):** e1000247.
3. World Trade Organization. (2001) Declaration on the TRIPS Agreement and public health. Available from www.wto.org/english/theWTO_e/minist_e/min01_e/mindecl_trips_e.htm (accessed May 5, 2011).
4. World Trade Organization General Council. (2003) Implementation of paragraph 6 of the Doha Declaration on the TRIPS Agreement and public health.

Available from www.wto.org/english/tratop_E/TRIPS_e/implem_para6_e.htm (accessed May 5, 2011).

5. Lee E. (2005) The World Health Organization global strategy on diet, physical activity, and health: Turning strategy into action. *Food Drug Law J* **60(4):** 569–602.

6. Reich N, Smith LJ. (1983) Implementation of the International Code of Marketing of Breast-Milk Substitutes by the EEC. *J Consum Policy* **6(3):** 355–364.

7. Spence M. (2009) *Negotiating Trade, Innovation and Intellectual Property: Lessons from the CARIFORUM EPA Experience from a Negotiator's Perspective.* UNCTAD–ICTSD Policy Brief No. 4. International Centre for Trade and Sustainable Development, Geneva. Available from http://ictsd.org/i/publications/54502 (accessed May 4, 2011).

8. United Nations Development Programme. (2010) *What are the Millennium Development Goals?* United Nations Development Program, New York City. Available from www.undp.org/mdg/basics.shtml (accessed May 4, 2011).

9. Hulme D. (2009) *Governing Global Poverty? Global Ambivalence and the Millennium Development Goals.* Brooks World Poverty Institute and Institute for Development Policy and Management, University of Manchester, UK. Available from www.eadi.org/fileadmin/MDG_2015_Publications/Hulme_PAPER.pdf (accessed May 5, 2011).

10. Lee K, Chagas LC, Novotny T. (2010) Brazil and the Framework Convention on Tobacco Control: Global health diplomacy as soft power. *PLoS Med* **7(4):** 1–5.

11. Bhagwati J. (2004) *In Defense of Globalization.* Oxford University Press.

12. Drahos P. (No date) *Developing Countries and International Property Standard-Setting.* Commission on Intellectual Property Rights Study Paper 8. Available from www.iprcommission.org/papers/pdfs/study_papers/sp8_drahos_study.pdf (accessed May 4, 2011).

13. Enyart J, quoted in Keayla BK. (1998) Conquest by patents. The TRIPS Agreement on patent laws: impact on pharmaceuticals and health for all. Centre for Study of Global Trade System and Development, New Delhi.

14. World Health Organization. (No date) The Doha Declaration on the TRIPS Agreement and Public Health. Available from www.who.int/medicines/areas/policy/doha_declaration/en/index.html (accessed May 15, 2011).

15. Çakmak C. (2007) Coalition building in world politics: Definitions, conceptions, and examples. *Perceptions* (Winter), pp. 1–20.

16. Tallberg J. (2010) The power of the chair: Formal leadership in international cooperation. *Int Stud Quart* **54(1):** 241–265.

17. Rockefeller Foundation. (2009) *Bellagio Center: The First 50 Years.* Rockefeller Foundation, New York City. Available from www.rockefeller-foundation.org/news/publications/bellagio-center-first-50-years (accessed May 5, 2011).

18. Nossal G. (2000) The Global Alliance for Vaccines and Immunization — A millennial challenge. *Prometheus* **18(1):** 33–37.

19. Vidal J, Stratton A, Goldenberg S. (2009) Low targets, goals dropped: Copenhagen ends in failure. *The Guardian*, December 19. Available from www.guardian.co.uk/environment/2009/dec/18/copenhagen-deal (accessed May 5, 2011).

20. Organisation for Economic Co-operation and Development. (2007) *2007 Development Co-operation Report.* Organization for Economic Co-operation and Development, Paris.

21. Fidler D. (2008) After the revolution: Global health politics in a time of economic crisis and threatening future trends. *Global Health Govern* **2(2):** 1–21.

22. Von Shirnding Y. (2005) The World Summit on Sustainable Development: reaffirming the centrality of health. *Globalization and Health* **1(8):** 1–6. Available from www.globalizationandhealth.com/content/pdf/1744-8603-1-8.pdf (accessed May 4, 2011).

23. Fisher R, Ury W, Patton B. (1991) *Getting to Yes: Negotiating Agreement Without Giving in*, 2nd edn. Random House, New York City.

24. Khruscheva N. (2000) The case of Kruschchev's shoe. *The New Statesman*, October 2. Available from www.newstatesman.com/200010020025 (accessed May 5, 2011).

25. Belford A. (2008) Indonesia's bird flu warrior takes on the world. *AFP*, October 12. Available from http://afp.google.com/article/ALeqM5hZw VUAJGlcX8VNojn0MB98vQb8Gg

26. Gaspers J. (2010) Putting Europe first. *The World Today* **66(1):** 20–22.

27. Collin J, Lee K, Bissell K. (2002) The Framework Convention on Tobacco Control: The politics of global health governance. *Third World Q* **23(2):** 265–282.

28. The Global Forum on MSM and HIV. (No date.) About MSMGF. Available from www.msmgf.org/index.cfm/id/4/About-Us/ (accessed May 10, 2011).

29. Women's Global Network for Reproductive Rights. (No date) Who we are. Available from www.wgnrr.org/who-we-are (accessed May 10, 2011).

30. Patel M. (2007) *New Faces in the Green Room: Developing Country Coalitions and Decision-Making in the WTO.* Global Governance Project (GEG) Working Paper 2007/33. University College, Oxford, UK. Available from www.globaleconomicgovernance.org/wp-content/uploads/Patel_Main%20text_new.pdf (accessed May 9, 2011).

31. Roberts I. (2010) Digital age diplomacy. *The World Today* **66(1):** 23–24.

11

Global Health Begins at Home: Policy Coherence

*Gaudenz Silberschmidt, MD**
and Thomas Zeltner, MD[†]

> If you want to go fast, go alone. If you want to go far, go together.
>
> — old African proverb

Introduction

Improvements in human health in the 20th century were based, to a large degree, on improvements in health care delivery, technological development, and general socioeconomic conditions. The major focus of health research during that century was on how to restore ill health through scientific development and advanced medical care. Health care delivery is a national, state, or local responsibility, and for most of the 20th century, debates on how to improve human health were oriented toward these jurisdictions. This is in contrast to the 19th century, when knowledge of infectious diseases grew rapidly and international sanitary conventions became necessary in order to stop cross-border spread of diseases such as cholera,

---

*Master of International Relations, Ambassador and Vice-Director, Swiss Federal Office of Public Health.

[†]Master in Law, Professor of Public Health, University of Bern, former Director General of the Swiss Federal Office of Public Health (1991–2009).

yellow fever, smallpox, plague, and typhoid. According to Kickbusch 2011[1] and Adams 2008,[2] global health diplomacy is rooted in the 19th century and in the colonial foreign policies of that period. Control of cross-border infectious diseases was necessary for sustaining colonial commerce and the movement of goods and people across borders as the global marketplace expanded rapidly.

In the 20th century, the international aspect of health policy was mostly focused on the exchange of scientific and technical information, which was of limited importance in foreign policy. As a result, the key multilateral health organization that originated in the 20th century, the World Health Organization (WHO), was designed to be a technical forum for health collaboration among ministries of health, without major political inputs or mandates from other sectors; consequently, it had very limited political impact, globally or domestically. During the Cold War period, international responsibilities within industrialized countries' governments were quite distinct. Technical health issues for industrialized countries were the responsibility of ministries of health, but health assistance to developing countries was the responsibility of development agencies or ministries. The end of the Cold War hastened major demographic and power shifts, and facilitated the most extensive globalization the world has ever known. Economic integration, trade liberalization, and the end of East–West proxy politics changed the complexion of health and development throughout the globe. In the first decade of the 21st century, the world witnessed the development of a multipolar international political system, with emerging powerhouses such as China, Brazil, and India ascending to economic importance, and with shifting responsibilities seen within the multinational organizations. In addition to many positive but unequally distributed benefits of globalization, several challenges to international health policy have emerged. These include the increased risk of global pandemics and spread of infectious diseases; the mass migration of health personnel; the expansion of both legal and illegal trade in health services and pharmaceuticals; the persistent threats to food security and food safety; the growth of unhealthy behaviors such as tobacco use and alcohol abuse; and the increasingly visible health effects of climate change. With such emergent, transborder issues, the health sector is no longer a purely technical and nationalistic enterprise. Health security is now more than ever a global mandate and, as such, a global public good that needs to be supported simultaneously at national, regional, and global levels.

The globalization of health issues has resulted in greater interdependence among countries and, along with the health system reforms now taking place in many countries, health is the source of major policy challenges for governments. Health policy concerns now extend across many other non-health ministries, with both national and international implications. For example, policies involving trade in health-related goods are the concern of trade agencies, and these agencies are not concerned about health outcomes as much as the maintenance of fair trade. Ministries of trade and agriculture are also involved in food security and safety policies. Economic development — as national commitments to the UN Millennium Development Goals (MDGs) — demands a more global political engagement of development agencies.[3] Threats to human security created by the growing number of global health crises such as natural disasters, conflict, and forced migration, also have demanded increased engagement of ministries of foreign affairs and sometimes of ministries of defense in response to these emergencies as well as to prevention efforts.

Why Policy Coherence is Important

While these developments reflect what health experts have advocated as "health in all policies," they also reflect a growing need for policy coherence across government agencies. Since health-related issues are now addressed in multiple international fora, not just in health organizations, the lack of national policy coordination becomes strikingly visible when different ministries of the same government defend different positions on the same health issue. This in turn leads to international policy incoherencies which may impede development, waste scarce resources, and burden recipient governments with competing agency agendas.

Policy coherence is now even more important with the increase in the number of global stakeholders engaged in health-related issues. Concerns about duplication of work, transparency of funding streams, goals to be achieved, and the desire of nongovernmental actors to gain political importance have undermined the influence of sovereign states and their agencies on the one hand, and on the other brought serious concerns about fragmentation. Some programs, such as the Global Alliance for Vaccine and Immunizations (GAVI) and Global Fund for AIDS, Tuberculosis, and Malaria (GFATM), with their billions in resources, have influence in both technical health issues and development politics. The traditional donors, such as the World Bank, the International Money Fund, and the donor countries of the so-called "Global North," no longer monopolize the global health political landscape. This situation then exposes the need for policy coherence and governance at the global level, for both nations and multilateral organizations. In addition, more and more interactions in global health, especially those of emerging economies, move away from the classical donor–recipient relationship.

The Campaign for Access to Essential Medicines was an early example of the need for policy coherence. This campaign was launched in 1998 after a court case involving the South African Pharmaceutical Manufacturers against the South African government,[4] and then embraced in 1999 by Medicins Sans Frontiers (MSF).[5] The multinational campaign's goals were to lower the prices of existing drugs, vaccines, and diagnostic tests; to stimulate research and development on new treatments for diseases that primarily affect the poor; and to overcome other barriers that prevent patients in poor countries from accessing effective treatments. These goals can be met only if there is policy coherence across trade and health sectors, both nationally and internationally.

Country Examples

Some countries have explicitly addressed gaps in global health policy coherence as a national strategic priority. Switzerland and the United Kingdom were the first to have fully endorsed national strategies aimed at strengthening coordination of national health, global health, and foreign policies. They were followed by Norway and Japan, which formulated some rather specific approaches to global health cooperation (for example, Japan focuses on achieving the health-related MDGs, and Norway focuses on goals it wishes to achieve during its membership on the Executive Board of the WHO). The United States' Global Health Initiative aims to bring together the different departmental efforts of the

US government in health development. We will now describe various national efforts at global health policy consistency, which we believe is necessary for successful outcomes in global health diplomacy. Several other countries are working explicitly or implicitly to improve policy coherence for global health but have not produced or published — to our knowledge — a formal government document.

Switzerland

In the late 20th century, global health issues were managed by two ministries within the Swiss government: health and development fell within the remit of the Swiss Development Cooperation (SDC), an agency of the Ministry of Foreign Affairs (MOFA), and all other global health issues were the responsibility of the Federal Office of Public Health (FOPH), a branch of the Ministry of Home Affairs (MHA). Often, even if various aspects of a specific health issue were addressed in one meeting (for example, the World Health Assembly), the two ministries acted independently. Other ministries with interests in a specific issue (such as trade in pharmaceuticals) limited their engagement in these fora, due to a lack of competence in the health technicalities.

Challenges to policy coherence for Switzerland emerged in 1973–1978 with the global concern for the international marketing of breast milk substitutes by the Swiss-based Nestle Corporation.[6] With international pressure to dramatically change established marketing practices (derided in a booklet entitled *The Baby Killer*), a third agency, the Ministry of Economics and Trade, was forced to take careful interest in health issues. The conflicts between health concerns surrounding this issue and economic concerns, accentuated by an international boycott against Nestlé, required the Swiss government to develop a coherent strategy across disparate ministries.

Similarly, with debates on intellectual property and access to medicines in the 1990 and 2000s,[7] a fourth ministry (Justice, which is responsible for intellectual property issues) was required to engage in health-related issues. The economic interests of Swiss-based pharmaceutical manufacturers were of course included in the government debates. Conflicts of interest among the different government ministries became more and more evident in interactions with multilateral negotiations, where Switzerland's positions on issues fluctuated, depending on which office represented the country in an international forum. These positions often reflected both the economic concerns of Switzerland's booming pharmaceutical industry and the traditional Swiss concerns for public health, human rights, and international development. The need for increased policy coherence in health across the government thus became very clear.

Switzerland's lack of policy coherence became apparent in several ways: (1) Switzerland was perceived by other international actors as an unreliable partner because of its fluctuating position on various health topics; (2) distrust developed between different Swiss ministries such that every ministry felt the need to be present at every international meeting to defend its position; these interministerial power games consumed substantial time and energy, and often resulted in interpersonal tensions between the representatives of the various ministries; (3) the lack of policy coherence opened the door for lobbyists to push their economic interests in the various international arenas using a divide-and-conquer approach within the Swiss government.

A debate on how to overcome this situation was initiated in 2000 by the FOPH and SDC. Such debates were still underway when the Swiss government decided in 2005 to elaborate foreign policy strategies in other policy sectors. Since preliminary discussions already had taken place, the health sector was an ideal arena in which to pilot a multi-agency strategy to assure policy coherence. The MOFA led strategy development among the MOFA, FOPH, and SDC, later expanding to other ministries. As a result of this process, Switzerland was the first country to formally adopt (in 2006) a national global health strategy, entitled the "Swiss Health Foreign Policy."[8] It constitutes an "internal agreement between the relevant services of the Swiss federal administration," the purpose of which is to improve the "instruments of internal cooperation." This agreement on health and foreign policy objectives was adopted by the MOFA and FOPH, and submitted to the Federal Council (the seven-member body which constitutes the federal government of Switzerland).

The document presents a clear determination to strengthen international coordination on health matters and asserts health as a fundamental component of sustainable development, foreign policy, and global security. It further asserts the role of all individual federal departments and offices that address health matters. The policy document describes five main areas of interest. The first relates to *protecting the health interests of the Swiss population*, through measures against the spread of communicable and noncommunicable diseases and ensuring consumer protection. This demands improved cooperation with both international organizations and the European Union (EU).

The second area involves *harmonization of national and international health policies* to both improve the Swiss health system and support international public health norms. International harmonization reduces the risk of non-tariff barriers to trade caused by health challenges, such as pandemic influenza. It also addresses the specific issue of the migration of health professionals, which affects both international development and the Swiss national health system.

The third area of interest addresses *the effectiveness of international collaboration in the area of health.* In particular, this would be achieved by strengthening the WHO's normative role as a multinational organization; supporting the coordination of the WHO, OECD, and EU on normative health issues; and promoting synergies with other global health actors that may improve the work of various multilateral organizations.

The fourth area of interest is to *improve the global health situation* by strengthening health systems in developing countries; specifically addressing HIV/AIDS, TB, and malaria; combating noncommunicable diseases by emphasizing prevention, health promotion, and reproductive health; and devoting health care assistance in conflict and crisis situations.

The fifth area of interest is to reinforce *Switzerland's role as a host country to international organizations and as an industrial center* for research and development of new therapeutics, emphasizing Geneva's role as an international center of excellence for public health and humanitarian action, and at the same time ensuring incentives for scientific development and appropriate protection of intellectual property (IP).

This list of objectives combines the concerns of the FOPH and SDC with foreign policy, trade, and IP, which had previously not appeared in a single document. The strategy explicitly acknowledges that conflicts of interest cannot be avoided in the development of foreign policy goals. It therefore strives for a coherent *health* foreign policy in order to ensure that

Switzerland supports positions in different international fora that are consistent with its national policies.

Since 2006, the MOFA has established *a coordinating unit for health foreign policy*, in charge of ensuring overall policy coherence and monitoring progress. An intranet platform allows the exchange and storage of information that may be used in preparation for negotiations and consultations on major global health issues. The platform is now in use across the entire administration to support communications on the majority of foreign policy issues. The health ministry took the lead in elaborating more detailed policy documents in consultation with all other relevant ministries, such as on the migration of health professionals or on fair access to medicines. An Interdepartmental Conference on Health Foreign Policy is cochaired by the Secretary of State for Foreign Affairs and the Director General of Health. Staff exchange between the ministries is another way to establish policy coherence in global health. Because of budget constraints no new resources could be directly associated with the implementation of the Swiss Health Foreign Policy, but the already existing resources can be used more efficiently and more effectively.

A common foreign policy approach to health improved relationships among the different ministries. It stimulated a cultural shift toward mutual understanding, not least to understand why other ministries may have opposing positions on some issues. The one-voice principle now employed by Swiss delegations made the country a stronger actor in international settings and has given the Swiss position on global health issues a sharper profile nationally and internationally.

United Kingdom

In part because of its long colonial history, the United Kingdom has developed a sense of responsibility to ensure the well-being of former colonial subjects. This is reflected in the UK's work as a traditional aid donor and its strong antipoverty foreign policy agenda. This is highlighted in the International Development Act (June 2002), the authorizing legislation for the Department for International Development (DFID), which makes poverty reduction the prime focus of DFID's work. DFID's funding for health and healthcare-related projects is substantial, and thus there is a need for coherence in the UK's international aid policies and global health engagement, especially since the two often overlap. Additionally, national health policies, and the activities of the National Health Service (NHS), need to be coordinated with international policies, especially with respect to the migration of health professionals to work in the NHS.

The UK strategy was devised by an interministerial group led by Chief Medical Officer Liam Donaldson and published in 2007 in a document entitled "Health Is Global: Proposals for a UK Government-wide Strategy".[9] Upon approval of this discussion paper by Prime Minister Gordon Brown and his Cabinet, the interministerial group led further development of the strategy. This involved numerous government departments and civil society representatives, such as the editor of *The Lancet,* the Dean of the London School of Hygiene and Tropical Medicine, and the President of the Royal College of Surgeons.

The strategy asserts health as a human right and global public good; it is rooted in the understanding of globalization and its effects on health, and it brings together the UK's foreign relations, international development, trade, and investment policies in conjunction with health. Specific strategies are established for five years, while the overall vision covers a 10–15-year period. The first strategy included an estimated £400 million for global health research. In order to respond to the changing global health environment, the recommendations of the first annual review, as well as cross-government consultation and informal input from partners, the new government published a second document in 2011, entitled "Health is Global: An Outcomes Framework for Global Health 2011–2015."[10] It reaffirms a set of guiding principles underpinning the original strategy, and focusing on outcomes it prioritizes three areas for action, each of which includes a more detailed set of actionable goals. It builds on the 31 "differences in 5 years' time" (outcome indicators) and the 41 "we wills" (process indicators) from the first strategy to identify 12 high-level outcomes to be achieved by 2015. A monitoring process through various departments' annual delivery plans is integrated into this strategy. The outcomes framework confirms the aim to honor commitments made at the launch of the original strategy, despite pressure from the financial situation, as well as to hold an annual partners forum to review progress and reflect on new challenges and opportunities. The following discussion elaborates on the three focus areas as well as key elements related to implementation.

The first area focuses on *global health security*, encompassing issues related to the MDGs and food and water security, climate change and the environment, the effects of conflict on health, emergency preparedness, and research.

The second area of action is devoted to *international development*, highlighting the determination "to help reduce the inequalities of opportunity" as well as to continue to honor the UK's international commitments. In the context of the MDG targets, resources will be used *to support health system strengthening to ensure greater coverage and access*. Attention is also given to reducing the global crisis in the healthcare workforce; stronger actions and support for international agencies in the fight against NCDS and their drivers; learning from international experience; better coordination between UK and EU global health research agencies; and enhanced access to research knowledge for researchers and policymakers in developing countries.

The third area of action is dedicated to *trade for better health*. This focus concerns access to medicines, trade policy, research investment, and partnerships to scale up innovation and interventions to achieve universal coverage. It also calls for enhancing the UK as a market leader in health services and medical products. The outcomes framework clearly describes the need for improved collaboration between the various health actors and seeks to engage and work more effectively with NGO partners, international organizations, and partner nations. It builds on the useful support and expertise provided in the development of the original strategy and the success of the first partners' forum. At the same time, the dynamic nature of global health challenges continues to highlight the need for a coherent and consistent cross-Government approach. It requires identifying "when and where departments can add value to one another's efforts." Effective communication across different institutions and organizations within and beyond the Government is essential. A strengthened cross-Government steering group is to provide leadership, support coherence and consistency across departments, and track the progress toward departments' own deliverables.

EU Commission

The European Union (EU), as it stands today, was initially designed around economic integration and as a means of ensuring peace and cooperation in Europe. As such, it has a strong tradition in striving for coherence of economic policies within and between nations. However, health was initially not one of the topics on the economic integration agenda of the EU. The core treaty of the EU — as initially signed by the six founding members (France, Germany, Italy, The Netherlands, Belgium, and Luxembourg) — aimed at ensuring a free single market in the Western Europe for free movement of people, goods, services, and capital. Public health was first included in the EU agenda through the Maastricht Treaty in November 1993, as a separate article.[11]

Over the years, health matters have become more important for the EU. The most pressing issues included a series of food crises and the spread of emerging and re-emerging infectious diseases in Europe. Nonetheless, health policies focused primarily on European public health issues. In 2007, the European Commission published a White Paper entitled "Together for Health: A Strategic Approach for the EU 2008–2013," where one of the four principles for action was "strengthening the EU's voice in global health."[12] Based on an enlarged foreign policy agenda established by the Lisbon Treaty (the latest version of the EU treaty), the Commission in 2010 released a communication to the European Parliament, the European Economic and Social Committee, and the Committee of the Regions on "The EU Role in Global Health." This communication was taken up by member states by adopting (on 10 May, 2010) the council conclusions on the EU's role in global health. It is worth noting that the council conclusions were adopted by the Foreign Affairs Council and address, in the same document, development cooperation, public health, foreign affairs, trade, and research aspects.[13]

Norway

In line with this emerging pattern of policy coherence, the Government of Norway published a global health strategy paper in 2010, focusing on a narrower remit through its tenure as a member of the WHO executive board for 2011–2013. The "Norwegian WHO Strategy — Norway as a member of WHO's Executive Board 2010–2013" supports the WHO's central role in coordinating global health efforts in collaboration with Member States.[14] The strategy was endorsed by the Ministers of Foreign Affairs, of Health and Care Services, of Environment, and of International Development. With this strategy, Norway specifically calls for strengthening the leadership role of the WHO as part of its national strategy, thereby emphasizing the need for coherence among Member States as well as nonstate actors globally.

Japan

Japan announced in 2010 a new global health policy for 2011–2015, strongly focused on the health-related MDGs.[15] The three areas for action were: (1) maternal, newborn, and child health; (2) major infectious diseases; and (3) the response to global public health emergencies, such as pandemic influenza. The Japanese global health policy aims to protect human security and to improve coordination for its substantial development assistance activities. The policy reflected public support for international involvement and cooperation, and a dialogue among the various national stakeholders in global health helped to achieve this national policy coherence. The policy emphasizes how international coordination could be improved, notably by "strengthening multi-stakeholder partnerships with other governments, multilateral agencies, philanthropic donors, NGOs, civil society and businesses."

United States

The US Global Health Initiative (GHI) was announced in May 2009 by President Barack Obama.[16] Building on the previously authorized President's Emergency Plan for AIDS Relief (PEPFAR) program, it sought to expand existing financial appropriations (US$45 billion) for HIV/AIDS to a six-year commitment of US$63 billion. This is the largest financial commitment to global health ever proposed and, in addition to funding, it asserted a "whole of government" approach to health development assistance. This approach was meant to coordinate and consolidate health assistance under high-level leadership within the Department of

State (the US Ministry of Foreign Affairs). Previously, the global health architecture for the US Government involved 42 different agencies with differing agendas and reporting requirements.[17] The GHI brings together the US Agency for International Development (USAID); the Office of the Global AIDS Coordinator (OGAC); the Centers for Disease Control and Prevention (CDC); the National Institutes of Health (NIH); and other agencies from the Departments of Health and Human Services (HHS), the Department of Defense (DOD), and the Peace Corps, among others, to work together under the Deputy Secretary of State. Under a revised plan, the GHI is now administered by a new Office of Health Diplomacy within the US Department of State. This Department is also informed by the CDC, USAID, and OGAC, the main health-related international assistance agencies in the US Government.

Despite presidential leadership, congressional authorization has not been forthcoming, due to the current political divisions within the US Government and to the economic downturn which has severely impacted the US economy. Should this program be fully funded, the GHI sets ambitious global targets in eight health/disease arenas: HIV/AIDS, malaria, TB, maternal health, child health, nutrition, family planning, and neglected tropical diseases. The GHI also includes seven principles to achieve these targets, including a focus on women, girls, and gender equality; encouraging country ownership and investment in country-led plans; building sustainability through health systems strengthening; leveraging key organizations; partnerships across all sectors; increasing impact through strategic coordination and integration; improving metrics, monitoring, and evaluation; and promoting research and innovation.

However, the GHI, as with the Japanese Global Health Policy 2011–2015, does not seem to address the issue of global cooperation in health funding, nor does it seek sufficient coherence between national activities and multinational organizations, non-state actors, and the private sector.

Foreign Policy and Global Health

In 2006 the ministers of foreign affairs of seven countries — Brazil, France, Indonesia, Norway, Senegal, South Africa, and Thailand — embarked on promoting a health lens on foreign affairs by agreeing on the

Oslo Ministerial Declaration on Foreign Policy and Global Health.[18] This initiative has clearly put global health on the radar of the foreign ministries, whose core mission is to work toward a coherent foreign policy. This is also reflected in the UN General Assembly resolution initiated by the same countries every year since 2008.[19-22] The resolution of 2009 requested the UN Secretary General to provide a report which "examines ways in which foreign and health policy coordination and coherence can be strengthened at the national, regional and international levels." This examination is still an active concern for the WHO and thus a focus for research, training, and further development among Member States, donors, and NGOs, collectively and as individual actors in global health.

Discussion

Physicists understand how entropy in our universe permits chaos to be the norm and that any attempt at ordering this situation needs constant investment of energy and resources. With the growing complexity of global health issues and the interplay of these issues with foreign policy, governments are increasingly confronted with the challenges of policy consistency and coherence. Most government ministries or agencies are bound by their primary missions as well as the authorizing legislation for financing these missions; thus, noncoherence is the norm, and policy coherence in global health needs specific attention through legislation, leadership, and cooperative efforts, both within and outside of national governments.

Policy coherence for health and development means that diverse organs of government not only sustain their core mandates but also see interagency coordination as an essential element of their mission. This requires negotiations to find synergies and compromises in the overlapping areas of agency mandates and competencies. When consensus cannot be achieved at the agency level, these agencies must bring the issue to the next level of decision, with leadership at this level necessary to assure policy coherence as well as the success of individual agencies' agenda.

Most industrialized countries separate policies for health (as mainly a domestic focus) and development (as mainly a developing country focus), even though health development and global interdependence in health issues are closely linked; thus, there is a need for sovereign nations to address both issues with a coherent global health policy. Health ministries generally take the lead in representing their countries in multilateral health fora such as the WHO, while development agencies have much larger budgets for their nation's global health activities. This creates a challenge for policy coherence at the interface of health and development ministries, notwithstanding the concerns for trade, security, and other sectors. Health and development leaders may in fact oppose agencies responsible for intellectual property protections for their domestic health-related industries, which are a core economic interest for many countries.

Policy coherence in global health is a concern at all levels of decision-making and within different departments of a single ministry. A coherent global health policy should involve the following elements: (1) interministerial coherence between foreign policy and the international positions of different sectors within governments; (2) coherence between national and international health policies; and (3) coherence among the multilevel global health actors. With regard to the last, many Member States blame multilateral organizations for lack of coherence, while at the same time these countries (especially donor countries) may be forcing this incoherence through their own incoherent positions within the respective governing bodies of these organizations.

Global health programs aim to achieve long-term goals, and thus there is a need for long-term policy commitments for these programs. This is a challenging task in a political world geared toward short-term successes. For example, most ministers of health have terms of only a few years, and during this time they will be evaluated on the basis of accomplishments within their term. Even with short-term accomplishments, countervailing actions of other agencies may neutralize these efforts later. Long-term global health policy coherence must therefore come from a national or multinational conviction that conflicting policies are inefficient and do not serve the global public good in an interconnected world. The concept of "health in all policies" is increasingly applied to foreign policy by a growing roster of donor and recipient countries.

Establishing policy coherence consumes time and resources. Therefore a balance has to be achieved between these efforts and the bureaucratic paralysis that may get in the way of any such negotiations. Policy coherence must bring added value to participating agencies, and must be considered a two-way process. Ministries of health can only expect other ministries to assume responsibility in health policy if the health ministries also understand their own cross-government responsibility in other policy arenas. Further, coherence in international development objectives can only succeed if conflicting foreign policy objectives can be negotiated across government; politics may trump global health commitments unless these issues can be translated into political objectives common with foreign policy. See the case study on vaccine diplomacy by Kaufman and Feldbaum in this volume for an example of such translation.

How can policy coherence be achieved in global health? Governments have started to experiment with different instruments to achieve this end. Examples of these processes are:

- Establishing interministerial coordination platforms specific to global health.
- Assigning a focal point for global health issues in the Ministry of Foreign Affairs.
- Establishing a global health affairs unit in the Ministry of Health, led by a senior, experienced official (director general, assistant secretary, or a similar high-level administrator).
- Developing a published, coordinated national global health strategy.
- Including training in global health issues in the basic training of diplomats.
- Including training in foreign affairs and negotiation skills for staff members of global health units in ministries of health.
- Assigning health attachés to multilateral and bilateral diplomatic missions (especially those in Geneva and New York).
- Supporting staff exchange between ministries of health and of foreign affairs.
- Promoting curriculum content on health diplomacy in global health academic programs.

While lenses through which global health policy are viewed may differ between foreign policy and public health disciplines, the underlying purpose of national global health strategies is common to both: health is global and therefore a key element of foreign policy, and foreign policy is a key mechanism through which cross-border health challenges are addressed by sovereign nations. Some countries now focus on defining common health and foreign policy objectives, while others seek more consistency internally so that their representation in multinational fora such as the WHO may be more effective. The key feature of all national global health strategies is that they are the product of an intentional, interagency collaborative process that recognizes the interdependence of nations, multilateral organizations, NGOs, and the private sector in addressing 21st century health challenges.

Acknowledgment

This chapter reflects the personal views of the authors and not necessarily the position of the Swiss government. The analysis in it is based on the available policy documents as of July 2011.

References

1. Kickbusch I. (2011) Global health diplomacy: How foreign policy can influence health. *BMJ* **342:** d3154. doi:10.1136/bmj.d3154
2. Adams V, Novotny TE, Leslie H. (2008) Global health diplomacy [editorial], *Med Anthropol* **12(4):** 315–323.
3. Anonymous. (2010) The Millennium Development Goals: Global targets, local ingenuity. *The Economist*, September 23. Available from http://www.economist.com/node/17090934 (accessed August 6, 2011).
4. High Court of South Africa. (1998) Case number 4183/98, the Pharmaceutical Manufacturers' Association of South Africa *et al.* v. the President of the Republic of South Africa, the Honorable Mr. N. R. Mandela *et al.*
5. Medicins sans Frontiers. (2011) Access to Essential Medicines Campaign. Available from http://www.msfaccess.org (accessed July 30, 2011).
6. Prakash SS. (1994) Multinational corporations and the impact of public advocacy on corporate strategy: Nestlé and the infant formula controversy. *J Int Bus Stud* **25(3):** 658–660. doi: 10.1057/jibs.1994.41. (6) US Government. The US Global Health Intiative. Available from http://www.ghi.gov (accessed July 30, 2011).

7. Tempest B. (2011) The structural changes in the global pharmaceutical marketplace and their possible implications for intellectual property. Policy Brief No. 10, July 2011. International Centre for Trade and Sustainable Development, Geneva.

8. Swiss Agency for Development and Cooperation (2008). Swiss Coordination GAP/Swiss Foreign Health Policy. Available from http://www.sdc-health.ch/priorities_in_health/good_governance/swiss, (accessed August 6, 2011).

9. Donaldson L. (2007) Health is global: Proposals for a UK government-wide strategy. Available from http://www.dh.gov.uk/prod_consum_dh/groups/dh_digitalassets/documents/digitalasset/dh_072696.pdf (accessed July 31, 2011).

10. Health is global: An outcomes framework for global health 2011–2015. Available from http://www.dh.gov.uk/en/Publicationsandstatistics/Publications/PublicationsPolicyAndGuidance/DH_125605 (accessed October 2011).

11. European Union. (1993) Maastricht Treaty. Eurotreaties. Available from http://www.eurotreaties.com/maastrichtext.html (accessed August 6, 2011).

12. Commission of the European Communities. (2007) Together for health: A strategic approach for the EU 2008–2013 [White Paper]. Brussels, 23.10.2007, COM(2007) 630 final. Available from http://ec.europa.eu/health/ph_overview/Documents/strategy_wp_en.pdf (accessed July 31, 2011).

13. European Union. (2010) Summary: 10 May 2010, Brussels — Council of the European Union 3011th Foreign Affairs Council meeting, conclusions on the EU role in global health. Available from http://www.europa-eu-un.org/articles/en/article_9727_en.htm (accessed July 31, 2011).

14. Norwegian Ministry of Health and Care Services, Norwegian Ministry of Foreign Affairs. (2010) Norwegian WHO strategy: Norway as a member of WHO's Executive Board 2010–2013. Available from http://www.helsedirektoratet.no/vp/multimedia/archive/00307/Norwegian_WHO_Strat_307109a.pdf (accessed July 31, 2011).

15. Okada K. (2010) Japan's new global health policy: 2011–2015. *Lancet* **376:** 938–940. Available from http://ec.europa.eu/health/eu_world/docs/ev_20101013_rd06_en.pdf (accessed July 31, 2011).

16. The United States Government. (2009) Global Health Initiative. Strategy document. Available from http://www.ghi.gov/documents/organization/157796.pdf (accessed August 6, 2011).

17. Kates J, Fischer J, Lief E. (2009) *The U.S. Government's Global Health Policy Architecture: Structure, Programs, and Funding.* Henry J. Kaiser Family Foundation, Washington DC.

18. Ministers of Foreign Affairs of Brazil, France, Indonesia, Norway, Senegal, South Africa, and Thailand. (2007) Oslo Ministerial Declaration — Global health: A pressing foreign policy issue of our time. *Lancet* **369(9570):** 1373–1378. doi:10.1016/S0140-6736(07)60498-X).

19. United Nations. (2008) Resolution adopted by the United Nations General Assembly on "Global Health and Foreign Policy," A/Res/63/33.

20. United Nations. (2009) Resolution adopted by the United Nations General Assembly on "Global health and Foreign Policy," A/Res/64/108.

21. United Nations. (2009) Global health and foreign policy: Strategic opportunities and challenges. Note by Secretary-General, A/64/365.

22. United Nations. (2010) Resolution adopted by the United Nations General Assembly on "Global Health and Foreign Policy," A/Res/65/95.

12

The Way Forward in Global Health Diplomacy: Definitions, Research, and Training

*Thomas E. Novotny, MD, MPH**
and Sebastian Kevany, MA, MPH†

Introduction

This volume has covered a wealth of historical, political, diplomatic, and technical information in an attempt to describe the deepening links between health and foreign policy and the architecture that characterizes 21st century health diplomacy. Since we began our work, considerable progress has been made in further defining, applying, and expanding our understanding of the growing field of "global health diplomacy" (GHD). An overriding question that arises from our attempts to define this field is: How does foreign policy serve health or how does health serve foreign policy?

Kickbusch and others have asserted that diplomats are no longer concerned only with matters of national power, security, and trade; they also need to deal with global challenges such as development, health, environment, water, and

---

*Professor and Associate Director for Border and Global Health, Graduate School of Public Health, San Diego State University, 5500 Campanile Drive, Hardy Tower 119, San Diego, California, 92182, USA
E-mail: tnovotny@mail.sdsu.edu, Tel.: 619-594-3109.
†Institute for Health Policy Studies, University of California, San Francisco.

food security.[1] Likewise, global health practitioners must look to international agreements, negotiations, and collaborations in order to assure the health of their domestic populations. The skills necessary for success in such activities are not taught in health sciences programs, nor are the in-depth technical health issues normally covered in foreign service training institutes. Nevertheless, such collaborative global engagement by foreign policy professionals, health professionals, and nongovernmental actors is essential not only in sustaining the health of national populations but also in assuring the effectiveness of the substantial investments in global health that have been made in the last two decades.

Increasingly, evidence-based outcomes of investments are demanded by donors and international health financing organizations, and these outcomes rightly depend on the success of the collaborations necessary for fully implementing these interventions. Yet the array of actors participating in global health negotiations, philanthropies, and health diplomacy has also grown enormously over the last two decades.[2] This final chapter will summarize the efforts to define GHD, present research questions that have been formulated by various scholars related to GHD, and briefly describe training scenarios and curricular content for GHD.

Defining Global Health Diplomacy

Feldbaum and Michaud[3] assembled helpful definitions for foreign policy, diplomacy, and global health as a baseline for developing a definition of GHD (Box 1).

In particular, diplomacy is a set of methods used by national governments to "implement their [own] foreign policy." Today, this diplomacy encompasses "hard power" (military and economic sanctions), "soft power" (co-option and cooperation), and "smart power" (which utilizes all modalities to achieve foreign policy objectives). These concepts help to set the stage for refining our notion of GHD not only as soft power but also as a part of smart power for governments; such an approach includes nongovernmental organizations, multilateral organizations, and a wide variety of donors and private sector actors. Recently, several authors have

Box 1. Definitions: Foreign Policy, Diplomacy, Global Health*

- Foreign policy is the "substance, aims and attitudes of a state's relations with others," and may be defined as the "activity whereby state actors act, react and interact" between the "internal or domestic environment and an external or global environment."[4]
- Diplomacy is the art and practice of conducting international relations, and "provides one instrument that international actors use to implement their foreign policy."[5]
- Global health "places a priority on improving health and achieving equity in health for all people worldwide... emphasizes transnational health issues, determinants, and solutions [and] involves many disciplines within and beyond the health sciences."[6]

*Adapted from Ref. 3.

provided definitions of GHD (Box 2). These definitions in fact all relate to the question of whether health drives foreign policy or vice versa. Perhaps, in the end, it does not matter which is the driving force, but certainly this question lends itself to research on several levels. It also lends itself to expanded training needs for health professionals, diplomats, and their non-state partners.

Health as a Driver of Foreign Policy

Although global health advocates view improving global health as a critical objective of foreign policy in and of itself, and that health diplomacy can "shape and manage the global policy environment for health,"[8] government action on health is motivated by foreign policy interests as well as by health or humanitarian goals. However, Feldbaum and Michaud argue that GHD must be linked to core economic, foreign policy, or security interests if health is to be prioritized in foreign policy. They emphasize that "foreign policy interests are of *primary* [italics added] and enduring

Box 2. Definitions of Global Health Diplomacy*

- *A political change activity that meets the dual goals of improving global health while maintaining and strengthening international relations abroad, particularly in conflict areas and resource-poor environments.*
- *Multi-level, multi-factor negotiation processes that shape and manage the global policy environment for health.*
- *Winning hearts and minds of people in poor countries by exporting medical care, expertise, and personnel to help those who need it most.*
- Health diplomacy is the chosen method of interaction between stakeholders engaged in public health and politics for the purpose of representation, cooperation, resolving disputes, improving health systems, and securing the right to health for vulnerable populations.
- *Health diplomacy is a means of self-preservation in an increasingly interconnected global community... health diplomacy also offers a much-needed opportunity for building bridges between the governments of the world and the private sector, synergizing efforts of nongovernmental organizations (NGOs) and allowing them to work together to improve public health.*

*Adapted from Ref. 7.

importance to understanding the potential and limits of health diplomacy." GHD is important in 21st century international relations (and hence smart power) because of the transcendent relevance of health to the following foreign policy priorities: (1) *security*, owing to the fear of global pandemics; bioterrorism; and the health consequences of humanitarian conflicts, natural disasters, and emergencies; (2) *economy*, owing to the economic effects of poor health on global development, of pandemic outbreaks on global trade, and of the growing global market in health goods (especially pharmaceuticals) and services; and (3) *social justice*, which reinforces health as a social value and as a human right, and calls for high-income countries to invest in a broad range of initiatives that benefit the poor.[1]

Katz *et al.*[2] reviewed the contexts, practice, and components of GHD in an operational context and proposed taxonomy to reflect the diversity of the field of GHD. They separated health diplomacy into three categories of interaction around global public health issues: (1) core diplomacy, including formal negotiations among nations; (2) multi-stakeholder diplomacy, involving negotiations among nations and non-state actors; and (3) informal diplomacy (or "freelance" diplomacy), which might include governments, nongovernmental organizations, private sector groups, international actors, and the public.

Lee and Smith[7] distinguished the "new diplomacy," dealing with health and globalization as a public health enterprise, from "traditional diplomacy," as practiced strictly in foreign policy circles. They *further* defined GHD, in concert with Kickbusch *et al.*,[4] as "negotiations on population health issues that require global collective action" to effectively address these problems.

GHD is now characterized by diverse actors, and different processes of interaction among these actors. These elements were included in a more concise definition of GHD for use in an international discourse funded by the Rockefeller Foundation at its Bellagio Conference Center in 2009–11. GHD, according to Smith and Fidler[9] in this forum, is "…policy-shaping processes through which state, non-state and other institutional actors negotiate responses to health challenges, or utilize health concepts or mechanisms in policy-shaping and negotiation strategies, to achieve other political, economic or social objectives."

In all these descriptions and definitions, health diplomacy is consistently and strongly recognized as a key foreign policy practice at multiple levels and in multiple fora that requires collective negotiations. This is especially necessary in an increasingly globalized world with growing economic disparities and with reduced capacity for official development assistance (ODA) among traditional donor nations. What is becoming clear, however, is that evidence is needed that GHD can demonstrate efficacy and effectiveness as a 21st century political investment for donors, multinational organizations, and governments. Such "investments" may include personnel, training, and the extra time commitments required for negotiations, collaborations, and convening activities. Instruments and procedures are available for traditional negotiations, as described by

Bertorelli *et al.* in this volume (Chapter 4), and governance structures and their limitations have been discussed in detail by Hein (Chapter 3). However, research is now needed as to how GHD works, what it can accomplish, and how it can be evaluated. Based on this research agenda and the reviews we have presented in this volume, we can think more about the design of GHD training programs, support networks and learning communities, and then continue to look critically at the outcomes of GHD practices going forward as a research agenda.

A Research Agenda in Global Health

First, let us consider the current state of research activities in GHD. Most scholars involved in such research are part of the Global Health Diplomacy Network (GHD-NET), which had its first formal meeting in June 2011 at Chatham House in London.[10] GHD-NET is an international organization of members that engage in research, training, and the practice of GHD (http://www.ghd-net.org). Founded in 2009 through the Rockefeller Bellagio Dialogue mentioned above, it is currently hosted at the Centre for Trade Policy and Law in Ottawa, Canada. GHD-NET's overall objective is "to build capacity for stakeholders to participate in, inform, and influence diplomatic negotiations in ways that reflect public health principles and evidence and improve collective action on global health."

At this writing, the future of the Network is somewhat tenuous; nevertheless, the individuals and institutions involved remain active in both GHD training and research activities. For example, GHD-Net commissioned researchers at the London School of Hygiene and Tropical Medicine to help define the research agenda in GHD. As a result of this commission, Smith, Fidler, and Lee[9] suggested that GHD research should:

- Focus on the processes (rather than the content) through which diplomatic activities address health problems or utilize health concepts or mechanisms to achieve other political, economic, or social objectives.
- Pay particular attention to challenges faced by low- and middle-income countries.

- Inform efforts that GHD-Net stakeholders make to provide policy-relevant input to foreign policy, diplomatic, and advocacy activities on global health issues.

Lee and Smith[8] further proposed a set of more specific research questions in order to move the health diplomacy discourse away from only normative advocacy toward an evidence-based agenda. These issues were discussed as part of the Chatham House meeting cited above (Boxes 3–5). These questions point out the importance of *evaluation* of GHD as a critical part of the research agenda and include the following approaches:[10]

- To measure the impact (both positive and negative) of GHD, on health and on other sectors.
- To establish and track qualitative and quantitative outcome measures.
- To increase understanding of the stages of getting to an outcome, and then how (and whether) the outcomes of diplomacy get implemented on the national level.
- To inform the global health and foreign policy sectors of each other's perspectives, in order to bridge the gap between two

---

Box 3. Global Health Diplomacy and Globalization

- What role does GHD play in addressing the particular challenges that globalization poses for global health and the broader global community as a whole?
- How does the shifting balance of power in world politics affect GHD?
- How can GHD play a role in maintaining global health as a high policy priority among world leaders in the coming decades?
- What can GHD teach us about the challenges of strengthening collective action in an increasingly global world?

Box 4. The Role of Diverse Actors in Global Health Diplomacy

- Who is responsible for undertaking or engaging in GHD?
- How do specific actors (and types of actors) participate in GHD? How do they influence GHD individually and collectively?
- What are the relative roles of state and non-state actors in GHD?
- What are the relative roles of health and non-health actors in GHD?
- Why do certain actors participate in GHD? What are their interests and what goals/interests do they seek to pursue?
- What determines the power and influence of specific actors in GHD?
- Who holds authority in GHD and from where does this authority derive? How does this change by issue area and over time?
- Does authority/legitimacy in GHD coincide with responsibility?
- Which actors are underrepresented in GHD and why? What can be done to improve the representativeness, of GHD?
- How can we assess the quality of GHD in terms of accountability, transparency, representativeness, and effectiveness?

communities that come together in times of crisis but with different contexts — for one group, health is the issue, while for the other, health is just one of many issues that need to be pursued, and not always the central one.

- To better equip those engaged in GHD, in coherence with the Network's training objectives; research processes that include the participation of GHD actors might yield more relevant information, forming a closer loop between research findings and practice.
- To learn lessons from diplomacy not related to health.
- To gain a better understanding of the role of the WHO in GHD, relative to other processes, both bilateral and multilateral.

Box 5. Venues and Forms of Global Health Diplomacy

- How can we assess the quality of GHD in terms of accountability, transparency, representativeness, and effectiveness?
- How much GHD takes place? How would it be measured?
- How does GHD actually work or not work? How would this be assessed?
- Which institutions formally conduct GHD and how effectively do they function?
- Are certain venues more effective at conducting GHD than others?
- At what different institutional levels does GHD take place? How do they function together?
- Can we distinguish between formal and informal GHD?
- What are the principles of decision making in GHD?
- What channels and processes of "new diplomacy" could be used for GHD?
- To what extent is GHD facilitated or hindered by netpolitik? How might this be changing the nature of GHD?
- What institutional mechanisms are needed to support GHD?
- Is there such a thing as new public diplomacy in global health?
- What is the relationship between new public diplomacy and global health?

Evaluating Global Health Programs from the Diplomatic and Foreign Policy Perspectives

In the increasingly constrained global health funding environment, the measurement of implicit and explicit outputs, outcomes, and impacts of global health financing has assumed great importance. In keeping with the principles of performance-based funding demanded by organizations such as the World Bank, the President's Emergency Plan for AIDS Relief (PEPFAR), the US Millennium Challenge Corporation, the Global Fund to Fight AIDS, Tuberculosis and Malaria (GFATM), and the Bill and

Melinda Gates Foundation, development programs are now expected to provide tangible and transparent data on outcomes of donor investments. Traditionally, evaluation measures have been confined to a relatively narrow range of programmatic results, focusing on health outputs and financial disbursements (e.g., cost-effectiveness analysis), and not necessarily on the more implicit, long-term, indirect, or collateral outputs, outcomes, and impacts of program activities. These measures may no longer be sufficient to reflect the actual gains made that are relevant to recipients, donors, or governments — of which the last are increasingly expected to assume responsibility for internationally funded interventions.

Traditional foreign policy interventions include those characterized by hard power (military force), economic sanctions or incentives, and these may be questioned or analyzed as to their efficacy and effectiveness. The old as well as new economic powers are now seeking alternative — and more inclusive — forms of international engagement both to sustain national interests and to assure global security in the world.[11,12] Thus, these GHD practices will need to be evaluated according to their "peace and stability" dividends, as well as for their economic, political, and of course global health dividends.

How can global health programs contribute to "political economy"? While global health programs provide recipient countries with significant international assistance, they also have the potential to support the "enlightened self-interest" of donors. On the economic level, both donor and recipient states — and, indeed, large corporations that may have more significant international investments than many donor nations — are increasingly interested in the role of GHD in supporting their international development objectives and economic interests.[3] The role of health and development programs in ensuring the well-being of the international labor force, in generating international business opportunities, in assuring free trade, and in facilitating access to commodity resources from LMICs complements altruism with hard-nosed economic reasons for development assistance. In a sense, these 21st century GHD efforts hark back to elements of colonial history as articulated by Adams in this volume (Chapter 2).

Today, however, the competition between national economic priorities and foreign aid commitments raises important ethical questions for

High-Income Countries (HICs).[13] Global health resources more than quadrupled from US$5.6 billion in 1990 to US$25 billion in 2011, and the rate of growth accelerated sharply after 2002, when the Millennium Development Goals were launched by UN Member States. However, the alleviation of suffering abroad is seen by many as discretionary in times of fiscal crisis, and therefore such assistance may be subordinated to other domestic economic priorities. The research question then involves showing the current and potential, both implicit and explicit, and national and global benefits of international assistance and how this assistance may more meaningfully serve critical foreign policy objectives when "diplomatically sensitized." These objectives include the high ideals of world peace, prosperity, and security — goals that may transcend the inherent idealism of global health programs.

The need for evaluation studies on the outcomes of GHD and related assistance programs from the economic, political, international relations, diplomatic, and human rights standpoints is evident in the 21st century, smart power era. The following discussion attempts to frame the evaluation of GHD.

Foreign assistance reform: Demands for advanced evaluation techniques

The need for the evaluation of GHD is reflected in the growing integration between departments of development assistance and ministries of foreign affairs across donor countries (HICs). Fidler[14] described this progression as the "high politics" of global health insofar as HICs may leverage development programs to support their foreign policy goals. This "progressive" approach was noted in a report by the US Global Leadership Coalition,[a] such that "...over the past decade, the importance of using all our foreign policy tools to shore up our national security — development and

---

[a]The US Global Leadership Coalition (USGLC) is a network of 400 businesses and NGOs; national security and foreign policy experts; and business, faith-based, academic, and community leaders who support a smart power approach that can elevate diplomacy and development alongside defense to assure global security. See http://www.usglc.org/about/our-mission/

diplomacy, alongside defense — has had strong bipartisan support" in the US Congress.[15]

In the United States, closer alignment between the activities of the United States Agency for International Development (USAID) and the Department of State (DOS) has become a central feature of foreign assistance reform under both the current (Obama) and the prior (Bush II) administration; this was further articulated by President Obama in 2009 as the US Global Health Initiative (GHI). The joint DOS and USAID Quadrennial Diplomacy and Development Review (QDDR) set institutional priorities and provided strategic guidance as a framework for efficient allocation of foreign assistance resources under the GHI, and this realignment was intended to be a post-partisan political effort. However, recent political obstructionism has precluded full funding of the GHI, and the initiative has now been moved to a new Office for Health Diplomacy embedded within the DOS.[16] At this writing, the outcome of the GHI's restructuring is not yet clear, though the broader trend of interdepartmental integration remains evident in the initiative. As a part of the DOS, it can be expected that health will be serving as an important component of US foreign policy and smart power in the "whole of government" approach going forward.

In the United Kingdom, the Department for International Development (DFID) has been recognized as a key element of modern British foreign policy.[17] In fact, it is a cabinet-level entity rather than a department within a ministry; while, in the European Union, the Common Foreign and Security Policy makes explicit reference to the role of development programs such as global health under a smart power framework.[18] These structures represent a determined effort to link global health programming and foreign policy priorities, helping to provide meaningful and effective alternatives to hard power interventions, and have been described earlier in this volume by Silberschmidt and Zeltner (Chapter 11) with a focus on Switzerland.

Fidler notes that "the implications of successful global health programs without foreign policy considerations are just as dangerous to human dignity as the reverse."[14] In all countries, the demands for key personnel with appropriate qualifications and experience in both the global health and foreign policy spheres are evident. Special, transdisciplinary skills are necessary in order align the mutual objectives of the foreign policy and foreign assistance communities in GHD.[2] In addition, new infrastructures in which to practice these skills may be necessary. For example, "political analysis liaison units" within multilateral health-related donor organizations such as the GFATM would complement the development of health expertise among foreign policy professionals. Equally important, systems of evaluation that "speak a language that people with power really understand,"[19] as well as systems of evaluating the success of such integration efforts within donor governments, will be necessary for cohesive foreign policy and global health assistance programs.

Diplomatic evaluation concepts

How then can the benefits of GHD be more explicitly measured in the foreign policy enterprise?[12] A good starting point may be to examine the distinction between "diplomatically sensitized" global health programmatic outcomes and "global-health-sensitized" foreign policy outcomes. On one hand, diplomatically sensitized global health programs may incorporate foreign policy considerations such as partnership development, recipient perceptions and priorities, strategic geographic issues, social justice and equity, and, of course, effectiveness and efficacy. On the other hand, global-health-sensitized foreign policy may influence the *realpolitik* of global affairs, including traditional foreign policy issues such as balance of power, peacekeeping, geostability, international prestige, economic stability, and other strategic objectives (Ref. 20 and Chapter 8 of this volume). Diplomacy is a tool of foreign policy, and GHD is a specialized version of diplomacy now recognized by many established as well as emerging economies as critically important to their national priorities.

In the more nuanced realm of humanitarian assistance in conflict and post-conflict settings (see Chapter 9), GHD considerations may be even more important (if not mission-critical), even if no formal method of quantifying their effectiveness is currently available. Internationally supported humanitarian or military interventions in settings such as South Sudan, Iraq, and Afghanistan may, intentionally or unintentionally, support (or undermine) peacekeeping, geopolitical, and "nation-building" goals[21,22] to an extent far beyond their stated purview. Perhaps most important in the evaluation of GHD in such settings is the contextual understanding and responsiveness that is necessary for successful program implementation. This means that while core elements of the intervention protocol are adhered to, these programs are also sensitized to the fundamental needs of recipient communities and the geopolitics of the region.[23]

There remains a need for criteria and associated tools by which global health programs can be monitored and evaluated from a foreign policy perspective. These tools would not aim to evaluate the interventions in terms of their primary health program goals, as numerous metrics already exist to do this, but rather to evaluate their value from a foreign policy perspective. Since "…the top priorities of foreign policy are national security and economic growth…,"[10] the health sector must consider how health policy can also have a negative impact on foreign policy goals, just as how foreign policy can have a negative impact on health. This has been described in policy discussions regarding the economic ramifications of different interventions — from the perspective of both the donor and recipient countries, at the national, community, and individual levels.[24] Quantification of such outcomes using standard statistical or epidemiological approaches, however, seems unlikely. Nonetheless, existing rapid assessment tools, such as the on-site data verification (OSDV) and routine service quality assessment (RSQA) tools employed by the GFATM,[25] may suggest opportunities for evaluation of program outcomes from a broader foreign policy perspective. Through the identification of the threats and benefits to foreign policy or diplomatic objectives using an amended rapid assessment tool (SYSRA[26]), policy-makers may be provided with tangible evidence of the relative diplomatic utility of GHD activities in different settings. Such data can help inform strategic decision-making and resource allocation around foreign assistance; in this sense, GHD may in fact fuel foreign policy development or modification.

Criteria to evaluate the utility of GHD must be responsive to the ever-changing global political environment and thus may be objectionable to those who believe that GHD should focus exclusively on global health objectives. These criteria may be developed using *political philosophy* perspectives on GHD as articulated by Fidler.[14] These perspectives include:

- Utilitarian or "neo-utilitarian" considerations: "Does the program possess a culture of measurement and accountability? Is it being utilized, as well as being cost-effective?"

- Rawlsian considerations: "Is there a concern for social justice in the health program? Is the program sustainable, and does it contribute to broader development goals?"
- Kantian considerations: "Has this program contributed to regional stability, nation-building, international relations, helping us move towards world peace?" And even
- Machiavellian considerations: "Does the program assist access to strategic resources or markets? Is the donor's regional or international influence and prestige enhanced?"

Implications for resource allocation

The rise of evidence-based decision-making in global health programs has, among its other effects, promulgated a dramatically enhanced role for cost-effectiveness analysis. However, this is not just an analysis of technical efficiency (how to best implement an agreed strategy), but also, perhaps more contentiously, includes assessments of allocative efficiency, i.e., informing decisions about how to divide funding among projects which target different populations, geographical areas, and program goals.[27] While such an approach can help to optimize program outcomes in constrained resource environments, it also has the potential to erode general health budgeting — and therefore overall health gains — through a narrow focus on specific program outcomes to the exclusion of broader political and diplomatic considerations. Is it possible, then, that through the channeling of donor funding to interventions, the value of which is judged solely on medical effectiveness, the broader diplomatic and foreign policy dividends of global health programs may be lost? Valentino[28] notes that "in all cases, these are political choices, and they are likely to be made badly if governed chiefly by philanthropic considerations. Instead, it is necessary to think about the two-in-one character of humanitarian aid."

If Valentino is correct, the implications for resource allocation decisions based on political realities are significant. Decisions about which interventions to support — and in which regions and target populations these interventions are applied — would need to take into account several often-competing criteria: foreign policy objectives, diplomatic considerations, *and* health needs. A recent example is the growing movement toward treatment of HIV-positive individuals with antiretroviral drugs. Cost-effectiveness analysts had claimed that many more lives might be saved if these funds were reprogrammed toward HIV prevention,[27] but this conclusion does not consider the humanitarian, international relations, and foreign policy dividends that result from the provision of life-saving treatment to those most in need. While such analyses did find that the emotional force of a focus on treatment could leverage overall funding for HIV/AIDS, the analysis concluded that even a 10-fold growth in funding would not justify a strong treatment approach if *the sole evaluation criterion is aggregate health status.* The analysis did not, however, examine other non-health outcomes, such as winning "hearts and minds." Perhaps more importantly, the risks associated with the suspension of treatment programs on economic or cost-effectiveness grounds have already been flagged as a possible threat both to national political stability and to relations between donor and recipient countries.[29]

With the development of more appropriate GHD evaluation criteria, resource allocation decisions across global health programs may, in the future, be made with favorable diplomatic outcomes included as part of expected program results. Resource allocation decisions will, in turn, need to be made on a more collaborative basis, combining inputs from scientists, economists, and the more "real world" considerations of foreign policy experts and recipient nations.

GHD research agenda conclusions

Policy-makers are increasingly aware of the special value of global health in the international relations sphere.[30] While agricultural and educational programs may provide compelling gains in measurable outcomes to donors and recipients alike, the specific additional value of GHD components of these programs, including their capacity to win hearts and minds, is perhaps even more important in today's globalized world. This is a world where pandemics may threaten economic stability and where disease challenges do not recognize national borders. Hence, the challenging task of evaluating global health programs from the diplomatic, international relations, and foreign policy standpoints may provide significant dividends — not only to foreign policy professionals but also to global health advocates. In the future, when policymakers ask "What is the return on our investment?" in GHD, they will be better informed about and therefore better understand the range of benefits — from national security to domestic economic gains to international prestige — that result from the blending of health and foreign policy objectives. Further, the need for international economic homeostasis achieved through the new global "balance of power" and multinationalism are essential elements of GHD that both transcend and support national foreign policy priorities. The emerging powers (Brazil, China, India, Russia,[b] and South Africa) in fact call for further research to evaluate how notions of "south-to-south" cooperation affect global stability and international economic development.

It is not just policymakers in the traditional donor governments that need to be provided with evidence for the efficacy of GHD. Foreign assistance may be considered by the public as an unnecessary holdover from the 20th century. However, the evidence is accumulating to show that such assistance is not simply a justifiable expenditure of tax dollars but also a critical foreign policy and security concern in the globalized economy.[30] If the public can be provided with compelling evidence that *they themselves* benefit from such investments through domestic economic, security, humanitarian, and national prestige dividends, there will be public support for global health investments and GHD. Thus, the disseminating results of GHD research will play a critical role in informing public opinion as well as national decision-making.

Training in Global Health Diplomacy

The response to global health challenges is heavily dependent on diplomats and health professionals understanding not only the health burden of these challenges but also the interwoven nature of foreign policy and health. Thus, training in GHD requires grounding in global health science as well as in foreign policy practices. It further requires integration at different levels of practice: among governments and non-state implementers

---

[b]Russia in fact has explicitly stated that its international development programs are to be designed and used with foreign policy as a primary consideration — see http://www.guardian. co.uk/global-development/2011/may/25/russia-foreign-aid-report-influence-image

in the field; among national governments and their various implementing agencies; and among multinational organizations, NGOs, and non-state actors in the global arena. Case-based learning has been increasingly used for understanding GHD. Cases studies are now appearing in published format,[31] but training programs using these cases will benefit from involvement of experienced professionals with expertise in both health and negotiations.

Global health educational programs have proliferated across both north and south, with curriculum content spanning research skills, cultural studies, social sciences, and basic sciences.[32] Skill building in GHD further requires more nuanced understanding of negotiation processes, economic and trade policy, global governance, cultural complexities, and political science. Scientists do not generally possess these skills, and diplomats may need broader understanding of public health principles and the integration of these with human rights regimes. Thus, cross-disciplinary training is critical to the field of GHD.[33] Case studies can illustrate the complexity of negotiations, which involve multi-level, multi-factor and multi-actor repercussions for science, health, trade, security, and ethics that make for complicated negotiations.[34]

Approaches to GHD Training

Different formats of GHD training may be needed to serve different audiences. The original training model of the Global Health Program of the Graduate Institute of International and Development Studies (Geneva) is a week-long summer course (http://graduateinstitute.ch/corporate/executive/training-workshops/global-health-diplomacy_fr.html). This flagship course now uses standardized training materials for capacity building in GHD based on accumulated experiences in Geneva and worldwide. The target audience for this executive training activity includes decision-makers and representatives from governments, international organizations, global health initiatives, and other stakeholders in global governance for health, such as civil society, foundations, the private sector, platforms, and alliances. Additional similar courses have been conducted in partnership with the Graduate Institute in Washington, Ottawa, Nairobi, Beijing, and Jakarta. Partners have included the US Centers for Disease Control and

Prevention (CDC), San Diego State University, Peking University, Mahidol University in Bangkok, the University of Nairobi and Government of Kenya, the Swiss Federal Office of Public Health, the Oswaldo Cruz Foundation of Brazil, the World Health Organization, and other international institutions.

Tailored, one-to-three–day training sessions may also be appropriate for upper- and mid-level participants who cannot take the time to travel to such executive courses. Modules on GHD may now be included in academic global health training programs and evaluated as to specific learning objectives. In addition, foreign service training programs may make use of case studies such as those found in other titles in this book series.[31] Based on lessons learned from such activities, all training models could be followed by refreshers or long-term leadership development programs that keep the learning community in touch and allow continued learning from the experiences of training program alumni.

Curricular Content

Although curricular content will vary according to the participating audience, venue, and training objectives, the Graduate Institute has developed and refined curricular content along with GHD. NET partners in Thailand, China, Kenya, and the United States.[35] Based on lessons learned during various training programs, the following curricular items have been included in GHD training programs:

(1) *Introduction to Health Diplomacy.* This covers the definition of health diplomacy, the multilayered processes involved in GHD, and the various actors involved in GHD today.
(2) *Historical Perspectives on Health Diplomacy.* This covers the historical and cultural underpinnings of GHD, including colonialism, trade policy, power asymmetries and recent power shifts, and the development of multinational health and development organizations.
(3) *Global Health Governance.* This covers the complexities of the various global health organizations, including recent changes in funding sources, philanthropies, development organization priorities, private–public

partnerships, south-to-south collaboration, and the various government global health initiatives.

(4) *International Health Law.* This module extends the previous discussion to cover theoretical and practical applications of international health law. It sets the stage for the *Instruments* discussion to follow.

(5) *Global Health Diplomacy Instruments.* This covers "hard law," "soft law," consensus agreements, bilateral agreements, country groupings, and new economic arrangements such as the Global Fund for AIDS, TB, and Malaria. Cases studies involve the International Health Regulations, the Framework Convention on Tobacco Control, and other instruments.

(6) *The Art and Practice of Negotiations.* After basic information on negotiation practices, a series of hands-on negotiation exercises is performed. If possible, these exercises take place in the actual physical settings used for real-life negotiating bodies.

(7) *Cultural, Ethical, and Legal Challenges in Global Health Diplomacy.* Using case studies, ethical issues are explored, including power asymmetries, global public goods, health and trade, intellectual property rights, and corruption.

(8) *Evaluating Global Health Diplomacy.* Using case studies, participants are asked to analyze the success, challenges, and lessons learned that can improve the practice of GHD.

(9) *Specific Global Health Diplomacy Issues.* Depending on the audience's needs, the following specific issues are addressed through additional lectures and case studies:

(a) *Military Health Diplomacy.* This covers recent patterns, development objectives, pratfalls, and case studies of how militaries have engaged in health programs.

(b) *Humanitarian Diplomacy.* This module presents a review of how humanitarian groups function in health development and how post-conflict and post-disaster relief activities interface with political, economic, and security issues.

(c) *The role of Private Sector Actors in Global Health.* Participants will gain understanding of business practices, marketing issues, and the potential for public–private partnerships in global health.

(d) *Rise of the BRICS in Health Diplomacy.* Participants will under-stand the power shifts that have led to the increased diplomatic strength of emerging economies such as Brazil, China, and South Africa. South-to-south health diplomacy (including Cuba) and extractive diplomacy (China) are cases to consider.

(e) *Policy Consistency in Global Health.* Participants will evaluate the impact of the Oslo Declaration, the Paris Declaration on Development Assistance, World Bank policies, and other government policies that attempt to place health in the forefront of foreign policy.

(f) *Participant-Provided Health Diplomacy Cases.* Participants will prepare a case study based on their home agency programs and agendas. These are then discussed by small learning groups in order to establish a pattern of collaboration and group learning.

Conclusion

We have provided an overview of the efforts to define the field and tax-onomy of GHD, a review of some of the key research challenges in this growing field, and suggestions as to how training in GHD might be approached. Certainly, the evaluation of GHD outcomes is the most criti-cal need on the research agenda; it is important for leaders in both foreign policy and health disciplines, as well as in the agencies responsible for these sectors, to have a sense of what works in GHD, who should conduct the GHD, and what skills are needed to prepare for GHD practice. Global health programs are now part of many, many schools of public health, medicine, and political science. However, the integration of training in foreign affairs and public health and the coverage of the transdisciplinary skills necessary for negotiating within the dynamic arena of GHD have not yet been included in most curricula of these programs. We have pro-posed some training scenarios geared more toward executive, profes-sional, or on-the-job training programs, but the content of these programs may well be translated to the formal academic environment or to the preparatory training of diplomats as well as global health providers. What is clear is that GHD has grown from a notion to a critical need in research and training. The success and sustainability of the complex, heavily funded, and extremely important global health assistance programs that have emerged over the last 20 years depends on the skills and evidence that must be incorporated into 21st century health diplomacy.

References

1. Kickbusch I. (2011) Global health diplomacy: how foreign policy can influence health. *BMJ* **342:** d3154. doi:10.1136/bmj.d3154.
2. Katz R, Kornblet S, Arnold G, *et al.* (2011) Defining health diplomacy: Changing demands in the era of globalization. *Milbank Q* **90(3):** 503–523.
3. Feldbaum H, Michaud J. (2010) Health diplomacy and the enduring relevance of foreign policy interests. *PLOS Med* **7(4):** e1000226. doi:10.1371/journal.pmed.1000226.
4. Evans G, Newnham J. (1998) *The Penguin Dictionary of International Relations.* Penguin, London, p. 623.
5. White B. (2001) Diplomacy. In: Baylis J, Smith S (eds.), *The Globalization of World Politics: An Introduction to International Relations.* Oxford University Press, pp. 317–330.
6. Koplan JP, Bond TC, Merson MH, *et al.* (2009) Towards a common definition of global health. *Lancet* **373:** 1993–1995.
7. Lee K, Smith R. (2011) What is "global health diplomacy"? A conceptual review. *Global Health Govern* **V(I):** 1–12. Available from http://www.ghgj.org
8. Kickbusch I, Silberschmidt G, Buss P. (2007) Global health diplomacy: The need for new perspectives, strategic approaches and skills in global health. *Bull World Health Organ* **85:** 243–244.
9. Smith R, Fidler D, Lee K. (2011) Global health diplomacy research. WHO Network on Global Health Diplomacy Trade, Foreign Policy, Diplomacy and Health Draft Working Paper Series. Accessed August 1, 2012, from http://www.ghd-net.org/sites/default/files/Navigating%20the%20Global%20Health%20Terrain%20Preliminary%20Considerations%20on%20Mapping%20Global%20Health%20Diplomacy.pdf
10. Chatham House. Global health diplomacy: A way forward in international affairs — inaugural conference of the Global Health Diplomacy Network, June 28–29, 2011. Available from http://www.chathamhouse.org/sites/default/files/public/Research/Global%20Health/280611summary.pdf

11. Center for Strategic and International Studies. (2007) CSIS Commission on Smart Power. Accessed through http://csis.org/files/media/csis/pubs/071106_csissmartpowerreport.pdf

12. Center for Strategic and International Studies. (2007) Report of the CSIS Commission on Smart Global Health: A safer, healithier and more prosperous world. Accessed through http://csis.org/files/publication/100318_Fallon_SmartGlobalHealth.pdf

13. Johri M, Chung R, Dawson A, Schrecker T. (2012) Global health and national borders: The ethics of foreign aid in a time of financial crisis. *Globalization and Health* **8:** 19. doi:10.1186/1744-8603-8-19.

14. Fidler D. (2007) Architecture amidst anarchy: Global health's quest for governance. *Global Health Govern* **I(1):** 1–17. Available from http://diplomacy.shu.edu/academics/global_health

15. US Global Leadership Coalition. (2012) Smart Power 2.0: America's global strategy. Accessed through http://www.usglc.org/2012/05/23/what-is-smart-power-2-0

16. Mungcal I. (2012) Clinton tightens grip on Global Health Initiative. Accessed through http://www.devex.com/en/news/blogs/new-office-takes-ghi-s-place-at-state-department?blog_id=development-assistance-under-obama

17. Lords Select Committee. (2011) Does UK aid make the right difference? Accessed through http://www.parliament.uk/business/committees/committees-a-z/lords-select/economic-affairs-committee/news/aid-inquiry — evidence-session-5-july/

18. European Commission. (2010) The EU role in global health. Brussels, March 2010, COM (2010)128 final.

19. Nye J. (2004). The decline of America's soft power. *Foreign Aff*, June 2004.

20. Bonventre E. (2008) Monitoring and evaluation of Department of Defense humanitarian assistance programs. *Mil Rev*, January, pp. 66–72.

21. Kevany S. (2012a) Diplomatic and operational adaptations to global health programmes in post-conflict settings: Contributions of monitoring and evaluation systems to health sector development and "nation-building" in South Sudan. *Med Conflict Surviv* (in press).

22. Eldon J, Waddington C, Hadi Y (2008). *Health System Reconstruction: Can It Contribute to State-Building?* Health & Fragile States Network. HLSP Institute, London. Available from http://www.healthandfragilestates.org/index2.php?option=com_docman&task=doc_view&gid=32&Itemid=38.

23. Kevany S. (2012b) Health diplomacy and adapting global health interventions to local needs in sub-Saharan Africa and Thailand: Findings from Project Accept (HPTN 043). *BMC Public Health* (in press).

24. Committee on Foreign Affairs. (2011) Assessing US foreign policy priorities and needs amidst economic challenges. Accessed through http://www.gpo.gov/fdsys/pkg/CHRG-112hhrg64869/pdf/CHRG-112hhrg-64869.pdf

25. The Global Fund. (2012) M&E tools and documents. Accessed through http://www.theglobalfund.org/en/me/documents/

26. Atun R. (2010) Interactions between critical health system functions and HIV/AIDS, tuberculosis and malaria programmes. *Health Policy Plann* **25:** i1–i3.

27. Marseille E. (2002) HIV prevention before HAART in sub-Saharan Africa. *Lancet* **359:** 1851–1856.

28. Valentino B. (2011) The true costs of humanitarian intervention: The hard truth about a noble notion. *Foreign Aff*, December 2011.

29. Lyman NP, Wittels SB. (2010) No good deed goes unpunished: The unintended consequences of Washington's HIV/AIDS programs. *Foreign Aff*, July–August. Accessed through http://www.foreignaffairs.com/articles/66464/princeton-n-lyman-and-stephenb-wittels/no-good-deed-goes-unpunished

30. Knight R. (2012) The Chatham House–YouGov Survey 2012: Hard choices ahead. Accessed through http://www.chathamhouse.org/publications/papers/view/184631

31. Rosskam E, Kickbusch I (eds.). (2011) *Negotiating and Navigating Global Health: Case Studies in Global Health Diplomacy*. World Scientific, Singapore.

32. Novotny TE. (2007) Global health education and careers. In: Markle W, Fisher M, Smego R (eds.). *Understanding Global Health*. McGraw-Hill, New York.

33. Kickbusch I, Novotny TE, Drager N, *et al.* (2007) Global health diplomacy: Training across disciplines. *Bull World Health Organ* **85(12):** 971–973.

34. Low-Beer D. (2011) *Innovative Health Partnerships: The Diplomacy of Diversity*. World Scientific, Singapore.

35. Kickbusch I, Drager N, Told M. (2012) *Textbook on Global Health Diplomacy*. Springer, New York (in press).

Author Biographies

(in alphabetical order, including editorial team)

Vincanne Adams, PhD, is Professor and Vice Chair, Department of Anthropology, History and Social Medicine, University of California, San Francisco, and Director, Program in Medical Anthropology. Her most recent books include *Sex and Development: Science, Sexuality and Morality in Global Perspective* (with Stacy Pigg) (Duke), *Medicine Between Science and Religion*: *Exploration on Tibetan Grounds* (with Mona Schrempf and Sienna R. Craig) (Berhahn), and *Markets of Sorrow, Labors of Faith: New Orleans in the Wake of Katrina* (Duke).

Santiago Alcázar is the first and current Brazilian Ambassador to Azerbaijan. He joined the Brazilian Ministry of External Relations in 1982. He has had a distinguished career, with previous postings to Ouagadougou, Belgrade, Washington, and Asunción. In Washington he was posted to the Brazilian Mission to the OAS. From 1989 till 1994, he was the Deputy at the Division of American States, Ministry of External Relations, and in the period 2001–2002 he held the position of Head of Division of Social Themes, also at the Ministry of External Relations. In 2003, he became the Special Adviser to the Minister of Health in Brazil. He left this position when he became the first Brazilian Ambassador to Burkina Faso in 2008.

Sir George Alleyne, MD, FRCP, FACP (Hons), DSc (Hons), is Director Emeritus of the Pan American Health Organization. A native of Barbados, Dr. Alleyne became Director of the Pan American Sanitary Bureau (PASB),

Regional Office of the World Health Organization (WHO) on February 1, 1995 and completed a second four-year term on January 31, 2003. In 2003, he was elected Director Emeritus of the PASB. From February 2003 until December 2010, he was the UN Secretary General's Special Envoy for HIV/AIDS in the Caribbean. In October 2003, he was appointed Chancellor of the University of the West Indies. He currently holds an adjunct professorship at the Bloomberg School of Public Health, Johns Hopkins University. Dr. Alleyne has received numerous awards in recognition of his work, including prestigious decorations and national honors from many countries of the Americas. In 1990, he was made Knight Bachelor by Her Majesty Queen Elizabeth II for his services to medicine. In 2001, he was awarded the Order of the Caribbean Community, the highest honor that can be conferred on a Caribbean national.

Kristofer Bergh is a researcher with the SIPRI Armed Conflict and Conflict Management Programme. He joined the Stockholm International Peace Research Institute (SIPRI) as an intern in January 2009 and has since worked with the SIPRI Global Health and Security Programme. He has a bachelor's degree in Political Science with a minor in International Relations from the University of Stockholm and is currently finishing his master's thesis on "Peace and Conflict Research" at the University of Uppsala. In April 2011, he joined the Armed Conflict and Conflict Management Programme as a researcher for its new project Arctic Futures, a joint effort of the Conflict Programme and the SIPRI China and Global Security Programme.

Ebony Bertorelli is an international development researcher and practitioner interested in multisectoral policymaking, capacity development, social/technological innovation for poverty and inequality, and how the developed world approaches issues of development. These interests have led her to her current position as the Global Health Diplomacy Program Officer at the McGill World Platform for Health and Economic Convergence (MWP) at McGill University. Her work at the MWP is focused on conducting research, capacity development, and advisory projects for policymaking and negotiation processes in the areas of trade and health, health and foreign policy, global health governance, and globalization and health. She has held fellowships at the Institute for Health and Social Policy and the Institute for the Study of International Development. She holds a Master's in Comparative Politics of the Developing World from McGill University and a BA in Film and Political Science from the University of British Columbia.

Eugene V. Bonventre, MD, is a senior consultant specializing in the intersection of global health and national security. He assists governmental agencies, academia, international and nongovernmental organizations to deal more effectively with militaries in complex emergencies, post-conflict reconstruction, and health diplomacy. He is an Adjunct Assistant Professor of Surgery and of Preventive Medicine and Biometrics at the Uniformed Services University of the Health Sciences in Bethesda, Maryland. Dr. Bonventre retired from the US Air Force as a colonel in October 2008, completing a 25-year career. His final assignment was as a Senior International Health Policy Advisor in the Office of the Deputy Assistant Secretary of Defense for Partnership Strategy, where he supported policy oversight of the Department of Defense's Humanitarian Assistance Programs. He served on the staffs of two combatant commanders, and on the American ambassador's country team in Freetown, Sierra Leone.

Paulo Marchiori Buss, MD, MPH, has been a professor in the National School of Public Health at the Oswaldo Cruz Foundation (FIOCRUZ) since 1977. Currently he is Director of the FIOCRUZ Center for Global Health. In 2001, he was appointed as President of FIOCRUZ (2001–2008). He was elected twice as Director of the FIOCRUZ National School of Public Health (1989–1992 and 1998–2000). Dr. Buss was President of the Latin American and Caribbean Association of Public Health Education (1998–2000) and of the World Federation of Public Health Associations (WFPHA) (2008–2010). He founded (in 1979) and was the first Executive Secretary of the Brazilian Association of Collective Health (ABRASCO) (1979–1983). From March 2006 to March 2008, he served as Chair of the Brazilian Commission on Social Determinants of Health. He is a Member of the National Academy of Medicine and has represented Brazil on the Executive Board of the WHO (2004–2007 and 2008–2011).

Col. Valérie Denux earned her medical doctorate from the University of Bordeaux in 1995. In addition, she holds different academic diplomas from postgraduate courses: Catastrophic Medicine and Tropical Diseases (1995), Master of Management (2000), International Relations Certificate (2007), and Master of Strategy (2009). She attended the Joint Staff College Course in Paris (2008–2009) and the US Medical Strategic Leadership Program (2010). From 1996 to 2004, she served as a general practitioner and acquired a wealth of operational experience in the Balkans, French Polynesia, Lebanon, Djibouti, and Chad. From 2005 to 2008, she served as a Medical Staff Officer on the French Joint Surgeon General's Staff and was involved in the Military Health Organization at the national and international levels (NATO, EU). She is currently assigned to the NATO headquarters, being in charge of the Medical Support Transformation. She is a lecturer at international conferences and has published many articles on the multinational approach to military health care, and written a *mémoire* on military medicine and strategy/diplomacy.

Nick Drager, a former director of the Department of Ethics, Equity, Trade and Human Rights at the World Health Organization, is Honorary Professor, Global Health Policy at the London School of Hygiene and Tropical Medicine and Professor of Practice of Public Policy and Global Health Diplomacy at McGill University. His work focuses on current and emerging public health issues related to globalization and health, especially global health diplomacy/governance, foreign policy, and international trade and health. He is also Senior Fellow in the Global Health Programme at the Graduate Institute of International and Development Studies, Geneva. He serves as chair or keynote speaker at many international conferences; lectures at universities in Europe, North America, and Asia; and is the author of numerous papers, editorials, and books in the area of global health and development. He has an MD from McGill University and a PhD in Economics from Hautes Etudes Internationales, University of Geneva.

Harley Feldbaum was at the time of this writing, the Director of the Global Health and Foreign Policy Initiative and a Professorial Lecturer at the Johns Hopkins Nitze School of Advanced International Studies. He was a White House Fellow in 2011–2012, working on global health initiatives at USAID. After earning his PhD in Public Health Policy at the London School of Hygiene and Tropical Medicine, he consulted for the Nuffield Trust on health and security issues, was a program associate with the California Endowment, and worked as an interviewer and analyst on the Baltimore City needle exchange vans. He is currently Director, Global Health, Food Security and Development at the National Security Staff, United States Government. The analysis and views offered in this book are the author's own and do not represent the position of National Security Staff or the United States Government.

Bates Gill has a long record of research and publication on international and regional security issues, including about arms control, nonproliferation, peacekeeping, and military-technical development, especially with regard to China and Asia. In recent years, his work has broadened to encompass other contemporary security-related trends, including multilateral security organizations, the impact of domestic politics and development on the foreign policies of states, and the nexus of public health and security. Dr. Gill was appointed by the Swedish government to become the seventh Director of the Stockholm International Peace Research Institute (SIPRI), serving from 2007–2012.

Wolfgang Hein is Senior Fellow at the Hamburg-based GIGA Institute of Latin American Studies, and he is teaching International Relations and Development Studies at the University of Hamburg. Since 2002 he has been leading the GIGA research group on "Global Governance and Norm-Building" after having done research on various aspects of global governance and sustainable development (development strategies, environment, tourism).

Sebastian Kevany, MA, MPH, is a research associate at the Institute for Health Policy Studies at the University of California, San Francisco, and acts as M&E advisor to KPMG in their capacity as the local funding agent for the Global Fund to Fight AIDS, Tuberculosis and Malaria. He holds BA and MA degrees in Economics and Political Science from the University of Dublin (Trinity College) and a Master's in Global Health from the University of Cape Town.

Ilona Kickbusch is the Director of the Global Health Programme at the Graduate Institute of International and Development Studies, Geneva. She advises organizations, government agencies, and the private sector on policies and strategies to promote health at the national, European, and international levels. She has published widely and is a member of a number of advisory boards in both the academic and the health policy arena. She has received many awards and served as Adelaide Thinker in Residence at the invitation of the Premier of South Australia. She has recently launched a think tank initiative, "Global Health Europe: A Platform for European Engagement in Global Health" and the "Consortium for Global Health Diplomacy." Her key areas of interest are global health governance, global health diplomacy, health in all policies, the health society, and health literacy. She has had a distinguished career with the World Health Organization, at both the regional and the global level, where she initiated the Ottawa Charter for Health Promotion and a range of "settings projects," including Healthy Cities. From 1998 to 2003, she was with Yale University as the head of the Global Health Division, where she contributed to shaping the field of global health and headed a major Fulbright program. She is a political scientist with a PhD from the University of Konstanz.

Kelley Lee, DPhil, MPA, MA, FFPH, is Associate Dean, Research, Director of Global Health and Professor, Faculty of Health Sciences, Simon Fraser University, and Professor of Global Health Policy, London School of Hygiene and Tropical Medicine. Her research and teaching focuses on the impacts of globalization on communicable and noncommunicable diseases, and the implications for emerging forms of global governance. She has authored over 75 scholarly papers, 40 book chapters, and 9 books, including *The World Health Organization* (Routledge, 2008), *Global Health and International Relations* (Polity, 2012; with Colin McInnes), and *Asia's Role in Governing Global Health* (Routledge, in press; with Tikki Pang and Yeling Tan).

Thomas E. Novotny, MD, MPH, is Professor of Global Health, San Diego State University (SDSU) and the University of California, San Diego (UCSD). He is a graduate of the University of Nebraska Medical Center (MD, 1973) and Johns Hopkins Bloomberg School of Public Health

(MPH, Epidemiology; 1992). During a 23-year career in the US Public Health Service, he served as a family physician in northern California, as a CDC Epidemic Intelligence Service Officer in Denver, Colorado, as Medical Epidemiologist in the Office on Smoking and Health, and as CDC Liaison to the World Bank in Washington, DC. He served in the Clinton and Bush administrations as HHS Deputy Assistant Secretary for International and Refugee Health, and Assistant Surgeon General from 1999 to 2002. He was a Professor in Residence of Epidemiology at the University of California, San Francisco from 2002 to 2008, where he directed international programs for medical and other health sciences students. He now co-directs a unique joint PhD program in Global Health at SDSU/UCSD. His current research program includes global health diplomacy, tobacco control and noncommunicable diseases, and pandemic response; he collaborates with researchers in China, Brazil, Ethiopia, Vietnam, Canada, Switzerland, and the UK. He is a member of the Council on Foreign Relations.

Valerie Percival is Assistant Professor, Norman Paterson School of International Affairs, Carleton University. She received her BA from the University of Toronto, her MA from the Norman Paterson School at Carleton University, and her PhD from the London School of Hygiene and Tropical Medicine. She has worked on engagement in fragile states through positions at the Canadian Department of Foreign Affairs, the International Crisis Group, the United Nations High Commissioner for Refugees, and the Peace Research Institute Oslo. Her research interests include the relationship between conflict, peace, and health; and rebuilding health systems in post-conflict states.

Gaudenz Silberschmidt has headed the International Affairs Division of the Swiss Federal Office of Public Health since 2003. Until joining the Swiss administration in 2003, he directed the International Society of Doctors for the Environment (ISDE), an NGO. In his current position, the main achievements have been the successful chairmanships of the drafting groups for the World Health Assembly Resolutions WHA 5.3 (on the Adoption of the International Health Regulations) and WHA 59.24 (on Public Health, Innovation, Essential Health Research and Intellectual

Property Rights: Towards a Global Strategy and Plan of Action). He also initiated the OECD/WHO reviews of the Swiss health system, and led the elaboration of the Swiss Health Foreign Policy and the negotiation team for the procurement of pre-pandemic vaccine. He graduated as an MD from the University of Zurich in 1995, the Swiss Tropical Institute in Basel, took up studies in International Relations (Economics, Law and Political Science) in St. Gallen and Geneva, and graduated in 1999 with an MA (IR). In 2011, he was appointed as the first Ambassador within the Swiss Federal Office of Public Health, and he represents Switzerland on the WHO Executive Board.

Steven A. Solomon is Principal Legal Officer at the World Health Organization. He has served in that position since 2005, focusing on public international law issues, global public health negotiations, and WHO governing body matters. Prior to joining the WHO, he served as Deputy Legal Counsellor at the United States Mission to United Nations Organizations in Geneva. He was an Attorney-Adviser with the State Department for several years before that. After law school and a stint in private practice, he was a lawyer for the Arms Control and Disarmament Agency. He also worked on Capitol Hill. He has published numerous articles on various topics of public international law — in particular, international humanitarian law and the Convention on Conventional Weapons.

Michaela Told is currently Executive Director of the Global Health Programme at the Graduate Institute of International and Development Studies, Geneva. Prior to moving into academia, she had been working for more than 10 years with the Red Cross and Red Crescent Movement at the local, regional, and international levels in all continents, most recently heading the Principles and Values Department of the International Federation of Red Cross and Red Crescent Societies. Earlier in her career, she worked with the Austrian Ministry of Foreign Affairs, Division of Development Cooperation, and later served as secretary general of an international women's human rights NGO based in Geneva. In her current position as Executive Director of the Global Health Programme at the Graduate Institute, she is responsible for the successful implementation of all activities of the Global Health Programme. She holds an MSW

(International Social Work; School of Social Work, Vienna), an MCom (Development Economics; University of Economics and Business Administration, Vienna), and an MA in Development Studies (Women and Development; Institute of Social Studies, The Hague).

Thomas Zeltner is an international expert leader in public health and health system development. He is a 2010 fellow of the Advanced Leadership Initiative of Harvard University and is Co-founder of the Global Patient Safety Forum, a convening body of the world's leading patient safety organizations. He advises international organizations, national governments, NGOs, and the private sector on health policies. Since 1992, he has been Professor of Public Health at the University of Bern. He has been Director-General of the Federal Office of Public Health of Switzerland (from 1991 to 2009), the National Health and Public Health Authority, and former Secretary of State for Health. Prior to these functions, he was head of Medical Services at the University Hospital in Bern and held various positions in the Medical Faculty of the University of Bern and at the Harvard School of Public Health. He graduated with an MD and a master's degree in Law from the University in his native town of Bern. He also holds a specialist degree in Human Pathology and Forensic Medicine.

Index

CPSIA information can be obtained
at www.ICGtesting.com
Printed in the USA
LVHW081334100422
715714LV00035B/393

9 789814 355155